Noncarious Cervical Lesions and Cervical Dentin Hypersensitivity:
Etiology, Diagnosis, and Treatment

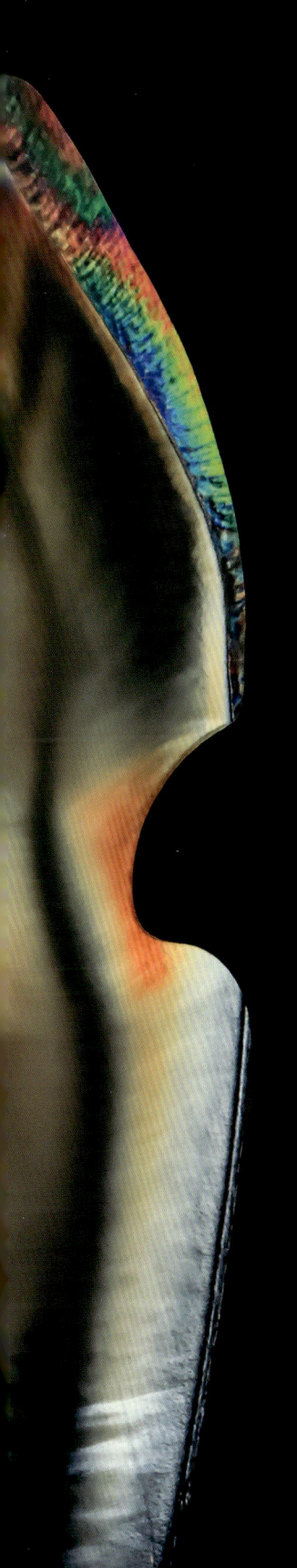

Noncarious Cervical Lesions and Cervical Dentin Hypersensitivity

Etiology, Diagnosis, and Treatment

Edited by

Paulo V. Soares, DDS, MS, PhD
Professor of Operative Dentistry and Dental Materials
Dental School, Federal University of Uberlândia
Coordinator of the NCCL Research Group and Public Ambulatory Center
 for the Treatment of NCCLs and CDH
Uberlândia, Brazil

John O. Grippo, DDS
Adjunct Professor Emeritus
Department of Biomedical Engineering
Western New England University
Springfield, Massachusetts

QUINTESSENCE PUBLISHING

Berlin, Barcelona, Chicago, Istanbul, London, Milan, Moscow, New Delhi, Paris, Prague, Sao Paulo,
Seoul, Singapore, Tokyo, Warsaw

Dedication

We dedicate this book to our families, our colleagues and patients, and to all of those who believe in the practice of dentistry based on scientific evidence.

Library of Congress Cataloging-in-Publication Data

Names: Soares, Paulo V., editor | Grippo, John O., editor
Title: Noncarious cervical lesions and cervical dentin hypersensitivity :
   etiology, diagnosis, and treatment / edited by Paulo V. Soares and
John O. Grippo
Description: Hanover Park, IL : Quintessence Publishing Co Inc, [2017] |
   Includes bibliographical references and index.
Identifiers: LCCN 2016055911 (print) | LCCN 2016057084 (ebook) | ISBN
   9780867157147 (hardcover : alk. paper) | ISBN 9780867157543
Subjects: | MESH: Tooth Cervix | Tooth Diseases | Dentin Sensitivity
Classification: LCC RK305 (print) | LCC RK305 (ebook) | NLM WU 210 | DDC
   617.6/3--dc23
LC record available at https://lccn.loc.gov/2016055911

QUINTESSENCE PUBLISHING USA

©2017 Quintessence Publishing Co, Inc

Quintessence Publishing Co Inc
4350 Chandler Drive
Hanover Park, IL 60133
www.quintpub.com

5 4 3 2 1

All rights reserved. This book or any part thereof may not be reproduced, stored in a retrieval system, or transmitted in any form or by any means, electronic, mechanical, photocopying, or otherwise, without prior written permission of the publisher.

Editor: Leah Huffman
Design: Erica Neumann
Production: Angelina Schmelter
Printed in Korea

Contents

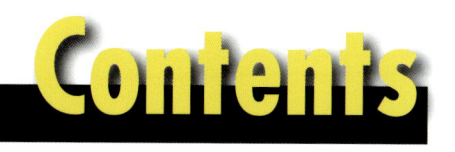

Forewords by John C. Kois and Luiz Narciso Baratieri vii
Preface viii
List of Coauthors ix
Acknowledgments xiv

SECTION I INTRODUCTION 1

1 History, Prevalence, and Etiology of NCCLs and CDH 3

2 Anatomical Considerations: *Enamel, Dentin, and Periodontium* 17

SECTION II MECHANISMS OF ACTION 29

3 Stress 31

4 Friction 43

5 Biocorrosion 51

SECTION III DIAGNOSIS AND TREATMENT   *73*

6   **Morphologic Characteristics of NCCLs**   *75*

7   **Clinical Analysis and Diagnosis of CDH and NCCLs**   *85*

8   **Nonrestorative Protocols:** *Occlusal, Chemical, and Laser Therapies*   *95*

9   **Restorative Protocols:** *Adhesive Bonding, Materials, and Techniques*   *125*

10   **Surgical Protocols:** *Periodontal Therapy and Root Coverage*   *167*

Future Perspectives   *183*
Appendix   *184*
Index   *190*

Forewords

It is difficult to imagine that such an enlightening textbook can be written about a seemingly focused topic. Noncarious cervical lesions (NCCLs) have been observed in both historical and current civilizations all over the world. Until recently, the relationship of NCCLs to cervical dentin hypersensitivity remained a misunderstood enigma in dentistry.

This textbook is the most comprehensive accumulation of data-driven science ever assembled. Drs Paulo V. Soares and John O. Grippo have organized their most important contributions to enable the reader to best understand this prevalent condition and offer solutions to their patients. The detailed level of documentation in the authors' stunning photographs provides a unique and necessary clarity to illustrate the clinical concepts presented.

Drs Soares and Grippo have orchestrated a body of work that allows us to move from passive observer to active investigator, making us capable of combining the clinical presentation with all the potential etiologic factors and thereby arriving at a multifactorial diagnosis. They reveal that these apparently simple notches in teeth require a great depth of understanding to resolve their progression and recommend definitive, successful treatment.

John C. Kois, DMD, MSD
Director of the Kois Center for Advancing Dentistry Through Science

---

At a time when dentistry (the "best" profession in the world) seems to have become, for some people, a new profession about facial appearance care, to receive an invitation to write a foreword for a book on any other subject is in itself a gift. But when the book topics are current and extremely relevant—what a precious gift. In fact, *Noncarious Cervical Lesions and Cervical Dentin Hypersensitivity: Etiology, Diagnosis, and Treatment* is much more than a gift expected by me; it is a gift expected by our profession, the profession of true dentistry. The one that values beyond beauty. The one that values the individual's overall health above all. With extensive clinical support and excellent photographs, the authors approach noncarious cervical lesions and cervical dentin hypersensitivity in 10 didactically organized chapters, providing practically everything that a student and/or clinician of any level needs to know and should know about these topics. I confess that I read the book without noticing the time. It was a real treat. I was extremely happy with the information I found and was very proud to see the name of a young and talented Brazilian teacher among the great team of authors and collaborators. In truth, I came to feel envy about not being part of the team. For all this, I would like to thank the authors and congratulate them on the excellence of the book.

Luiz Narciso Baratieri, DDS, MS, PhD
Professor, Federal University of Santa Catarina, Florianópolis, Brazil

Preface

Cervical dentin hypersensitivity (CDH) and loss of hard tooth substance at the cementoenamel junction (CEJ), designated as noncarious cervical lesions (NCCLs), are commonly encountered conditions in clinical practice. Yet most practitioners resort to treating the symptoms with various modalities rather than seeking an answer to their etiology.

Recent research findings have been published that have answered many of the questions surrounding the enigma of NCCLs. It has been concluded that NCCLs are a multifactorial condition that involves the three mechanisms of stress, biocorrosion, and friction, all of which play a role in its etiology. Unfortunately, the role of the dynamics of occlusion in the etiology of both NCCLs and CDH has been ignored or questioned, as little attention has been given to the effects of cervical stress concentration from occlusal loading. Simplistic answers have been commonly used by practitioners to explain to their patients the causes of these conditions, namely toothbrush/dentifrice abrasion or acid erosion.

NCCLs appear to be caries free and exist in various forms such as shallow grooves, broad dished-out lesions, or extensive wedge-shaped defects. The geometry at the depth of these lesions may range in shape from flat to round and may at times progress to be sharply angled like a notch, even progressing to the pulp chamber. For the past 75 years, attention has been focused on the etiology of NCCLs using photoelastic tests, strain gauges, finite element analysis, and electron microscopy, which verify that stress is a mechanism that is always occurring and a significant factor in the etiology of these lesions.

CDH appears to be a pathognomonic sign of the onset of NCCLs, as they both occur in the same area of stress concentration in the cervical region. An air indexing method is available to quantify the degree of CDH, and occlusal equilibration therapy has been found to eliminate the symptoms of CDH, avoiding the need for other treatment modalities to address the symptoms. Digital biomechanical and experimental studies corroborate the presence of cervical stress concentration at the CEJ resulting from occlusal loading forces. An awareness of the significance of stress as an etiologic factor for both CDH and NCCLs will assist in the understanding and treatment of these dental pathologies. Furthermore, the resolution of occlusal discrepancies improves the health and comfort of the masticatory system.

Treatment modalities for CDH commonly include but are not limited to the use of desensitizing agents, laser therapy, and/or periodontal surgical root coverage. Historically, NCCL applied therapies have involved restoring these defects with restorative materials. Little attention has been given to their mutual etiologic mechanisms of cervical stress concentration from occlusal loading and/or endogenous/exogenous biocorrosion. Frequency rates for both CDH and NCCLs are significant in modern populations. It is now time to involve greater diagnostic effort prior to treating these conditions. It is also time to alter treatment protocols to include a reduction in dietary intake or exposure to acids, management of reflux diseases, and consideration of the significance of occlusal therapies.

The authors have strategically accumulated their study, research, and clinical experiences to create this book. Since 2008, Professor Paulo V. Soares has been a coordinator of the NCCL Research Group and Public Ambulatory Center for treatment of patients with NCCLs and CDH at the Federal University of Uberlândia, Brazil. And John O. Grippo, Adjunct Professor Emeritus at the Western New England University Department of Biomedical Engineering, has dedicated the past 27 years of his life to the study and research of the etiology of NCCLs. The authors selected more than 70 collaborators to assemble all of the significant publications relating to NCCLs and CDH, according to their respective areas of expertise.

The book is divided into three sections totaling 10 chapters. Topics include an introduction and history of NCCLs and CDH, anatomical considerations, mechanisms of action, morphology, classification, diagnosis, and treatment. After reading this book, the reader will be able to understand the etiology of CDH and NCCLs and diagnose and treat clinical cases. This book is recommended to clinicians, scholars, researchers, and undergraduate and postgraduate students.

Paulo V. Soares
John O. Grippo

List of Coauthors

Thaiane Rodrigues Aguiar, DDS, MS, PhD
Adjunct Professor
Federal University of Bahia College of Dentistry
Salvador, Brazil
▶ Chapter 2

Guilherme de Araújo Almeida, DDS, PhD
Professor
Department of Orthodontics
Faculty of Dentistry
Federal University of Uberlândia
Uberlândia, Brazil
▶ Chapter 3

Raphael Monte Alto, DDS, MS, PhD
Professor
Department of General Dentistry
Implantology Specialization Course
Fluminense Federal University
Niterói, Brazil
▶ Chapter 8

Victor E. Arana-Chavez, DDS, MSc, PhD
Full Professor and Chairman, Department of Biomaterials and Oral Biology
President, Commission for Undergraduate Studies
School of Dentistry
University of São Paulo, Brazil
São Paulo, Brazil
▶ Chapter 2

Ana Cecilia Corrêa Aranha, MS, PhD
Associate Professor
Vice Coordinator of the Special Laboratory of Lasers in Dentistry
Department of Restorative Dentistry
School of Dentistry
University of São Paulo
São Paulo, Brazil
▶ Chapter 8

Ricardo Correa Barbuti, MD, PhD
Assistant Professor
Clinical Gastroenterology
Clinical Hospital University
São Paulo School of Medicine
São Paulo, Brazil
▶ Chapter 5

Bruno de Castro Ferreira Barreto, DDS, MSc, PhD
Biomechanics Applied to Dentistry
Katholieke Universiteit Leuven
Leuven, Belgium
▶ Chapter 2

Ana Bedran-Russo, DDS, MS, PhD
Associate Professor
Director of Applied Dental Materials and Interfaces
Program Director, Multi-Disciplinary Oral Sciences Program
Department of Restorative Dentistry
College of Dentistry
The University of Illinois at Chicago
Chicago, Illinois
▶ Chapters 2 and 5

André Luiz Fraga Briso, DDS, MS, PhD
Coordinator of the Postgraduate Program in Dentistry
Division of Restorative Dentistry
Araçatuba School of Dentistry
São Paulo State University
Araçatuba, Brazil
▶ Chapter 8

Andréa Brito, PhD
Coordinator of the Esthetic Dentistry Post-Graduate Program of the Brazilian Dentistry Association, Pernambuco Section
Adjunct Professor of Dentistry at the Federal University of Rio Grande do Sul (2005–2015)
Porto Alegre, Brazil
▶ Chapter 8

Maria Aparecida de Oliveira Campoli, DDS, MS
Assistant Professor
Department of Periodontics and Implantology
Faculty of Dentistry
Federal University of Uberlândia
Uberlândia, Brazil
▶ Chapter 10

Igor Oliveiros Cardoso, DDS
Master's Student
Member of the NCCL Research Group
Faculty of Dentistry
Federal University of Uberlândia
Uberlândia, Brazil
▶ Chapter 2

Bruno N. Cavalcanti, DDS, PhD
Associate Professor
Department of Endodontics
The University of Iowa College of Dentistry & Dental Clinics
Iowa City, Iowa
▶ Chapter 8

Neide Pena Coto, DDS, MS, PhD
Associate Professor
Department of Maxillofacial Surgery, Prosthetics and Traumatology
Division of Maxillofacial Prosthesis and Sports Dentistry
Coordinator, Laboratory of Sports Dentistry and Biomechanic Research
School of Dentistry
University of São Paulo
São Paulo, Brazil
▶ Chapter 5

Robert Carvalho da Silva, DDS, MS, PhD
Scientific Coordinator
ImplantePerio Institute
São Paulo, Brazil
▶ Chapter 10

Leticia Resende Davi, DDS, MS, PhD
Adjunct Professor
Department of Occlusion, Fixed Prostheses and Dental Materials
Faculty of Dentistry
Federal University of Uberlândia
Uberlândia, Brazil
▶ Chapter 8

Paulo Fernando Mesquita de Carvalho, DDS, MS, PhD
Scientific Coordinator
ImplantePerio Institute
São Paulo, Brazil
▶ Chapter 10

Ramon Corrêa de Queiroz de Gonzaga, DDS
Master's Student
Member of the NCCL Research Group
Faculty of Dentistry
Federal University of Uberlândia
Uberlândia, Brazil
▶ Chapter 6

Denildo de Magalhães, DDS, MS, PhD
Full Professor
Department of Periodontics and Implantology
Faculty of Dentistry
Federal University of Uberlândia
Uberlândia, Brazil
▶ Chapter 10

Jan De Munck, DDS, PhD
Researcher
Biomaterials
Katholieke Universiteit Leuven
Leuven, Belgium

Private Practice
Diest, Belgium
▶ Chapter 2

Foued Salmen Espindola, PhD
Full Professor of Biochemistry
Institute of Genetics and Biochemistry
Federal University of Uberlândia
Uberlândia, Brazil
▶ Chapter 5

Newton Fahl, Jr, DDS, MS
Clinical and Scientific Director
Fahl Center
Curitiba, Brazil
▶ Chapter 9

Juliana Jendiroba Faraoni, DDS, MSc, PhD
Department of Restorative Dentistry
Ribeirão Preto School of Dentistry
University of São Paulo
Ribeirão Preto, Brazil
▶ Chapter 4

André Luis Faria-e-Silva, DDS, MD, PhD
Professor
Department of Dentistry
School of Dentistry
Federal University of Sergipe
Aracaju, Brazil
▶ Chapter 9

Lorraine Braga Ferreira, DDS, PhD
Oral Biology and Biomaterials
University of São Paulo
São Paulo, Brazil
▶ Chapter 2

Alexia da Mata Galvão, DDS
Master's Student
Member of the NCCL Research Group
Faculty of Dentistry
Federal University of Uberlândia
Uberlândia, Brazil
▶ Chapter 7

Vinicius Rangel Geraldo-Martins, DDS, MSc, PhD
Professor
Department of Clinical Dentistry
University of Uberaba
Uberaba, Brazil
▶ Chapter 4

Rafaella Rodrigues Gomes, DDS, MS
Member of the NCCL Research Group
Faculty of Dentistry
Federal University of Uberlândia
Uberlândia, Brazil
▸ Chapter 6

João César Guimarães Henriques, DDS, MS, PhD
Chairman of Stomatology and Dentomaxillofacial Radiology
School of Dentistry
Federal University of Uberlândia
Uberlândia, Brazil
▸ Chapter 2

Cristian Higashi, DDS, MS, PhD
Ilapeo College
Curitiba, Brazil
▸ Chapter 9

Ronaldo Hirata, DDS, MS, PhD
Clinical Assistant Professor
Department of Biomaterials
NYU College of Dentistry
New York, New York
▸ Chapter 9

Siegfried Jaecques, PhD, MScEng
Coordinator
KU Leuven Medical Technology Centre
Department of Mechanical Engineering
Biomechanics Section
Katholieke Universiteit Leuven
Heverlee, Belgium
▸ Chapter 2

Julio Cesar Joly, DDS, MS, PhD
Coordinator of the Master of Science Programs of Implantology and Periodontology
São Leopoldo Mandic Dentistry Research Center
Campinas, Brazil

Scientific Coordinator
ImplantePerio Institute
São Paulo, Brazil
▸ Chapter 10

Paulo Cézar Simamoto Júnior, DDS, MSc, PhD
Professor
Department of Occlusion, Fixed Prostheses and Dental Materials
Faculty of Dentistry
Federal University of Uberlândia
Uberlândia, Brazil
▸ Chapter 8

Robert B. Kerstein, DMD
Private Practice in Prosthodontics
Boston, Massachusetts
▸ Chapter 7

Éverton Ribeiro Lelis, DDS, MSc, PhD
Department of Orthodontics, Brazilian Dental Association of Uberlândia
Uberlândia, Brazil
▸ Chapter 3

Ariene Arcas Leme-Kraus, DDS, MS, PhD
Department of Restorative Dentistry
University of Illinois at Chicago
Chicago, Illinois
▸ Chapter 2

Cesar Penazzo Lepri, DDS, MSc, PhD
Associate Professor
Coordinator of Post-Graduate Program in Dentistry
Department of Biomaterials
University of Uberaba
Uberaba, Brazil
▸ Chapter 4

Alessandro Dourado Loguercio, DDS, MS, PhD
Full Professor
Restorative Department
State University of Ponta Grossa
Ponta Grossa, Brazil
▸ Chapter 9

Alexandre Coelho Machado, DDS, MS
PhD Student
Member of the NCCL Research Group
Faculty of Dentistry
Federal University of Uberlândia
Uberlândia, Brazil
▸ Chapters 3 and 9

Fabiano Carlos Marson, DDS, MS, PhD
Professor and Program Coordinator
Department of Operative Dentistry
UNINGÁ – Centro Universitário Ingá Maringá
Maringá, Brazil
▸ Chapter 8

Leandro Martins, PhD
Adjunct Professor
Federal University of Amazonas
Manaus, Brazil
▸ Chapter 8

Daniela Baccelli Silveira Mendonça, DDS, MSc, PhD
Clinical Assistant Professor
Department of Biologic and Materials Sciences
Division of Prosthodontics
University of Michigan School of Dentistry
Ann Arbor, Michigan
▸ Chapter 8

Gustavo Mendonça, DDS, MSc, PhD
Clinical Associate Professor
Department of Biologic and Materials Sciences
Division of Prosthodontics
University of Michigan School of Dentistry
Ann Arbor, Michigan
▸ Chapter 8

Atsushi Mine, DDS, PhD
Assistant Professor
Department of Fixed Prothodontics
Osaka University Graduate School of Dentistry
Osaka, Japan
▸ Chapter 2

Fabio Franceschini Mitri, DDS, MSc, PhD
Professor
Human Anatomy Department
Federal University of Uberlândia
Uberlândia, Brazil
▸ Chapter 2

Breno Mont'Alverne, MSc, PhD
Professor
Dental Materials and Operative Dentistry
Federal University of Maranhão
São Luís, Brazil
▸ Chapter 9

Tatiana Carvalho Montes, DDS
Master's Student
Department of Restorative Dentistry
Ribeirão Preto School of Dentistry
University of São Paulo
Ribeirão Preto, Brazil
▸ Chapter 7

Guilherme Faria Moura, DDS, MS
PhD Student
Member of the NCCL Research Group
Faculty of Dentistry
Federal University of Uberlândia
Uberlândia, Brazil
▸ Chapter 8

Alfredo Júlio Fernandes Neto, DDS, MS, PhD
Full Professor
Department of Occlusion, Fixed Prostheses and Dental Materials
Faculty of Dentistry
Federal University of Uberlândia
Uberlândia, Brazil
▸ Chapter 8

Pedro Yoshito Noritomi, PhD
Three-Dimensional Technologies Division
Renato Archer Information Technology Center
Campinas, Brazil
▸ Chapter 2

Veridiana Resende Novais, DDS, MSD, PhD
Adjunct Professor
Department of Operative Dentistry and Dental Materials
Faculty of Dentistry
Federal University of Uberlândia
Uberlândia, Brazil
▸ Chapter 5

Daniel S. Oh, PhD
Assistant Professor
Division of Oral & Maxillofacial Surgery
College of Dental Medicine
Columbia University Medical Center
New York, New York
▸ Chapter 1

Luana Oliveira-Haas, DDS, MS, PhD
Associate Professor
Department of Cariology and Restorative Dentistry
Health Professions Division
College of Dental Medicine
Nova Southeastern University
Fort Lauderdale, Florida
▸ Chapter 3

Regina Guenka Palma-Dibb, BDS, MSc, PhD
Professor
Department of Restorative Dentistry
Ribeirão Preto School of Dentistry
University of São Paulo
Ribeirão Preto, Brazil
▸ Chapter 4

Analice Giovani Pereira, DDS, MSc, PhD
Professor
Endodontics Department
Faculty of Dentistry
Federal University of Uberlândia
Uberlândia, Brazil
▸ Chapter 10

Fabrícia Araújo Pereira, PhD
Professor of Dentistry Clinic, Dentistry Course
State University of the Southwest of Bahia
Jequié, Brazil
▸ Chapter 6

Carmem S. Pfeifer, DDS, PhD
Assistant Professor
Biomaterials and Biomechanics
Oregon Health & Sciences University
Portland, Oregon
▸ Chapter 9

Marleen Peumans, PhD, DDS
Associate Professor
Biomaterials
Department of Oral Health Sciences
Katholieke Universiteit Leuven
Leuven, Belgium
▶ Chapter 2

Maria Elisabeth Machado Pinto-e-Silva, MS, PhD
Associate Professor
Nutrition Department
School of Public Health
University of São Paulo
São Paulo, Brazil
▶ Chapter 5

Paulo Sérgio Quagliatto, MS, DDS, PhD
Professor
Operative Dentistry and Dental Materials
Faculty of Dentistry
Federal University of Uberlândia
Uberlândia, Brazil
▶ Chapter 8

Vanessa Rahal, PhD
Department of Restorative Dentistry
Araçatuba School of Dentistry
São Paulo State University
Araçatuba, Brazil
▶ Chapter 8

Luís Henrique Araújo Raposo, DDS, MSc, PhD
Adjunct Professor
Department of Occlusion, Fixed Prosthesis and Dental Materials
Faculty of Dentistry
Federal University of Uberlândia
Uberlândia, Brazil
▶ Chapter 8

Alessandra Reis, DDS, PhD
Full Professor
Restorative Department
State University of Ponta Grossa
Ponta Grossa, Brazil
▶ Chapter 9

Bruno Rodrigues Reis, DDS, MS, PhD
Professor
Operative Dentistry and Dental Materials
Faculty of Dentistry
Federal University of Uberlândia
Uberlândia, Brazil
▶ Chapter 9

Cristianne Pacheco Ribeiro, DDS, MS
Assistant Professor
Department of Periodontics and Implantology
Faculty of Dentistry
Federal University of Uberlândia
Uberlândia, Brazil
▶ Chapter 10

Linda Rigali, DMD
Private Practice in Orthodontics
Springfield, Massachusetts
▶ Chapter 3

Renata Borges Rodrigues, DDS, MS
Department of Dentistry and Dental Materials
Faculty of Dentistry
Federal University of Uberlândia
Uberlândia, Brazil
▶ Chapter 5

Júlia Olien Sanches, DDS, MSc
PhD Student
Department of Restorative Dentistry
Ribeirão Preto School of Dentistry
University of São Paulo
Ribeirão Preto, Brazil
▶ Chapter 4

Carlos José Soares, DDS, MS, PhD
Professor
Chair of the Operative Dentistry and Dental Materials Department
Director of the CPBio – Research Center for Biomechanics,
 Biomaterials and Cell Biology
Faculty of Dentistry
Federal University of Uberlândia
Uberlândia, Brazil
▶ Chapter 3

Paola Gomes Souza, DDS
Master's Student
Member of the NCCL Research Group
Faculty of Dentistry
Federal University of Uberlândia
Uberlândia, Brazil
▶ Chapter 5

Pedro Henrique Rezende Spini, DDS, MS
Member of the NCCL Research Group
Faculty of Dentistry
Federal University of Uberlândia
Uberlândia, Brazil
▶ Chapter 3

Thaís Yumi Umeda Suzuki, DDS, MS, PhD
Department of Dental Materials and Prosthodontics
Araçatuba School of Dentistry
São Paulo State University
Araçatuba, Brazil
▶ Chapter 2

Daniela Navarro Ribeiro Teixeira, DDS, MS
Member of the NCCL Research Group
Faculty of Dentistry
Federal University of Uberlândia
Uberlândia, Brazil
▶ Chapter 10

Bart Van Meerbeek, DDS, PhD
Professor in Dental Biomaterial Sciences
Biomaterials, Department of Oral Health Sciences
Conservative Dentistry
Katholieke Universiteit Leuven
Leuven, Belgium
▶ Chapter 2

Jos Vander Sloten, PhD
Full Professor
Chairman, Leuven Medical Technology Centre
Vice Dean for International Affairs
Department of Mechanical Engineering
Faculty of Engineering Science
Katholieke Universiteit Leuven
Leuven, Belgium
▶ Chapter 2

Cristina M. P. Vidal, DDS, MS, PhD
Assistant Professor
Department of Operative Dentistry
College of Dentistry & Dental Clinics
University of Iowa
Iowa City, Iowa
▶ Chapter 5

Maria Carolina B. C. von Atzingen, MS, PhD
School of Public Health
University of São Paulo
São Paulo, Brazil
▶ Chapter 5

Livia Fávaro Zeola, DDS, MS
PhD Student
Member of the NCCL Research Group
Faculty of Dentistry
Federal University of Uberlândia
Uberlândia, Brazil
▶ Chapters 5 and 7

Acknowledgments

The authors of this book would like to thank the many universities, dental schools, and public agencies who provided funding opportunities and grants (NIH, CNPq, CAPES, FAPEMIG) as well as the companies and partners of the NCCL Research Group. We would also like to thank the following doctors for their support: Thomas A. Coleman, André V. Ritter, Liliane Parreira Tannús Gontijo, Cleudmar Amaral de Araújo, Henner Alberto Gomide, Luis Roberto Marcondes Martins, Márcio Teixeira Nunes, Paulo César Freitas Santos-Filho, Gisele Rodrigues Silva, Murilo Sousa Menezes, Roberto Elias Campos, Márcio Magno Costa, Flávio Domingues das Neves, Sonia Cristina de Sousa, Tiago Augusto, Priscilla Fernanda, Anaíra Ribeiro Guedes Fonseca Costa, Fernanda Guedes, Lorena Souza, Liliane Cecília, Alex Herval, Liliana Seger, Marcos Rogério Mendonça, Osmar Aparecido Cuoghi, Mathew T. Mathew, Lucas Araújo Queiroz, Natália Sousa Freitas Queiroz, Tomás Navarro Rodriguez, Ana Paula Gines Geraldo, Antonello M. Messina, Brennan P. K. Cassidy, and Keirsten D. Rapoza.

Paulo V. Soares
John O. Grippo

Section I

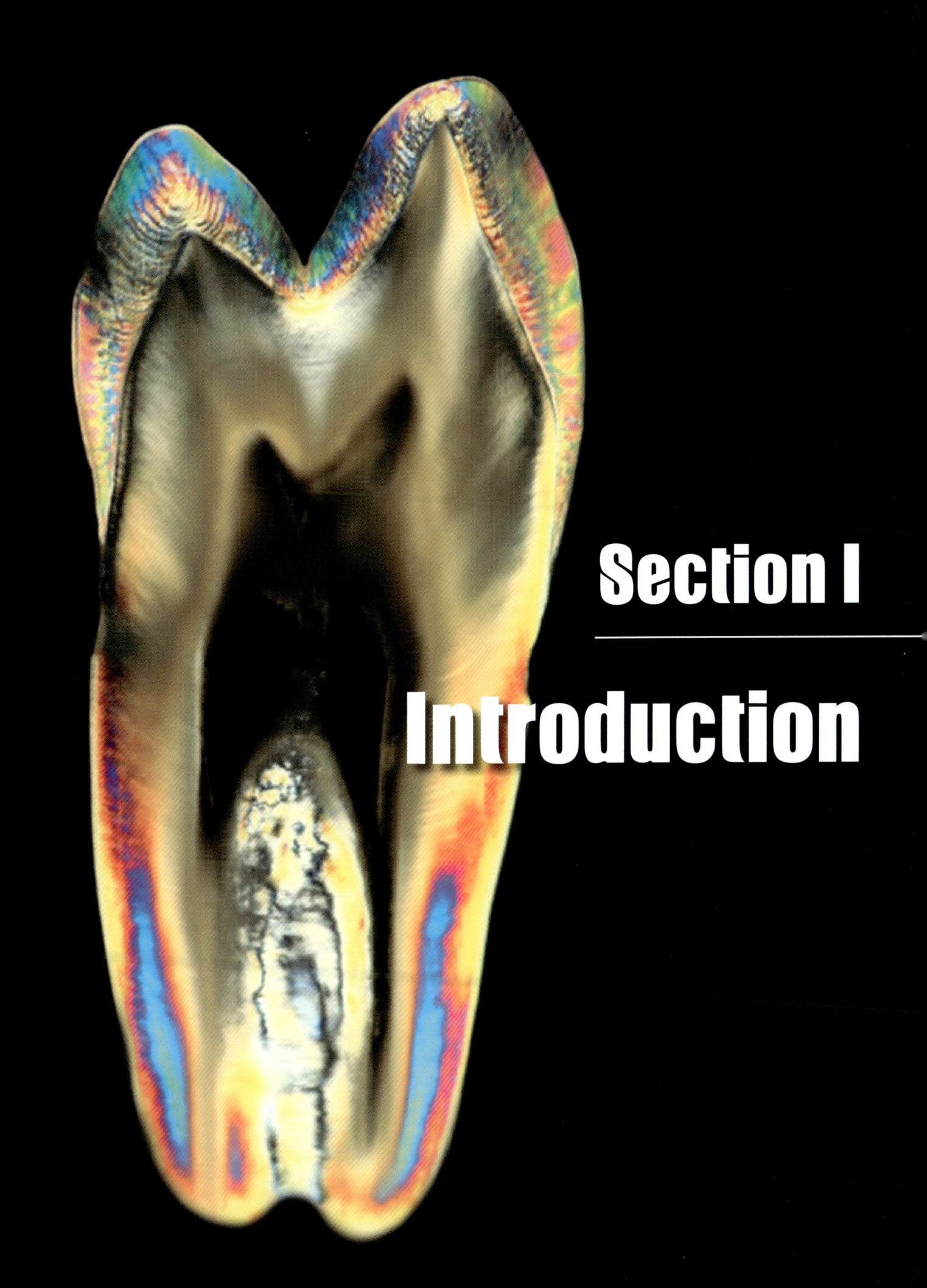

Introduction

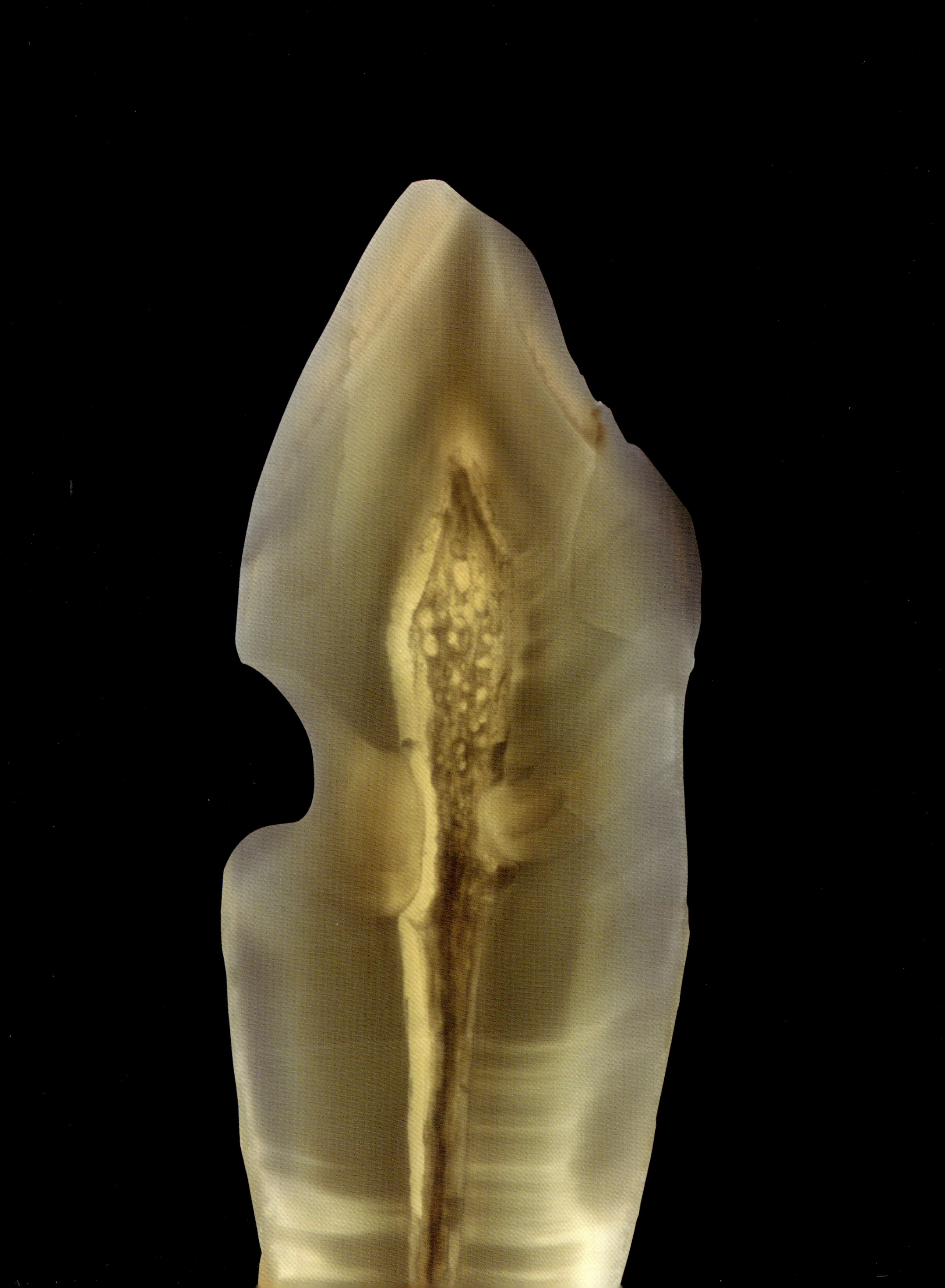

1

History, Prevalence, and Etiology of NCCLs and CDH

History of the Nomenclature and Etiology of NCCLs

The nomenclature and etiology of noncarious cervical lesions (NCCLs) have caused great consternation since the dawn of modern dental research (Table 1-1). From the beginning, the terms *erosion* and *abrasion* were often confused, and that confusion persisted throughout the 20th century.

Pierre Fauchard first used the terms *caries* and *erosion* in his *Le Chirurgien Dentiste, ou Traité des dents* (*The Surgeon Dentist, or Treatise on the Teeth*)[1] in 1728:

> The enamel of teeth is subject to disease which simulates caries, but it is however not caries. The external surface becomes uneven and rough like a grater but more irregular. I call this erosion of the surface of the enamel, or disposition to caries. From this it comes that the enamel is eaten away by some corrosive, in the same way that rust corrodes the surface of metals.

Fauchard was the first to use the term *erosion* as a chemical mechanism, mentioning that enamel is eaten away by a corrosive. Although Fauchard made no mention of NCCLs, his concept of erosion as a chemical mechanism has endured for nearly 300 years and is frequently implicated as a factor in the etiology of NCCLs.[9]

Fifty years after Fauchard introduced the concept of tooth erosion, English anatomist and physiologist John Hunter related the first distinct description of what we now refer to as *noncarious cervical lesions*:

> There is another decay of the teeth, much less common than that already described, which has a very singular appearance. It is a wasting of the substance of the tooth.... In all the instances I have seen, it has begun on the exterior surface of the tooth, pretty close to the arch of the gum. The first appearance is a want of enamel, whereby the bony part is left exposed, but neither the enamel, nor the bony part alter in consistence.... As this decay spreads, more and more of the bone becomes exposed ... and hence it may be called a denudation process. The bony substance of the teeth gives way, and the whole wasted surface has exactly the appearance, as if the tooth had been filed with a rounded file, and afterwards had been finely polished. At these places the bony parts, being exposed, become brown.[2]

Hunter interpreted these denudations as inherent weaknesses in the teeth.

In 1849, Chapin Harris, the father of American dental science, alluded to NCCLs and cervical dentin hypersensitivity

Table 1-1 Historical etiologic opinions regarding NCCLs

Author	Publication	Country	Etiology	Year
Fauchard[1]	Textbook	France	Erosion	1728
Hunter[2]	Textbook	England	Inherent tooth weakness	1778
Fox[3]	Textbook	England	Saliva and friction of lips	1803
Bell[4]	Textbook	England	Imperfections in enamel	1831
Harris[5]	Textbook	USA	Toothbrush abrasion, acidulated buccal mucosa	1839
Koch[6]	Dental Cosmos	USA	Mucous acids	1873
Darby[7]	Dental Cosmos	USA	Acid gouty diathesis	1892
Tomes, Sir John	—	England	Toothbrush/dentifrice abrasion	1892
Tomes, Charles	—	England	Mucous acids	1892
Kirk[8]	Dental Cosmos	USA	Mucous acids	1902

(CDH) in his definition for "Erosion" in the *Dictionary of Dental Science, Biography, Bibliography and Medical Terminology*[10]:

> Erosion, properly speaking, confines itself to the enamel, and is usually developed on a series of teeth at the same time. When the disease occurs subsequently to the eruption of the teeth, it generally manifests itself on their labial and outer surfaces near the margin of the gums, and the decomposed part of the enamel is generally white and of a soft chalky texture, though sometimes assumes other aspects. The eroded parts are usually very sensitive to the touch, and to impressions of heat and cold.

Like Hunter, Harris designated this "erosion" as a denuding of the teeth. He adopted the opinion that these lesions were produced by the action of acidulated buccal mucus and recommended that patients avoid stiff-bristled toothbrushes and brush up and down instead of across the front teeth. This is one of the first published citations alluding to toothbrush abrasion as a causative cofactor in the etiology of NCCLs.

In 1873, Charles R. E. Koch published a scholarly paper in *Dental Cosmos* describing and designating NCCLs as erosions.[6] He cited "an entirely revised view on erosion" from Charles S. Tomes that rejected the idea that all grooving was caused by the action of the toothbrush or mechanical force of some form and rather posited that this grooving could be the result of a chemical process. Koch had doubts that toothbrushes/dentifrice caused all lesions; he himself had tried every device that he could think of to produce the conditions seen in erosion by the use of brushes and brush wheels, but he was unsuccessful. Koch concluded that "At this time the most general belief undoubtedly is that the disease is a process of chemical dissolution."

In 1892, Edwin T. Darby[7] addressed the Dental Society of the State of New York and contended that erosion was caused by an acid condition of the fluids of the mouth, particularly the product of the labial and buccal mucous glands. He had most likely clinically observed what is now recognized as *gastroesophageal reflux disease* (GERD).

Two years later, a German dentist named U. Zsigmondy published a paper that described NCCLs in teeth, designating them macromorphologically as "keilformige Defekte," meaning *wedge-shaped defects*.[11] He characterized these defects as having the appearance of triangular fractures resulting from flexure.

At this time, Willoughby D. Miller was pursuing the study of microbiology in Robert Koch's microbiologic laboratory. In 1890, Miller formulated the chemoparasitic theory of caries. This theory held that caries is the result of acids produced by oral bacteria following fermentation of sugars. In 1907, Miller published his "Experiments and observations on the wasting of tooth tissue variously designated as erosion, abrasion, chemical abrasion, denudation, etc."[12] He noted that the term *erosion* had "given rise to considerable confusion" and instead used *wasting* in a collective sense to designate any kind of slow and gradual loss of tooth substance characterized by a smooth, polished surface, without reference to the cause of such loss. Thus emerged the "toothbrush/dentifrice theory of tooth abrasion," which exists to this day in the literature among some proponents as the sole cause of "wastings," now referred to as NCCLs.

In Miller's studies of wasting, he found that it was produced by mechanical action of the toothbrush combined with tooth powder. Miller conducted numerous studies using tooth powders concocted of various materials, including powdered oyster shell, cigar ashes, or prepared chalk with a small amount of pumice. All of these agents severely abraded the teeth, particularly in the cervical region whenever there was gingival recession. Miller concluded that "Anyone who brushes their teeth once daily thoroughly, using a gritty tooth-powder, will invariably wear away his teeth at the necks inside of a very few years, unless they are protected by healthy gums." Brushing without powder, on the other hand, resulted in no trace of wear.

Miller also conducted experiments with various acid solutions and designated the combined action of acid and friction from the toothbrush as *chemico-abrasion*. From his numerous experiments, Miller concluded the following: *(1)* Wasting of the teeth is a mechanical process of abrasion caused by brushing the teeth with tooth powder. *(2)* Acids that occur naturally in the mouth cannot produce wasting, although they do decalcify tooth structure. Erosion therefore is not the same as wasting. *(3)* Enamel is more susceptible to wasting after having been eroded by acid. That is, chemico-abrasion of the enamel is more readily produced than simple abrasion. *(4)* Substances that weaken organic tooth structure make the tooth more liable to wear and wasting. Despite the paucity of scientific instruments available to Miller during his research, his conclusions are mostly accepted to this day.

Greene Vardiman Black, a contemporary of Miller, recognized that Miller demonstrated the possibility and probability that teeth are often injured by vigorous brushing with gritty powders after many years, but he argued that Miller's evidence was not conclusive that all "erosions" are the result of wasting and that Miller's experiments did not explain all of the lesions Black had clinically observed. He further suggested that acids naturally present in the mouth could aid the degradation process. However, Black also concluded that "erosion" is caused by the toothbrush loaded with abrasive powders.[13] According to this view, erosion is not a disease but rather a purely mechanical injury. This confusion between the distinct mechanisms of abrasion and erosion lasted throughout the 20th century.

In 1932, Benjamin Kornfeld[14] shed light on the enigma of NCCLs as well as CDH (see "History of the Nomenclature and Etiology of CDH" below). He used the term *cervical erosions* to describe NCCLs as eroded areas that may be rounded, saucer shaped, or have a definite triangular notch. He further stated that erosion usually attacks the buccal and labial surfaces of the teeth at the gingival third, though it is not limited to these surfaces. Kornfeld also argued that erosion was far more prevalent than was generally considered, possibly as prevalent as the more common form of decay (ie, caries). He noted that in all cases of cervical erosion he had witnessed, the facets on the articulating surfaces of the teeth involved were worn. A study of these facets, he stated, will reveal that when the teeth are in occlusion, the resul-

Fig 1-1 Conceptual model of the elastic deformation of teeth: Flexural expansive *(a)* and strained compressive *(b)* bending and buckling are the results of occlusally applied loading forces. Their effects are located in the cervical region.[17]

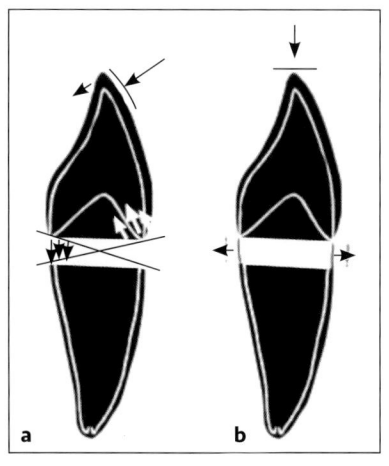

tant stress of the bite is not in a direction parallel with the long axes of the teeth.

In 1945, Charles F. Bodecker studied the gingival crevicular fluid and showed it to be acidic.[15] This fluid appears to cause erosion from its chemical action on the mineral elements of the enamel, cementum, and dentin when in contact with teeth in the cervical region. Bodecker stated that abrasion was also a factor and argued that these cervical lesions must involve both erosion and abrasion. Concluding that his investigation demonstrated the presence of an acidic crevicular exudate, he suggested that in many instances the toothbrush hastens the physical removal of the superficially softened tooth structure.

In 1962, as the dawn of biodental engineering was emerging, Körber[16] described and computed the elastic deformation of teeth. He concluded that forces applied horizontally give rise to flexion (causing tension and compression) in the cervical region, whereas forces applied vertically result in compressive stress to the cervical area (Fig 1-1). Three years later, Kohler[17] demonstrated the angular spread of foreign matter to the pulp by diffusion in connection with these defects, thus supporting the hypothesis that precarious activities are involved in the genesis of NCCLs.

Using tooth models, Grosskopf[18] concluded that misdirected or excessive loading of teeth may have a causal effect during clinical observations of cervical lesions. Lukas and Spranger[19,20] investigated the horizontal loading of teeth during lateral movements of the mandible and demonstrated that both torsion and translation (twisting and straight-line movement) take place at the cervix. In agreement with their studies, Vahl and Haunfelder[21] proposed the genesis of wedge-shaped lesions to be changes to the crystal structure of teeth. Spranger et al[22,23] described the genesis of hard tissue cervical lesions (NCCLs) as a multifactorial event with biodynamics related to stress.

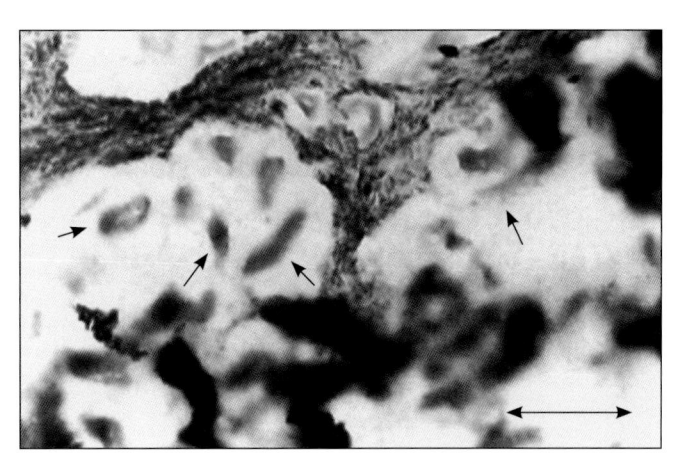

Fig 1-2 Electron microscopic examination of a dentinal surface just exposed within a wedge-shaped angular defect. Bacteria *(arrows)* can be seen colonizing the freshly exposed dentinal surface. (Arrowed bar = 1 μm.) (Reprinted with permission from Spranger et al.[22])

Spranger's numerous studies had a great influence in understanding the etiology of NCCLs. He recognized that NCCLs were multifactorial and that mechanisms of stress, biocorrosion, and friction were all involved in their genesis. His most significant finding was his observation that bacteria colonized the freshly exposed dentinal surface (Fig 1-2). Furthermore, this coating of microbes simultaneously triggers a local inflammatory reaction of the gingiva, which stimulates an increased rate of sulcular fluids to flow. This, in turn, provides nutrition for the microbes while the saliva produces buffering and remineralizing substances, resulting in an unstable equilibrium between defect formation and remineralization (Figs 1-3 and 1-4).

Following Körber's first photoelastic study, Lehman and Meyer[24] showed that wherever stress concentration occurs on teeth, caries will occur in the presence of a biocorrodent, such as plaque. Clinical observations support this hypothesis; other than in pits and fissures, caries is frequently observed at the interproximal contact areas as well as in the cervical area of teeth, where it progresses rapidly and is referred to as *root caries*. In 1968, Lebau hypothesized that stress resulting from occlusal forces played a role in the etiology of caries,[25,26] supporting the work done by Lehman and Meyer.[24] In 1974, Klähn et al[27] confirmed the results of these studies by demonstrating the distribution of lines of stress in loaded teeth (Fig 1-5). Other significant studies were done in the 1970s using finite element analysis (FEA), which demonstrated that eccentric loads applied to the occlusal surfaces of teeth generate stresses that are concentrated in the cervical region.[28-35]

Scanning electron microscopic (SEM) studies were also used to shed light on the etiology of so-called "cervical lesions." In 1977, Brady and Woody[36] postulated that cervical erosion may result from two different mechanisms: *(1)* a more common destructive process with angular and deep lesions from occlusal stress and *(2)* a less severe shallow process with rounded lesions from physical abrasion from toothbrush/dentifrice or oral fluids.

In 1982, Gene McCoy introduced clinical observations that associations existed between the presence of cervical regions of flexural stress and bruxism, temporomandibular joint problems, and cementoenamel junction (CEJ) hard tissue breakdown, all of which he termed *ablations*.[37] His landmark publication in 1983 introduced a conceptual relationship between FEA stress studies available at that time and his clinical observation of noncarious tooth substance loss.[38] As a clinician, he reported that cervical gingival notch formation resulted from tensile stress fatigue due to eccentric occlusal overload. He further implicated strain resulting from cervical stress as the reason for hard tissue loss in cervical regions. In 1979,[39] McCoy introduced the "dental compression syndrome," stating that off-loading of axial stresses during intercuspation produces cervical notching. McCoy expressed an opinion that the stress from clenching and bruxing contributed to the formation of abfractive lesions.

Shortly after McCoy averred that stress was a factor in the etiology of NCCLs, Lee and Eakle[40,41] published their hypothesis that tensile stresses were responsible for the loss of noncarious enamel in the cervical region. They observed that wedge-shaped lesions seem to indicate that occlusal stress on teeth is a major factor that initiates these lesions. At that time they termed them *cervical erosions* for a lack of a better term and to distinguish them from smooth, rounded acid erosions. Their hypothesis was that "the primary etiologic factor in cervical erosion is the tensile stress caused by mastication and malocclusion and that the local milieu plays a secondary role in dissolution of the tooth structure to create the lesion."

In 1991, John Grippo[42] introduced the term *abfraction* as the manifestation of the effects of the mechanism of stress, or the microstructural loss of tooth substance in areas of stress concentration. Up until this point, noncarious lesions were classified into the three categories of abrasion (loss of tooth structure by mechanical means), attrition (loss of tooth structure by wear), and erosion (loss of tooth structure by chemical or idiopathic process), so this became a new classification that joined all three mechanisms affecting tooth substance loss. Subsequently, Grippo et al[43,44] advocated that the term *erosion* be deleted from the dental lexicon and supplanted with the term *biocorrosion*, denoting the chemical, biochemical, and electrochemical dissolution of teeth.

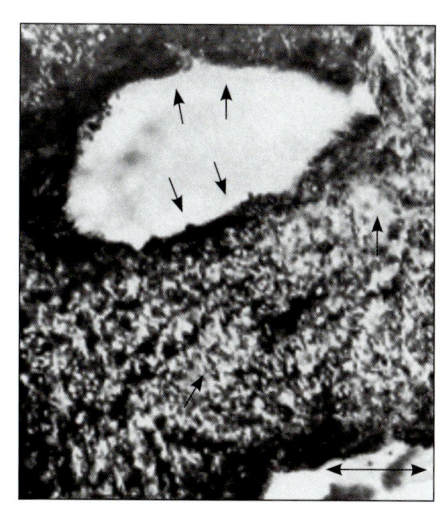

Fig 1-3 Electron microscopic examination of the superficial dentin of an angular lesion just after the abfractional phase. Note the demineralization *(arrows)* of the dentin and wide-open dentinal tubules. (Arrowed bar = 1 μm.) (Reprinted with permission from Spranger et al.[22])

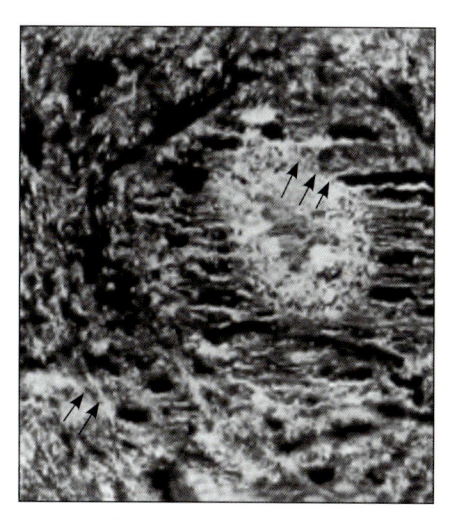

Fig 1-4 Electron microscopic examination of the dentin near the surface of an old angular lesion. Peritubular and intratubular remineralization and regular remineralized dentinal floor substance can be identified *(arrows)*. (Arrowed bar = 1 μm.) (Reprinted with permission from Spranger et al.[22])

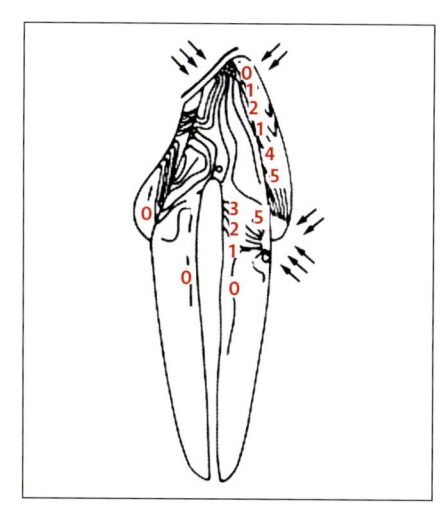

Fig 1-5 Stress lines in the model of a tooth from a photoelastic examination (adapted from Klähn et al[27]). Para-axial force induces flexure preferentially at the cervical region. 0, lines without any deformation; 1 to 5, lines of minimal to maximal deformation.

Once the concept of abfraction was introduced, much attention was given to the etiology of NCCLs. The mechanisms of abrasion and erosion, acting solely or combined, had been generally accepted in the literature and embraced by clinicians. Until the 1990s, there had been no documentation of the effects of stress on the acid dissolution of enamel or dentin, so Grippo and Masi[45] set out to investigate this. Their experiments demonstrated that teeth under a static load degraded more rapidly than unloaded teeth (Fig 1-6). Fatigue cracking (due to failure at the CEJ) was also observed because of the combined effects of stress and biocorrosion. They also determined that a tooth deformed in flexion, indicating that one side was in tension while the opposing side was in compression.

Palamara et al[46] also investigated the effects of stress on acid dissolution of enamel at the CEJ. Their experiments provided the first documentation of the interplay of cyclic loading force and acid on enamel loss in the laboratory under controlled conditions using extracted teeth. They showed that enamel dissolution is increased in sites subjected to cyclic tensile load, thus supporting the role of stress/biocorrosion in the etiology of NCCLs.

In 2005, in a series of in vitro fatigue-cycling experiments on human dentin cantilever beams, Staninec et al[47] showed that both mechanical stress and lower pH accelerated material loss of dentin surfaces. Compressive stresses generally led to more loss than tensile stress, and a change in pH from 7 to 6 nearly doubled the loss observed. Even at neutral pH, mechanical stresses caused some biocorrosion of exposed dentin surfaces.

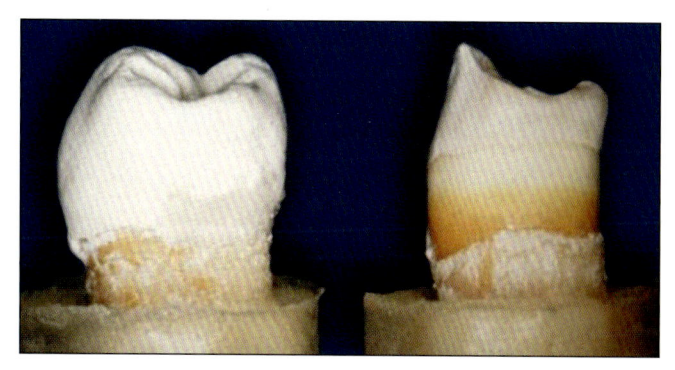

Fig 1-6 Experimental teeth demonstrate the effects of stress/biocorrosion. The tooth on the left is unstressed, while the tooth on the right shows the effects of a horizontal static load (150 pounds), resulting in stress/biocorrosion. The stylus from the loading device was placed 3 mm below the summit of the buccal cusp. Both teeth were immersed for 96 hours in citric acid (pH 3.5). The effects on dentin were not quantified.

Over the course of nearly 300 years, the nomenclature and our understanding of the etiology of NCCLs have changed dramatically, and our understanding will only continue to evolve as more studies are performed and more information comes to light.

Prevalence of NCCLs

The prevalence of NCCLs, regardless of form or etiology, varies from 5% to 85% in modern dentitions[48,49] (Table 1-2). These lesions are most commonly found in premolars and molars, and the prevalence and severity have been shown to increase

History, Prevalence, and Etiology of NCCLs and CDH

Table 1-2 Prevalence of NCCLs in the modern era

Author(s)	Year	Sample origin	Size of study	Type of lesion described	Age group	Prevalence
Kitchin[50]	1941	Dental clinic patients, students, staff	200	Abrasion	20–29 years 30–39 years 40–49 years 50–59 years	42% > 42% 76% < 76%
Ervin and Bucher[51]	1944	Adult dental patients from 40 practices	1,252	Abrasion	20–29 years 30–39 years 40–49 years ≥ 50 years	45% 68% 83% 87%
Shulman and Robinson[52]	1948	Boys entering freshman year	1,345	Erosion	14–15 years	2%
Zipkin and McClure[53]	1949	Dental clinic patients	83	Erosion	27–39 years ≥ 40 years	21% 32%
ten Bruggen Cate[54]	1968	British industrial workers	555	Erosion	15–65 years	32%
Sangnes and Gjermo[55]	1976	Dental clinic patients and factory workers	533	Abrasion	18–29 years ≥ 30 years	32% 50%
Radentz et al[56]	1976	Laboratory technician students enlisted in the military	80	Abrasion/erosion	17–45 years	50%
Brady and Woody[36]	1977	Dentists	900	Occlusal stress/abrasion	Not provided	5%
Bergström and Lavstedt[57]	1979	Stratified sample from Stockholm, Sweden	818	Abrasion	18–25 years 26–35 years 36–45 years 46–55 years 56–65 years	16% 38% 41% 40% 41%
Xhonga and Valdmanis[58]	1983	Dental clinic patients from two cities	527	Not provided	14–88 years	~25%
Hand et al[59]	1986	Noninstitutionalized rural and elderly Iowans	520	Abrasion	≥ 65 years	56%
Bergström and Eliasson[60]	1988	Dental clinic patients	250	Abrasion	21–30 years 31–60 years	67% 90%
Natusch and Klimm[61]	1989	Dental clinic patients	300	Erosion/abrasion	16–35 years	13% (erosion) 4% (abrasion)
Järvinen et al[62]	1991	Dental clinic patients	206	Erosion	13–83 years	5%
Lussi et al[63]	1991	Residents of Berne and Lucerne cantons, Switzerland	391	Erosion	26–30 years 46–50 years	16% (facial) ~5% (lingual)
Borcic et al[64]	2004	Inhabitants of Rijeka, Croatia	1,002	NCCLs	< 26 years 26–35 years 36–45 years 46–55 years 56–65 years > 65 years	4% 11.2% 18.7% 25.6% 25.6% 33%
Faye et al[65]	2006	Dental clinic patients in Senegal with leprosy	102	Biocorrosion/abfraction	20–77 years	47%
Bernhardt et al[66]	2006	Population of Pomerania	2,707	Abfraction	20–59 years	45.4% (maxilla) 54.6% (mandible)
Ommerborn et al[67]	2007	Dental clinic patients with sleep bruxism	58	NCCLs	20–39 years	25.8%
Smith et al[68]	2008	Dental clinic patients	156	NCCLs	16–64 years	62.2%
Hirata et al[69]	2010	Industrial workers	386	NCCLs	30–39 years 40–49 years 50–59 years	42.8% 63.5% 68.8%
Brandini et al[70]	2012	Students and workers	132	NCCLs	20–30 years	39%
Que et al[71]	2013	General population in China	1,023	NCCLs	20–29 years 30–39 years 40–49 years 50–59 years 60–69 years	30.1% 42.3% 58.6% 77.5% 81.6%
Bartlett et al[72]	2013	Population of Estonia, Finland, Latvia, France, the United Kingdom, and Italy	3,187	Erosion	18–25 years 26–35 years	26.5% 31.4%
George et al[73]	2014	Wine testers	25	Erosion	22–66 years	44%
Kumar et al[74]	2015	Schoolchildren in India	395	NCCLs	12–15 years	22.7%

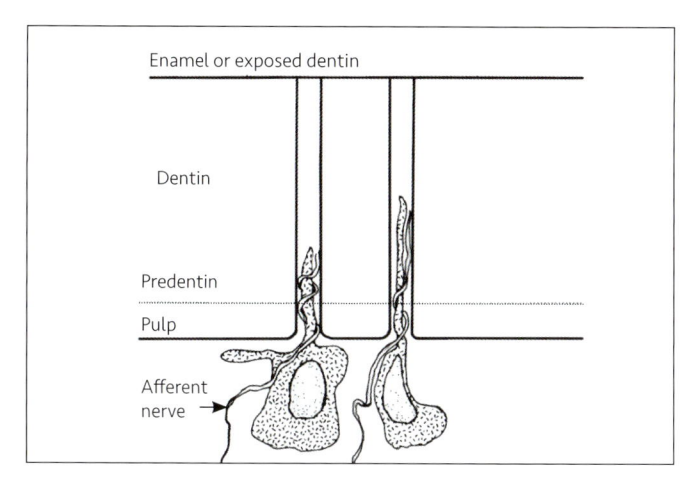

Fig 1-7 Illustration from Brännström's 1981 text, *Dentin and Pulp in Restorative Dentistry*. He theorized that fluid movement in dentinal tubules distorts odontoblasts and afferent nerves, leading to the sensation of pain. (Reprinted with permission.[101])

Fig 1-8 Illustration from Pashley's electron microscopy of a smear layer (SL) and smear layer plug (SP) in a dentinal tubule following a cutting procedure on the external root surface. (Reprinted from Pashley[107] with permission.)

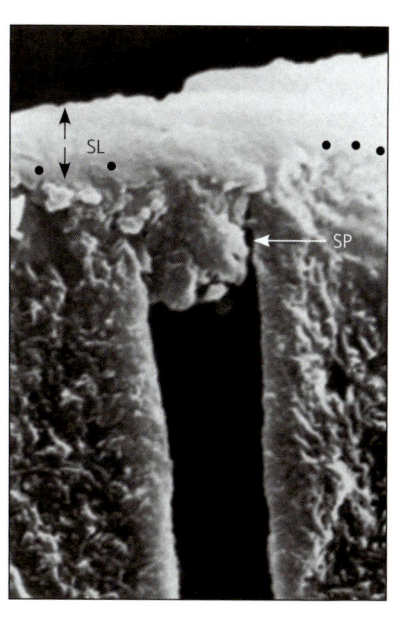

with age.[41] Prevalence data in the literature are highly discrepant and determined by the defect criteria of NCCL morphology. This high variance pinpoints the difficulty of defining what constitutes a single etiologic mechanism for NCCLs.[66] It would be a difficult task to arrive at a precise figure of prevalence of NCCLs for all populations because factors such as age and ethnic group create wide variations in figures.

History of the Nomenclature and Etiology of CDH

In 1932, Kornfeld reported the presence of CDH associated with occlusal overloading.[14] He found that this "sensitiveness" resolved within 10 days following minor occlusal adjustment (coronoplasty). Subsequent decades witnessed the use of the term *dentin hypersensitivity* to describe this sensitivity in the literature, and in the 1990s the more definitive term *cervical dentin hypersensitivity* was introduced.[75,76] CDH has been clinically detected as a pain distinct from that of postoperative dentin hypersensitivity.[77] The development of CDH has been attributed to a threshold of open dentinal tubules resulting from loss of the cementum, smear, and/or pellicle layer at cervical root surfaces.[78-81]

CDH has been described in the modern literature as a rapidly induced pain response to a stimulus from air, cold, touch, electric impulse, acid exposure, or a combination of these stimuli to dentin in the cervical area of the tooth.[78-99] The exact cause of the open dentinal tubules is not clear, but etiologic theories behind CDH point to stress and/or biocorrosion (see "Etiology of NCCLs and CDH" below). Further study is required to confirm these theories.

Because CDH presents with pain, professionals have followed a course of empirical treatment to eliminate the problem rather than scientific investigations into its etiologic factors: cervical stress concentration, biocorrosion, and friction. The following chapters present the proposed mechanisms for CDH and its impact on the development of NCCLs.

Brännström et al's hydrodynamic theory, based on Gysi's postulates of 1900, is likely the most widely accepted explanation for the presence of CDH.[82-85,100,101] According to this theory, mechanoreceptors at the pulp-dentin interface stimulate the conduction of A-δ myelinated nerves to produce pain in response to a given stimulus. CDH pain is the result of the inward and outward flow of dentinal tubular fluid (Fig 1-7). The presence of free nerve endings extending 100 microns from the pulp-dentin interface into the dentinal tubules have also been implicated as cofactors in the nociception of CDH pain.[101] These mechanoreceptors and free nerve endings have been extensively studied in the literature.[102-108] Pashley added support to the hydrodynamic theory of Brännström by his 1989 SEM illustration of a smear layer plug of a dentinal tubule[107] (Fig 1-8). To this day, the flow of dentinal tubular fluid is considered responsible for stimulating pulp receptors, thereby producing CDH pain.

Another theory that cannot be entirely discounted is the contribution of the neural transmission of molecular mediators to CDH pain.[109] These molecular mediators produced in or by the pulp tissues as a response to stimuli can produce odontoblast stimulation/reaction.[108]

Berkowitz et al investigated pulp nociception before and after placement of resin-based composites.[110] In pa-

Table 1-3 Prevalence of CDH

Authors	Year	Country	Age group	Prevalence
Flynn et al[115]	1985	Scotland	11–74 years	29%
Rees et al[116]	2003	China	11–90 years	67.7%
Rees et al[117]	2004	United Kingdom	11–90 years	2.8%
Colak et al[120]	2012	Turkey	University students (young adults)	64.2% (1 week); 87% (occasional)
Wang et al[119]	2012	China	20–69 years	34.5%
Ye et al[118]	2012	China	20–69 years	34.1%
Cunha-Cruz et al[114]	2013	United States	18–64 years	4.6%–95%
Davari et al[121]	2013	Canada	Variable	2%–85%
Rahiotis et al[122]	2013	Greece	31–59 years	21.3%–38.6%
Splieth et al[123]	2013	Various	Unspecified	3%–98%
West et al[99]	2013	France, Italy, Spain, Finland, Latvia, Estonia, United Kingdom	18–35 years	41% (air stimulation); 56.8% (Schiff scale); 26.8% (questionnaire)
Costa et al[125]	2014	Brazil	> 34 years	33.4% (air probe); 34.2% (probe)
Naidu et al[124]	2014	India	Young adults	32%

tients without preoperative hypersensitivity, they found a 10% increase in hypersensitivity at 4 weeks. Because resin-restored teeth do not have dentinal tubules open to the oral environment, acidic conditions could not initiate fluid flow in these tubules, nor could the dentinal fluid evaporate. In 2013, Chung et al reported that neurotransmitters released by odontoblasts are a part of the neurogenic inflammatory process producing dentin hypersensitivity and CDH.[108,111] These studies suggest that dentin hypersensitivity does not require open dentinal tubules to initiate pulp pain.[108,110] In addition, neurogenic inflammation can lower the nociceptive induction threshold for CDH. However, further investigation is required to enhance our understanding of CDH induction.

The concept of frictional dental hypersensitivity as proposed by Yiannios has also been advanced as a potential cause of CDH resulting from the biomechanical flexure of enamel and dentin.[112] In an FEA study, Linsuwanont et al[113] reported rapid biphasic temperature transduction in pulp tissues resulting from occlusal force. Because friction produces heat, and stress results from hyperfunction or parafunction, the concept of dentin hypersensitivity arising from chronic microtrauma is plausible. Further study is required to investigate the contributions of these mechanisms in CDH.

Prevalence of CDH

The prevalence of CDH has been found to vary from 2% to 98% in specific populations[99,114–125] (Table 1-3). Unlike NCCLs, CDH cannot be identified visually. Therefore, methodology for CDH detection has varied from subjective patient reporting to in vivo placebo/study group investigation with air, cold, or tactile stimuli.[126–128] The use of an air blast stimulus during CDH study has become an accepted nonsubjective investigative means.[129] However, differences in investigative design (eg, distance from air source to root, volume of air, etc) can impact the reported prevalence of CDH.[78] In addition, acidic diets common to modern populations, societal variations of alcohol intake, coarseness of foods, and environmental exposure to abrasives that affect the integrity of the smear and pellicle layers/cementum can also influence the prevalence rates of CDH.[41,56,130,131] Analysis of several studies investigating the incidence rate of CDH shows that it appears most frequently among 20- to 40-year-old populations, with a mean age of approximately 25 to 30 years.[90,98,114,132] It is rarely detected among younger groups and less frequently in older individuals.[133]

Etiology of NCCLs and CDH

It is now generally accepted that NCCLs have a multifactorial etiology comprising stress, friction, and biocorrosion (Figs 1-9 and 1-10 and Box 1-1). However, the etiology of CDH related to occlusion has remained an enigma, since most attention has been given to the modalities of treatment rather than the cause. The authors of this book contend that there is a strong relationship between the two pathologies of CDH and

Etiology of NCCLs and CDH

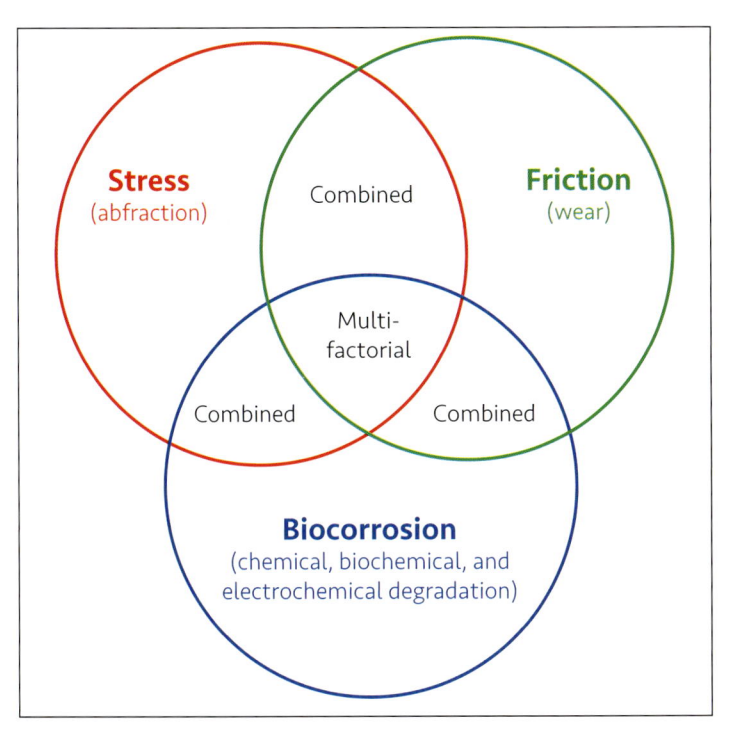

Fig 1-9 Mechanisms of the initiating and perpetuating etiologic factors of CDH and NCCLs (see Box 1-1 for more details).

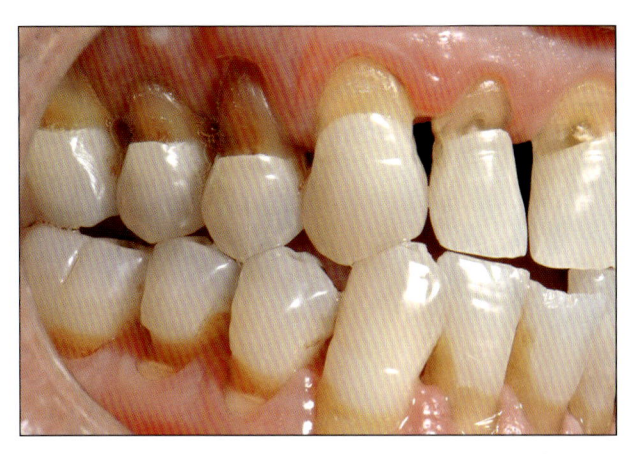

Fig 1-10 A Brazilian orange grower with advanced abfractions caused by stress and biocorrosion in the cervical region. He sucks between 9 to 12 oranges per day, and the citric acid acts as an exogenous biocorrodent. He does not use a toothbrush or dentifrice. (Courtesy of the NCCL Research Group, Uberlândia, Brazil.)

Box 1-1 Etiologic factors for CDH and NCCLs

Stress
Endogenous
- Parafunction: bruxism, clenching
- Occlusion: premature contacts or eccentric loading
- Deglutition
- Mastication of hard and resistant foods

Exogenous
- Habits: biting objects such as pencils, pipe stems, and fingernails
- Occupations: holding nails with teeth, playing a wind instrument
- Dental appliances: orthodontic appliances, partial denture clasps, bite guards

Friction
Exogenous (abrasion)
- Dental hygiene: overzealous brushing, use of gritty toothpaste
- Erosion (flow of liquids)
- Dental appliances (eg, metal clasps)

Biocorrosion
Endogenous (acids)
- Plaque acidogenic bacteria
- Gingival crevicular fluid
- Gastric juice in patients with GERD, bulimia

Exogenous (acids)
- Consumption of acidic citrus fruits, juices, and beverages
- Occupational exposures to acidic industrial gases and other environmental factors

Proteolysis
- Enzymatic lysis (caries)
- Proteases (pepsin and trypsin)
- Crevicular fluid

Electrochemical
- Piezoelectric effect in dentin

NCCLs and that they both stem from eccentric loading forces to teeth. These forces result in stress to the periodontium and the cervical region of the tooth and are perceived by the pulp as pain. Whereas stress is the prime etiologic factor for CDH (see section below), friction and biocorrosion also play a role.

Friction

This physical mechanism refers to the loss of substrate from the effect of flow induced by solid, liquid, or gas. Interaction in the mouth by toothbrush/dentifrice abrasion as well as ingested foods or liquid flow over teeth has the potential to result in loss of pellicle/smear layer or cementum. However, flow in the mouth is also moderated and buffered by saliva, which contains organic protein/glycoprotein and inorganic salts. These substances readily cover and protect exposed dentinal surfaces from tubule liquid pressure change but not necessarily from abrasion.

A common assumption exists that the etiology of CDH is related to abrasion from dentifrice and toothbrush.[134] The authors of this text could not locate scientific in vivo investigations by literature review to support or refute the concept that toothbrush/dentifrice use removes cementum and/or the smear layer. Further, in vitro studies cannot replicate oral salivary conditions of root dentin loss or nociception of CDH during short-term abrasion investigation. However, some studies have suggested that dentifrice and toothbrush, whether used alone or in conjunction, cannot be an initiating factor for CDH.[135-138] The reduced rate of wear associated with modern soft-bristle toothbrushes and smaller abrasive grain size in dentifrices seems to indicate a minor or secondary influence upon CDH.[139] Toothbrush and dentifrice are indicated to play a "contributing" role, not an etiologic role, for CDH.

Biocorrosion

The presence of biocorrosion is a cofactor during the production of CDH. Acidic endogenous or exogenous conditions in the mouth produce smear and/or pellicle layer loss from exposed dental surfaces. The action of acids and proteases over time produces dissolution of glycoprotein and other components that otherwise occlude dentinal tubules. Oral conditions of biocorrosion, including reduced salivary flow related to aging and use of pharmaceuticals to control depression, hypertension, and other chronic systemic conditions with oral manifestations, may unavoidably increase the likelihood of CDH by lowering oral pH. Any condition that produces xerostomia will carry a risk of CDH from biocorrosion.[121,140]

Stress

Chronic stress to cervical regions is the result of minor regions of force upon occlusal surfaces, as introduced by Kornfeld in 1932.[14] Cervical stress has been implicated by numerous clinicians and FEA researchers to cause pellicle/smear layer, cementum, and enamel/dentin loss in the CEJ region.[78,81,96,98,141-146] When the rate of this loss exceeds the salivary speed of smear/pellicle layer re-formation, open dentinal tubules reach a threshold of nociception, that of CDH. The presence of CDH is therefore indicated as an early sign and symptom during the stress-induced clinical formation of the abfractive lesion (or NCCL).

The clinical and FEA studies presented in this text disclose the concomitant etiologic foundation of stress during NCCL and CDH development. The authors do not intend to debate the contributory mechanisms of CDH nor their etiology for the NCCL. Rather, the information presented will illustrate an intimate relationship between CDH and NCCLs.

Cervical Root Caries

Root caries results from the same two mechanisms (stress and biocorrosion) as do NCCLs in that stress as well as bacterial plaque and proteolytic enzymes acting as biocorrodents degrade the tooth substance. The dentin is particularly susceptible to root caries because its surface is rougher than enamel and retains plaque. The only distinction between NCCLs and root caries is the degree of oral hygiene maintained by the patient.

Conclusion

Let's review what we have covered in this chapter:
- The etiology of NCCLs is multifactorial.
- CDH is the initial pathognomonic sign of cervical stress concentration resulting from occlusal disharmony.
- The rapid progression of root/cervical caries is closely related to NCCLs.

The mechanisms of stress, friction, and biocorrosion as well as their cofactors are further described in chapters 3, 4, and 5.

References

1. Fauchard P. The Surgeon Dentist, or Treatise on the Teeth, ed 2. Lindsay L (trans). London: Butterworth, 1946:20–21,40,46–47.
2. Hunter J. The Natural History of Human Teeth: Explaining Their Structure, Use, Formation, Growth, and Diseases. London: J. Johnson, 1778:98–100.
3. Fox J. The Natural History of the Human Teeth. London: Cox, 1803.
4. Bell T. The Anatomy, Physiology, and Diseases of the Teeth, ed 3. Philadelphia: Carey, Lea & Blanchard, 1837.
5. Harris CA. The Principles and Practice of Dentistry, ed 10. Philadelphia: Lindsay and Blakiston, 1871:245–263.
6. Koch CRE. Abrasion and erosion. Dental Cosmos 1873;15:461–475.
7. Darby ET. Dental erosion and the gouty diathesis: Are they usually associated? Dental Cosmos 1892;34:629–640.
8. Kirk EC. A contribution to the etiology of erosion. Dental Cosmos 1887;2850–58.
9. Grippo JO. Biocorrosion vs erosion: The 21st century and a time to change. Compend Contin Educ Dent 2012;33:e33–e37.

10. Harris CA. Dictionary of Dental Science, Biography, Bibliography and Medical Terminology. Philadelphia: Lindsay & Blakiston, 1849.
11. Zsigmondy U. Über die keilförmigen Defekte an den Facialflächen der Zähne. Österr Ungar Vjhrschr Zahnärzte 1894;1:439–442.
12. Miller WD. Experiments and observations on the wasting of tooth tissue variously designated as erosion, abrasion, chemical abrasion, denudation, etc. Dental Cosmos 1907;49:1–23,109–124,225–247.
13. Black GV. A Work on Operative Dentistry. Vol 1: Pathology of the Hard Tissues of the Teeth. Chicago: Medico-Dental, 1908:39–59.
14. Kornfeld B. Preliminary report of clinical observations of cervical erosions: A suggested analysis of the cause and the treatment for its relief. Dent Items Interest 1932;54:905–909.
15. Bodecker CF. Local acidity: A cause of dental erosion-abrasion—Progress report of the erosion-abrasion committee of the New York Academy of Dentistry. Ann Dent 1945;4:50–55.
16. Körber KH. Die elastische Deformierung menschlicher Zähne. Dtsch Zahnarztl Z 1962;17:691–698.
17. Kohler E. Experimentelle Untersuchungen uber die Ausbreitung von Fremdstoffen in den menschlichen Zahnartzgeweben. Dtsch Zahnartzl Z 1965;20:721–736.
18. Grosskopf G. Untersuchungen zur Entstehung der sogenannten keilförmigen Defekte am organum dentale [thesis]. Frankfurt-am-Main, 1967.
19. Lukas D, Spranger H. Untersuchungen uber die Horizontabelastung des zahnes bei definierten Unterkiefer- lateralbewegungen. Dtsch Zahnartzl Z 1973;28:280.
20. Lukas D, Spranger H. Experimentelle Untersuchungen uber die Auswirkungen unterschiedlich gemessener Gelenkbahn und Benntwinkel auf die Horizontalbelastung des Zahnes. Dtsch Zahnartzl Z 1973;28:755–758.
21. Vahl J, Haunfelder D. Feinstrukturuntersschungen von Zahnschaden bei Substanzverlust im Zahnhalsbereich (keilförmige Defekte). Dtsch Zahnartzl Z 1974;29:266–275.
22. Spranger H, Weber G, Kung YS. Untersuchungen uber die Ätiologie Pathogenese und Therpiekonsequenzen der zervikalen Zahnhartsubstanzdefekte. Hessische Zahnarzt Separatum Otto-Loos Preis 1973;12:328–341.
23. Spranger H. Investigations into the genesis of angular lesions at the cervical region of teeth. Quintessence Int 1995;26:149–154.
24. Lehman ML, Meyer ML. Relationship of dental caries and stress: Concentration in teeth as revealed by photoelastic tests. J Dent Res 1966;45:1706–1714.
25. Lebau GI. The primary cause and prevention of dental caries. Bull Union Cty Dent Soc 1968;47:11–13.
26. Lebau GI. The primary cause and prevention of dental caries. (II). Bull Union Cty Dent Soc 1968;57:13–16.
27. Klähn KH, Köhler KU, Kreter F, Motsch A. Spannungsoptische Untersuchungen zur Entstehung der sogenannten keilförmigen Defekte am Organum dentale. Dtsch Zahnartzl Z 1974;29:923–927.
28. Thresher RW, Saito GE. The stress analysis of human teeth. J Biomech 1973;6:443–449.
29. Selna LG, Shillingburg HT Jr, Kerr PA. Finite element analysis of dental structures—Axisymmetric and plane stress idealizations. J Biomed Mater Res 1975;9:237–252.
30. Yettram AL, Wright KW, Pickard HM. Finite element stress analysis of the crowns of normal and restored teeth. J Dent Res 1976;55:1004–1011.
31. Bowen RL, Rodriguez MS. Tensile strength and modulus of elasticity of tooth structure and several restorative materials. J Am Dent Assoc 1962;64:378–387.
32. Rubin C, Krishnamurthy N, Capilouto E, Yi H. Stress analysis of the human tooth using a three-dimensional finite element model. J Dent Res 1983;62:82–86.
33. Goel VK, Khera SC, Ralston JL, Chang KH. Stresses at the dentinoenamel junction of human teeth—A finite element investigation. J Prosthet Dent 1991;66:451–459.
34. Hood JA. Experimental studies on tooth deformation: Stress distribution in class V restorations. N Z Dent J 1972;68(312):116–131.
35. Powers JM, Craig RG, Ludema KC,. Frictional behavior and surface failure of human enamel. J Dent Res 1973;52:1327–1331.
36. Brady JM, Woody RD. Scanning microscopy of cervical erosion. J Am Dent Assoc 1977;94:726–729.
37. McCoy G. The etiology of gingival erosion. J Oral Implantol 1982;10:361–362.
38. McCoy G. On the longevity of teeth. J Oral Implantol 1983;11:248–267.
39. McCoy G. Bruxism, ablation and distribution of occlusal stress. Presented at the 9th International Meeting of Dental Implants and Transplants, Bologna, 22-24 May 1979.
40. Lee WC, Eakle WS. Possible role of tensile stress in the etiology of cervical erosive lesions of teeth. J Prosthet Dent 1984;53:374–380.
41. Lee WC, Eakle WS. Stress-induced cervical lesions: Review of advances in the past 10 years. J Prosthet Dent 1996;75:487–494.
42. Grippo JO. Abfractions: A new classification of hard tissue lesions of teeth. J Esthet Dent 1991;3:14–19.
43. Grippo JO, Simring M. Dental 'erosion' revisited. J Am Dent Assoc 1995;126:619–620,623–624,627–630.
44. Grippo JO, Simring M, Schreiner S. Attrition, abrasion, corrosion and abfraction revisited: A new perspective on tooth surface lesions. J Am Dent Assoc 2004;135:1109–1118.
45. Grippo JO, Masi JV. Role of biodental engineering factors (BEF) in the etiology of root caries. J Esthet Dent 1991;3;71–76.
46. Palamara D, Palamara JE, Tyas MJ, Pintado M, Messer HH. Effect of stress on acid dissolution of enamel. Dent Mater 2001;17:109–115.
47. Staninec M, Nalla RK, Hilton JF, et al. Dentin erosion simulation by cantilever beam fatigue and pH change. J Dent Res 2005;84:371–375.
48. Levitch LC, Bader JD, Shugars DA, Heymann HO. Non-carious cervical lesions. J Dent 1994;22:195–207.
49. Becker C, Freesmeyer WB. Der Keilförmige Defekt—Epidemiologie un Äitologie im Literaturvergleich ZWR 1999;108:732–739.
50. Kitchin PC. Cervical exposure and abrasion in human teeth for different age classes. Science 1941;94(2429):65–66.
51. Ervin JC, Bucher EM. Prevalence of tooth root exposure and abrasion among dental patients. Dent Items Interest 1944;66:760–769.
52. Shulman EH, Robinson HB. Salivary citrate content and erosion of the teeth. J Dent Res 1948;27:541–544
53. Zipkin I, McClure FJ. Salivary citrate and dental erosion: Procedure for determining citric acid in saliva—Dental erosion and citric acid in saliva. J Dent Res 1949;28:613–626.
54. ten Bruggen Cate HJ. Dental erosion in industry. Br J Ind Med 1968;25:249–266.
55. Sangnes G, Gjermo P. Prevalence of oral soft and hard tissue lesions related to mechanical toothcleansing procedures. Community Dent Oral Epidemiol 1976;4(2):77–83.
56. Radentz WH, Barnes GP, Cutright DE. A survey of factors possibly associated with cervical abrasion of tooth surfaces. J Periodontol 1976;47:148–154.
57. Bergström J, Lavstedt S. An epidemiologic approach to toothbrushing and dental abrasion. Community Dent Oral Epidemiol 1979;7(1):57–64.
58. Xhonga FA, Valdmanis S. Geographic comparisons of the incidence of dental erosion: A two centre study. J Oral Rehabil 1983;10:269–277.
59. Hand JS, Hunt RJ, Reihardt JW. The prevalence and treatment implications of cervical abrasion in the elderly. Gerodontics 1986;2:167–170.
60. Bergström J, Eliasson S. Cervical abrasion in relation to toothbrushing and periodontal health. Scand J Dent Res 1988;96:405–411.
61. Natusch I, Klimm W. Chronic loss of dental hard substance in early and middle adulthood [in German]. Zahn Mund Kieferheilkd Zentralbl 1989;77:123–127.
62. Järvinen VK, Rytömaa II, Heinonen OP. Risk factors in dental erosion. J Dent Res 1991;70:942–947.
63. Lussi A, Schaffner M, Holtz P, Suter P. Dental erosion in a population of Swiss adults. Community Dent Oral Epidemiol 1991;19:286–290.
64. Borcic J, Anic I, Urek MM, Ferreri S. The prevalence of non-carious cervical lesions in permanent dentition. J Oral Rehabil 2004;31:117–123.
65. Faye B, Kane AW, Sarr M, Lo C, Ritter AV, Grippo JO. Noncarious cervical lesions among a non-toothbrushing population with Hansen's disease (leprosy): Initial findings. Quintessence Int 2006;37:613–619.
66. Bernhardt O, Gesch D, Schwahn C, et al. Epidemiological evaluation of the multifactorial aetiology of abfraction. J Oral Rehabil 2006;33:17–25.
67. Ommerborn MA, Schneider C, Giraki M, et al. In vivo evaluation of noncarious cervical lesions in sleep bruxism subjects. J Prosthet Dent 2007;98:150–158.

68. Smith WA, Marchan S, Rafeek RN. The prevalence and severity of non-carious cervical lesions in a group of patients attending a university hospital in Trinidad. J Oral Rehabil 2008;35:128–134.
69. Hirata Y, Yamamoto T, Kawagoe T, Sasaguri K, Sato S. Relationship between occlusal contact pattern and non-carious cervical lesions among male adults. J Stomat Occ Med 2010;3:10–14.
70. Brandini DA, Pedrini D, Panzarini SR, Benete IM, Trevisan CL. Clinical evaluation of the association of noncarious cervical lesions, parafunctional habits, and TMD diagnosis. Quintessence Int 2012;43:255–262.
71. Que K, Guo B, Jia Z, Chen Z, Yang J, Gao P. A cross-sectional study: Non-carious cervical lesions, cervical dentine hypersensitivity and related risk factors. J Oral Rehabil 2013;40:24–32.
72. Bartlett DW, Lussi A, West NX, Bouchard P, Sanz M, Bourgeois D. Prevalence of tooth wear on buccal and lingual surfaces and possible risk factors in young European adults. J Dent 2013;41:1007–1013.
73. George R, Chell A, Chen B, Undery R, Ahmed H. Dental erosion and dentinal sensitivity amongst professional wine tasters in South East Queensland, Australia. ScientificWorld Journal 2014;2014:516975.
74. Kumar S, Kumar A, Debnath N, et al. Prevalence and risk factors for non-carious cervical lesions in children attending special needs schools in India. J Oral Sci 2015;57:37–43.
75. Gillam DG, Newman HN, Bulman JS, Davies EH. Dentifrice abrasivity and cervical dentinal hypersensitivity. Results 12 weeks following cessation of 8 weeks' supervised use. J Periodontol 1992;63:7–12.
76. Gillam DG, Newman HN, Davies EH, Bulman JS. Clinical efficacy of a low abrasive dentifrice for the relief of cervical dentinal hypersensitivity. J Clin Periodontol 1992;19:197–201.
77. Porto ICCM. Post-operative sensitivity on direct resin composite restorations: Clinical practice guidelines. Int J Restorative Dent 2012;1:1–12.
78. Pashley DH. Mechanisms of dentin sensitivity. Dent Clin North Am 1990;34:449–473.
79. Addy M. Etiology and clinical implications of dentine hypersensitivity. Dent Clin North Am 1990;34:503–514.
80. Kerns DG, Scheidt MJ, Pashley DH, Horner JA, Strong SL, Van Dyke TE. Dentinal tubule occlusion and root hypersensitivity. J Periodontol 1991;62:421–428.
81. Terry DA. Cervical dentin hypersensitivity: Etiology, diagnosis, and management. Dent Today 2011;30(4):61–62,64.
82. Gysi A. An attempt to explain the sensitiveness of dentin. Br J Dent Sci 1900;43:865–868.
83. Brännström M. Dentinal and pulpal response. III. Application of an air stream to exposed dentine; long observation periods. Acta Odontol Scand 1960;18:235–252.
84. Brännström M. Dentin sensitivity and aspiration of odontoblasts. J Am Dent Assoc 1963;66:366–370.
85. Anderson DJ, Hannam AG, Mathews B. Sensory mechanisms in mammalian teeth and their supporting structures. Physiol Rev 1970;50:171–195.
86. Dowell P, Addy M. Dentine hypersensitivity—A review. Aetiology, symptoms and theories of pain production. J Clin Periodontol 1983;10:341–350.
87. Dowell P, Addy M, Dummer P. Dentine hypersensitivity: Aetiology, differential diagnosis and management. Br Dent J 1985;158(3):92–96.
88. Absi EG, Addy M, Adams D. Dentine hypersensitivity. A study of the patency of dentinal tubules in sensitive and non-sensitive cervical dentine. J Clin Periodontol 1987;14:280–284.
89. Curro FA. Tooth hypersensitivity in the spectrum of pain. Dent Clin North Am 1990;34:429–437.
90. Pashley DH. Dentin sensitivity: Theory and treatment. Adult Oral Health 1993:1–7.
91. Tavares M, Depaola PF, Soparkar P. Using a fluoride-releasing resin to reduce cervical sensitivity. J Am Dent Assoc 1994;125:1337–1342.
92. Holland GR, Närhi MN, Addy M, Gangarosa L, Orchardson R. Guidelines for the design and conduct of clinical trials on dentine hypersensitivity. J Clin Periodontol 1997;24:808–813.
93. Dababneh RH, Khouri AT, Addy M. Dentine hypersensitivity—An enigma? A review of terminology, mechanisms, aetiology and management. Br Dent J 1999;187:606–611.
94. Taani DQ, Awartani F. Prevalence and distribution of dentin hypersensitivity and plaque in a dental hospital population. Quintessence Int 2001;32:372–376.
95. Ritter AV, de L Dias W, Miguez P, Caplan DJ, Swift EJ Jr. Treating cervical dentin hypersensitivity with fluoride varnish: A randomized clinical study. J Am Dent Assoc 2006;137:1013–1020.
96. Bartold PM. Dentinal hypersensitivity: A review. Aust Dent J 2006;51:212–218.
97. Ozen T, Orhan K, Avsever H, Tunca YM, Ulker AE, Akyol M. Dentin hypersensitivity: A randomized clinical comparison of three different agents in a short-term treatment period. Oper Dent 2009;34:392–398.
98. Shiau HJ. Dentin hypersensitivity. J Evid Based Dent Pract 2012;12(3 suppl):220–228.
99. West NX, Sanz M, Lussi A, Bartlett D, Bouchard P, Bourgeois D. Prevalence of dentine hypersensitivity and study of associated factors: A European population-based cross-sectional study. J Dent 2013;41:841–851.
100. Brännström M, Åström A. A study on the mechanism of pain elicited from the dentin. J Dent Res 1964;43:619–625.
101. Brännström M. Dentin and Pulp in Restorative Dentistry. Naka, Sweden: Dental Therapeutics AB, 1981.
102. Jyväsjärvi E, Kniffki KD. Cold stimulation of teeth: A comparison between the responses of cat intradental A delta and C fibres and human sensation. J Physiol 1987;391:193–207.
103. Närhi M, Jyväsjärvi E, Virtanen A, Huopaniemi T, Ngassapa D, Hirvonen T. Role of intradental A- and C-type nerve fibres in dental pain mechanisms. Proc Finn Dent Soc 1992;88(1 suppl):507–516.
104. Ikeda T, Nakano M, Bando E, Suzuki A. The effect of light premature occlusal contact on tooth pain threshold in humans. J Oral Rehabil 1998;25:589–595.
105. Abd-Elmeguid A, Yu DC. Dental pulp neurophysiology: Part 1. Clinical and diagnostic implications. J Can Dent Assoc 2009;75:55–59.
106. Henry MA, Luo S, Levinson SR. Unmyelinated nerve fibers in the human dental pulp express markers for myelinated fibers and show sodium channel accumulations. BMC Neurosci 2012;13:29.
107. Pashley DH. Dentin: A dynamic substrate—A review. Scanning Microsc 1989;3:161–174.
108. Chung G, Jung SJ, Oh SB. Cellular and molecular mechanisms of dental nociception. J Dent Res 2013;92:948–955.
109. Rapp R, Avery JK, Strachan DS. Possible Role of the Acetylcholinesterase in Neural Conduction Within the Dental Pulp. Birmingham: University of Alabama Press, 1968.
110. Berkowitz GS, Horowitz AJ, Curro FA, et al. Postoperative hypersensitivity in class I resin-based composite restorations in general practice: Interim results. Compend Contin Educ Dent 2009;30:356–358,360,362–363.
111. Cherkas PS, Dostrovsky JO, Sessle BJ. Activation of peripheral P2X receptors is sufficient to induce central sensitization in rat medullary dorsal horn nociceptive neurons. Neurosci Lett 2012;526:160–163.
112. Yiannios N. Occlusal Considerations in the Hypersensitive Dentition. Hershey, PA: IGI Global, 2015.
113. Linsuwanont P, Versluis A, Palamara JE, Messer HH. Thermal stimulation causes tooth deformation: A possible alternative to the hydrodynamic theory? Arch Oral Biol 2008;53:261–272.
114. Cunha-Cruz J, Wataha JC, Heaton LJ, et al. The prevalence of dentin hypersensitivity in general dental practices in the northwest United States. J Am Dent Assoc 2013;144:288–296.
115. Flynn J, Galloway R, Orchardson R. The incidence of 'hypersensitive' teeth in the West of Scotland. J Dent 1985;13:230–236.
116. Rees JS, Jin LJ, Lam S, Kudanowska I, Vowles R. The prevalence of dentine hypersensitivity in a hospital clinic population in Hong Kong. J Dent 2003;31:453–461.
117. Rees JS, Addy M. A cross-sectional study of buccal cervical sensitivity in UK general dental practice and a summary review of prevalence studies. Int J Dent Hyg 2004;2:64–69.
118. Ye W, Feng XP, Li R. The prevalence of dentine hypersensitivity in Chinese adults. J Oral Rehabil 2012;39:182–187.
119. Wang Y, Que K, Lin L, Hu D, Li X. The prevalence of dentine hypersensitivity in the general population in China. J Oral Rehabil 2012;39:812–820.
120. Colak H, Aylikci BU, Hamidi MM, Uzgur R. Prevalence of dentine hypersensitivity among university students in Turkey. Niger J Clin Pract 2012;15:415–419.
121. Davari A, Ataei E, Assarzadeh H. Dentin hypersensitivity: Etiology, diagnosis and treatment; A literature review. J Dent (Shiraz) 2013;14:136–145.

References

122. Rahiotis C, Polychronopoulou A, Tsiklakis K, Kakaboura A. Cervical dentin hypersensitivity: A cross-sectional investigation in Athens, Greece. J Oral Rehabil 2013;40:948–957.
123. Splieth CH, Tachou A. Epidemiology of dentin hypersensitivity. Clin Oral Investig 2013;17(1 suppl):S3–S8.
124. Naidu GM, Ram KC, Sirisha NR, et al. Prevalence of dentin hypersensitivity and related factors among adult patients visiting a dental school in Andhra Pradesh, southern India. J Clin Diagn Res 2014;8(9):ZC48–ZC51.
125. Costa RS, Rios FS, Moura MS, Jardim JJ, Maltz M, Haas AN. Prevalence and risk indicators of dentin hypersensitivity in adult and elderly populations from Porto Alegre, Brazil. J Periodontol 2014;85:1247–1258.
126. Ayad F, Ayad N, Zhang YP, DeVizio W, Cummins D, Mateo LR. Comparing the efficacy in reducing dentin hypersensitivity of a new toothpaste containing 8.0% arginine, calcium carbonate, and 1450 ppm fluoride to a commercial sensitive toothpaste containing 2% potassium ion: An eight-week clinical study on Canadian adults. J Clin Dent 2009;20:10–16.
127. Thrash WJ, Dorman HL, Smith FD. A method to measure pain associated with hypersensitive dentin. J Periodontol 1983;54:160–162.
128. Matthews WG, Showman CD, Pashley DH. Air blast-induced evaporative water loss from human dentine, in vitro. Arch Oral Biol 1993;38:517–523.
129. Bae H, Kim Y, Myung S. Desensitizing toothpaste versus placebo for dentin hypersensitivity: A systematic review and meta-analysis. J Clin Periodontol 2015;42:131–141.
130. Ritter AV, Grippo JO, Coleman TA, Morgan ME. Prevalence of carious and non-carious cervical lesions in archaeological populations from North America and Europe. J Esthet Restor Dent 2009;21:324–334.
131. Grippo JO, Simring M, Coleman TA. Abfraction, abrasion, biocorrosion, and the enigma of noncarious cervical lesions: A 20-year perspective. J Esthet Restor Dent 2012;24:10–23.
132. Cummins D. Dentin hypersensitivity: From diagnosis to a breakthrough therapy for everyday sensitivity relief. J Clin Dent 2009;20:1–9.
133. Tagami J, Hosoda H, Burrow MF, Nakajima M. Effect of aging and caries on dentin permeability. Proc Finn Dent Soc 1992;88(1 suppl):149–154.
134. Abrahamsen TC. The worn dentition—Pathognomonic patterns of abrasion and erosion. Int Dent J 2005;55(4 suppl):268–276.
135. Addy M, Hunter ML. Can tooth brushing damage your health? Effects on oral and dental tissues. Int Dent J 2003;53(3 suppl):177–186.
136. Ganss C, Hardt M, Blazek D, Klimek J, Schlueter N. Effects of toothbrushing force on the mineral content and demineralized organic matrix of eroded dentine. Eur J Oral Sci 2009;117:255–260.
137. Ganss C, Schlueter N, Preiss S, Klimek J. Tooth brushing habits in uninstructed adults—Frequency, technique, duration and force. Clin Oral Investig 2009;13:203–208.
138. Schlueter N, Klimek J, Saleschke G, Ganss C. Adoption of a toothbrushing technique: A controlled, randomised clinical trial. Clin Oral Investig 2010;14:99–106.
139. Lewis R, Dwyer-Joyce RS. Interactions between toothbrush and toothpaste particles during simulated abrasive cleaning. J Engineering Tribology 2006;220:755–765.
140. Jones JA. Dentin hypersensitivity: Etiology, risk factors, and prevention strategies. Dent Today 2011;30(11):108,110,112–113.
141. Pashley DH, Tao L, Boyd L, King GE, Horner JA. Scanning electron microscopy of the substructure of smear layers in human dentine. Arch Oral Biol 1988;33:265–270.
142. Soares PV, Machado AC, Zeola LF, et al. Loading and composite restoration assessment of various non-carious cervical lesions morphologies: 3D finite element analysis. Aust Dent J 2015;60:309–316.
143. Soares PV, Souza LV, Veríssimo C, et al. Effect of root morphology on biomechanical behaviour of premolars associated with abfraction lesions and different loading types. J Oral Rehabil 2014;41:108–114.
144. Soares PV, Santos-Filho PC, Soares CJ, et al. Non-carious cervical lesions: Influence of morphology and load type on biomechanical behaviour of maxillary incisors. Aust Dent J 2013;58:306–314.
145. Pereira FA, Zeola LF, de Almeida Milito G, Reis BR, Pereira RD, Soares PV. Restorative material and loading type influence on the biomechanical behavior of wedge shaped cervical lesions. Clin Oral Investig 2016;20:433–441.
146. Zeola LF, Pereira FA, Machado AC, et al. Effects of non-carious cervical lesion size, occlusal loading and restoration on biomechanical behaviour of premolar teeth. Aust Dent J 2016;61:408–417.

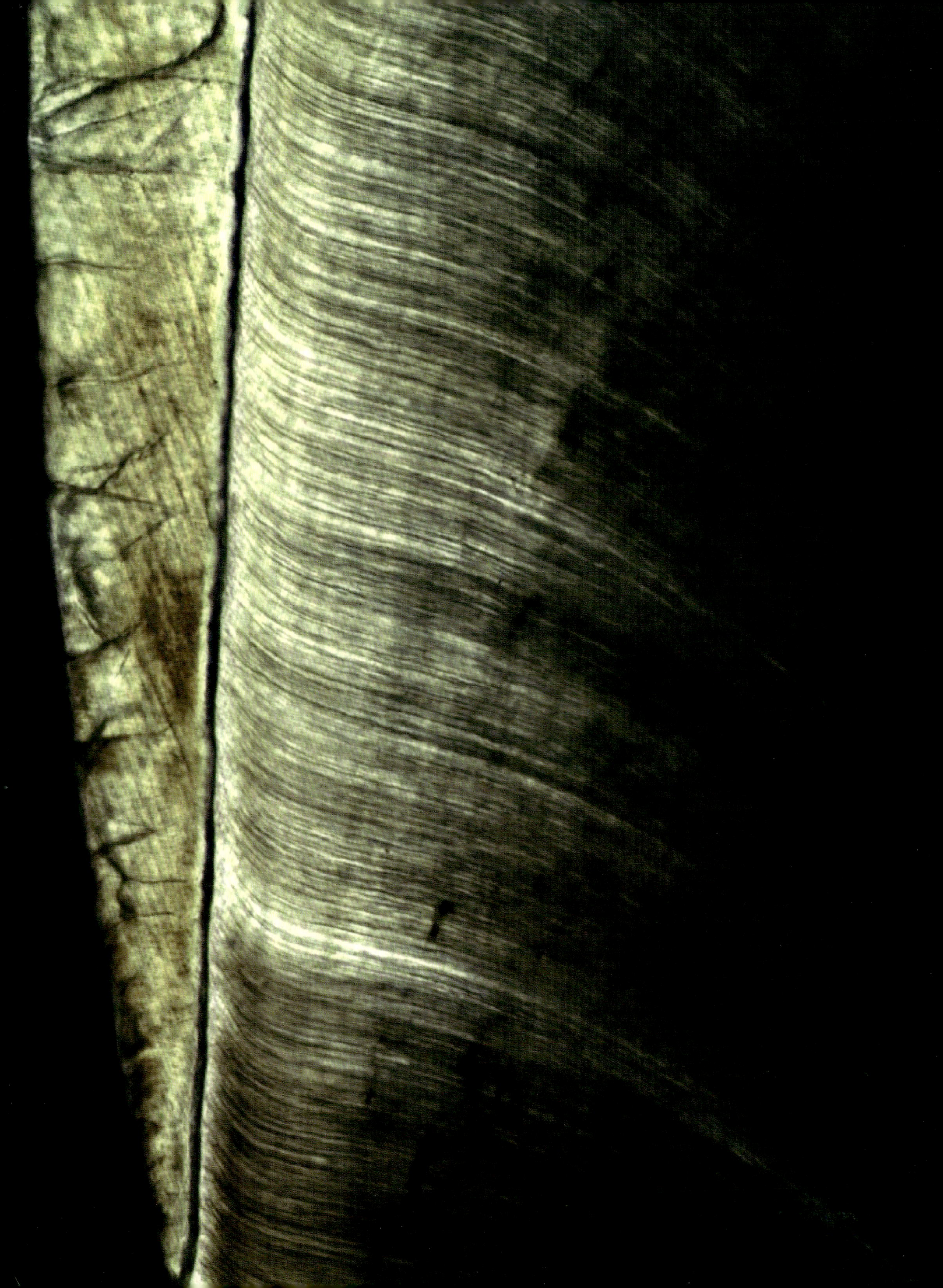

2

Anatomical Considerations: Enamel, Dentin, and Periodontium

Tooth Enamel

Enamel covers the entire anatomical crown of the tooth and protects the dentin and pulp against mechanical wear and biocorrosion.[1-3] Mature enamel is a nonvital tissue and has no ability to regenerate or repair itself if fractured, but it can remineralize.

Structural composition

Enamel is a mineralized epidermal tissue and represents the hardest material in the human body, consisting of approximately 96 wt% mineral (crystalline calcium phosphate in the form of hydroxyapatite), 3 wt% water, and 1 wt% organic material (noncollagenous proteins and enzymes).[1-4] The basic structural unit of enamel is the prism or rod, which is composed of stacked crystallites of hydroxyapatite oriented to optimize the mechanical properties of the material[5] (Fig 2-1). In human teeth, rods tend to be maintained in groups organized circumferentially around the long axis of the tooth. Normally, rods run in a perpendicular direction to the surface of the dentin, with a slight inclination to the cusp as they pass outward. Close to the cusp tip they run more vertically, and in cervical enamel they run mainly horizontally.[6] Interwoven with these cylinder-shaped rods is the interrod enamel (Fig 2-2). These two structures are bound by continuous crystals, providing a strong latticework to the enamel.[7]

Physical characteristics

Permeability

Tooth enamel is semipermeable, and various fluids, ions, and low-molecular weight substances can diffuse through its external micropores. This permeability allows for enamel remineralization because salivary ions can migrate back into the demineralized tooth surface. It also facilitates the uptake of fluoride to strengthen the enamel. At the same time, however, when teeth become dehydrated, the empty micropores make the enamel appear chalky and lighter in color. In addition, lifelong exposure of semipermeable enamel to the pigments from the oral environment can result in staining of the tooth.

2 Anatomical Considerations: Enamel, Dentin, and Periodontium

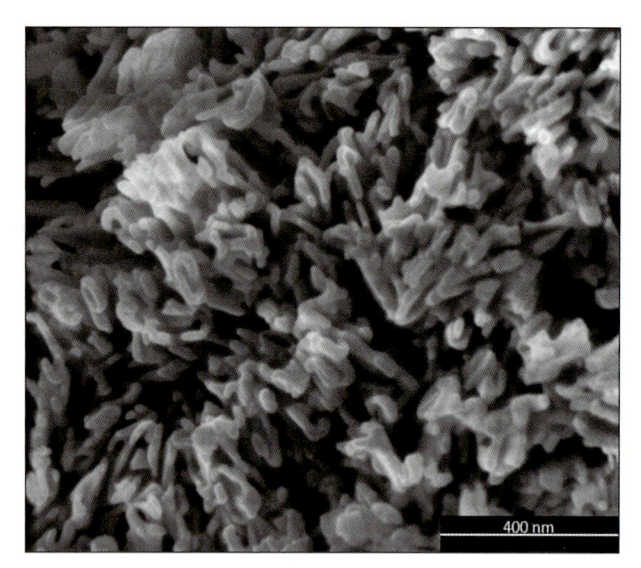

Fig 2-1 Nano-scanning electron micrograph of stacked hydroxyapatite crystals. (Courtesy of BIOMAT research group at KU Leuven, Belgium.)

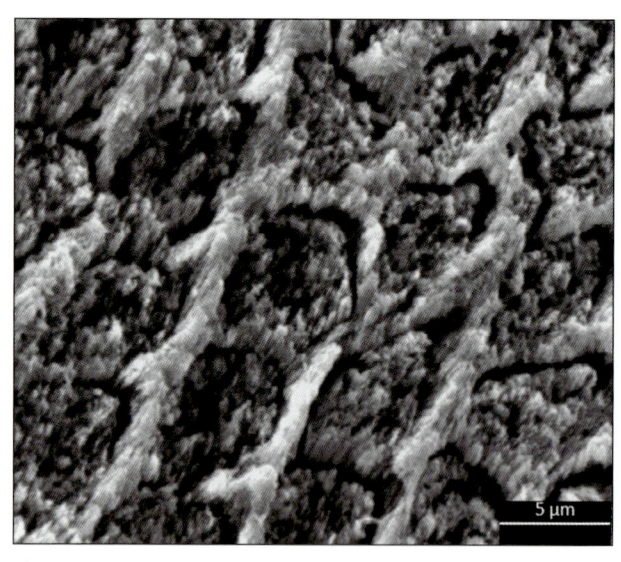

Fig 2-2 Scanning electron micrograph of divergent crystal orientations of enamel crystals with interrod enamel. (Courtesy of BIOMAT research group at KU Leuven, Belgium.)

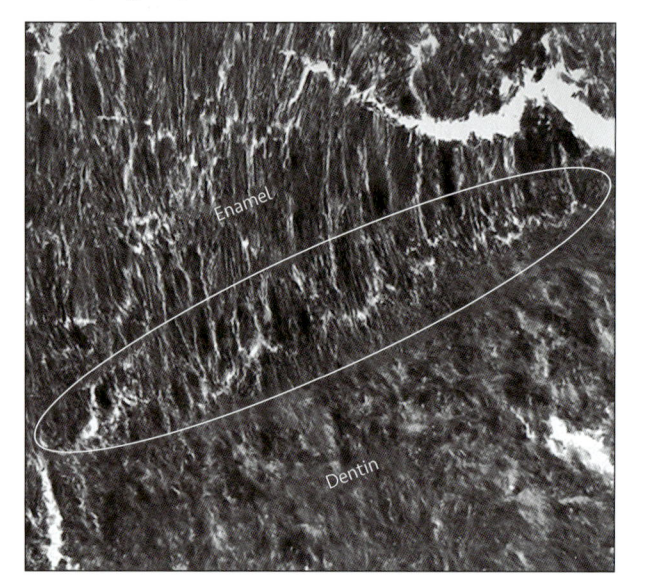

Fig 2-3 Before enamel forms, some developing odontoblast processes extend into the ameloblast layer and, when enamel formation begins, become trapped to form enamel spindles. The junction seems to be a series of ridges, the arrangement of which probably increases the adherence between dentin and enamel.

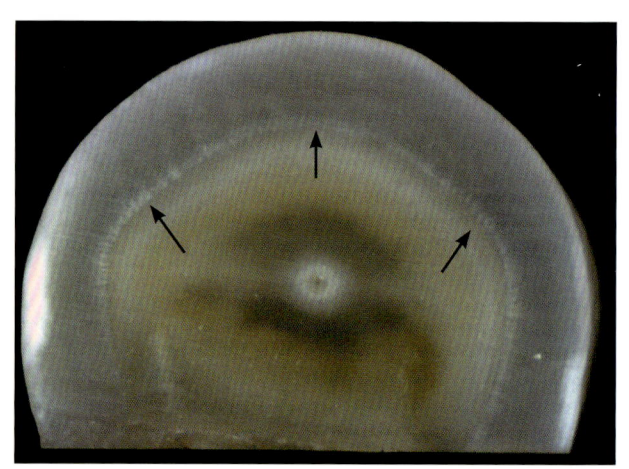

Fig 2-4 Macroscopic view of DEJ *(black arrows)*.

Thickness

The thickness of the enamel directly influences tooth color. Where the enamel is thicker, the underlying yellow dentin does not show through.[6] Enamel varies in thickness and density over the tooth surface; it is thickest over the cusps (2,500 microns) and thinnest at the fissures, base of pits, and cervical region of the crown (80 microns).[4,8,9] Enamel thickness decreases significantly below deep occlusal fissures and tapers to become very thin in the cervical area near the cementoenamel junction.[10] At the incisal edges, where there is no interposed layer of dentin, the enamel is more gray or slightly bluish.[11] The yellowing of older teeth may be attributed to thinning or increased translucency of enamel, accumulation of trace elements in the enamel structure, and perhaps the sclerosis of mature dentin.[10]

Dentinoenamel junction

The dentinoenamel junction (DEJ) is an interface between two mineralized tissues with different compositions and biomechanical properties (Fig 2-3). The shape and nature of the DEJ prevent crack propagation in the tooth that could cause fractures (Fig 2-4), and the resilient underlying dentin supports the integrity of the enamel during function.[12,13]

Tooth Enamel

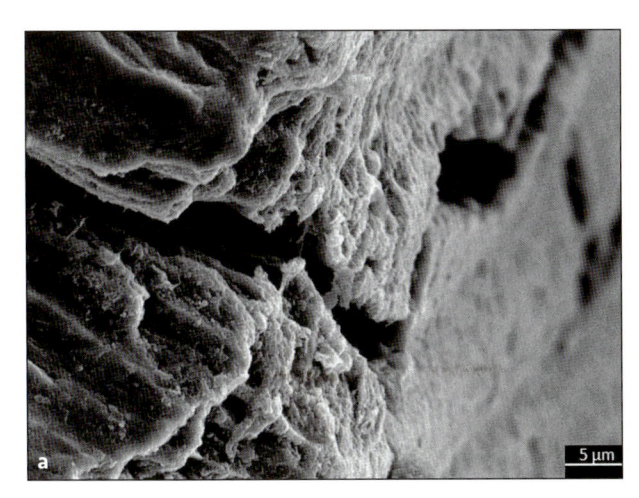

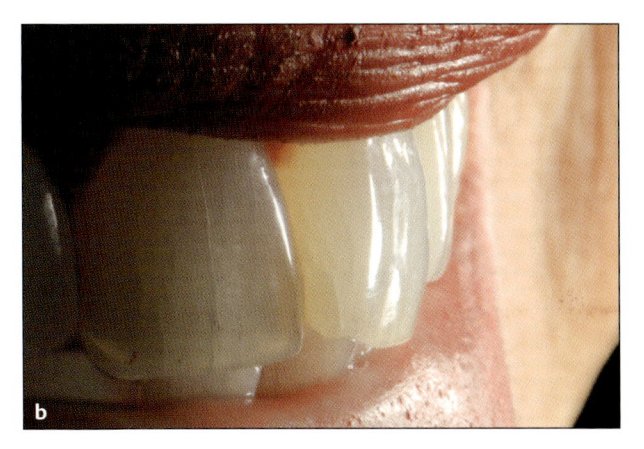

Fig 2-5 *(a)* Crack pathway in enamel. (Courtesy of BIOMAT research group at KU Leuven, Belgium.) *(b)* Clinical appearance of cracks in the enamel.

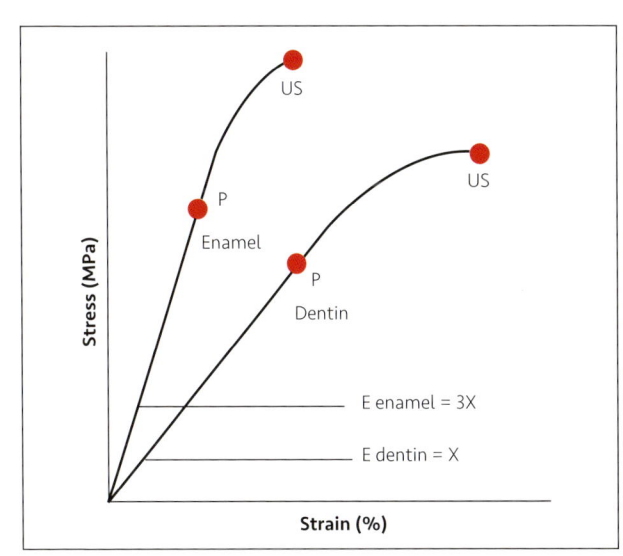

Fig 2-6 Stress/strain graph showing the elastic modulus (E), proportional limit (P), and ultimate strength (US) of enamel and dentin.

Biomechanical behavior

In the oral environment, tooth structures and restorative materials are exposed to chemical, thermal, and mechanical challenges. These challenges can cause deformation of the material, highlighted by mechanical interactions. The mechanical interactions involving biologic materials cause stress and strain in the bodies, which result in deformation.[14]

Despite its hardness and durability, enamel is susceptible to longitudinal fracture[12] (Fig 2-5) and damage accumulation through a lifetime of mechanical function. The fracture resistance between enamel rods is weakened if the underlying dentinal support is removed or pathologically destroyed.[15]

Elasticity

Elasticity is a term used to describe the characteristic in which a material changes in shape under an external force application and recovers to its initial form after the force is removed.

The elastic modulus (E) represents the inherent stiffness of a material within the elastic range. The proportional limit (P) is the point of transition between the elastic and plastic phase; above this point, even if the force ceases, the material does not recover from the deformation, instead suffering permanent plastic distortion.[16] The ultimate strength (US) of a material is the point at which it fractures. For human tooth enamel, E indicates the ability to elastically resist loads, and it is about three times that of dentin. However, the ultimate strength of dentin is higher than that of enamel, meaning that enamel is a stiffer and more brittle material than dentin and that unsupported enamel is more susceptible to fracture (Fig 2-6).

Hardness

Hardness is a mechanical property that can be defined as the resistance of the surface to permanent indentation or penetration.[14] The hardness of enamel, measured using nanoindentation, can vary between 2.5 GPa and 6.0 GPa depending on the location and thickness.[4]

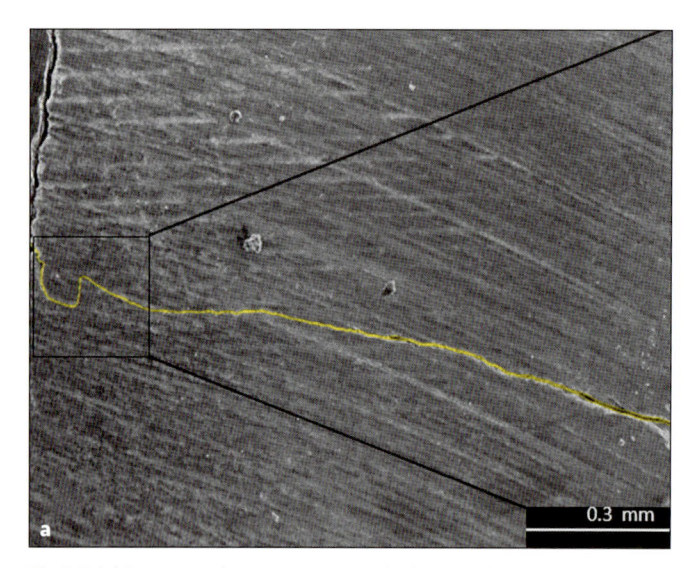

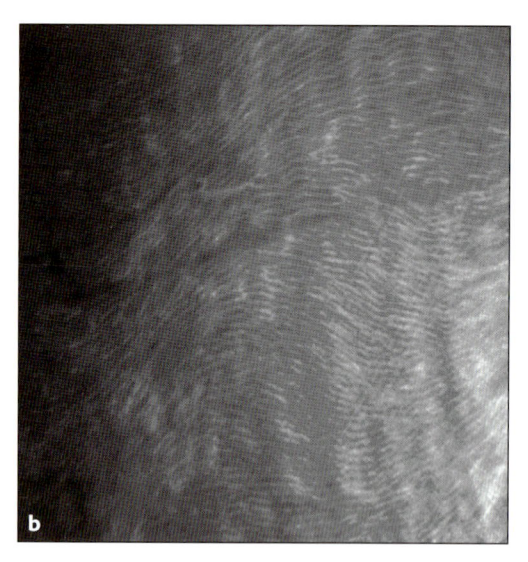

Fig 2-7 *(a)* Scanning electron micrograph showing the change in crack direction in the decussation area at the vicinity of the DEJ. *(b)* Inset of the decussation area in deep enamel. (Courtesy of BIOMAT research group at KU Leuven, Belgium.)

Hardness and elastic modulus interactions

Studies have observed that the mechanical properties of enamel are related to the location, chemical components, and arrangement patterns of the enamel rods.[4] In the enamel structure, the maximum hardness is located on the surface, and the hardness decreases gradually toward the DEJ.[17] The nanohardness and elastic modulus also decrease gradually from the surface of the enamel to the DEJ, and both are positively correlated with calcium content.[4] Age also has an influence on the enamel hardness and elastic modulus; as individuals age, the thickness of the enamel decreases due to abrasion of the cusps, and the mineral content increases, resulting in higher hardness and elastic modulus.[18]

Fracture behavior

The most common type of damage in enamel is fracture. *Fracture toughness* represents the ability of a material to absorb energy and resist plastic deformation without catastrophic failure. The higher the fracture toughness, the greater the resistance to fracture the material exhibits. There is a close relationship between the microstructure of enamel and its fracture toughness. The stacked cylindric rods of hydroxyapatite crystals that form the enamel tissue tend to radiate outward from the DEJ to the enamel surfaces and upward to the tooth crown. As a natural protection against stress, the rod bundles change orientation relative to their neighbors; for instance, hydroxyapatite crystals that are present in the interrod are obliquely inclined to 65 degrees in relation to the rods. Near the DEJ, the rods decussate (crisscross) one another like reeds in an interwoven basket (Fig 2-7), further shielding the tooth from crack growth and deformation.[19] Crack resistance increases externally to internally, meaning that crack growth becomes more difficult from outside to inside. Crack bridging, crack deflection, and crack bifurcation appear in regions of decussation.

Meanwhile, enamel has natural internal defects that serve as points of stress concentration and can promote the initiation of a crack. The most common defects inside the enamel are the hypocalcified, protein-dense fissures originating at the DEJ known as *tufts*. They tend to follow interrod paths and have the form of "closed cracks" filled with protein matter.[20] These tufts can act as crack fracture initiators in teeth.[21]

The second main source of crack initiation in enamel is yield deformation from hard, concentrated contacts.[22] Weak interfaces within the microstructures render enamel highly susceptible to shear-activated slippage along interrod boundaries. Shear stress can be a significant component of contact fields, typically three or more times greater in magnitude than tensile stress.

Fracture types

In brittle materials such as tooth enamel, cracks tend to start from internal or external flaws that represent defects in the microstructure and stress concentration points.[23] Once initiated, cracks are driven by tensile stresses perpendicular to the crack plane. Radial cracks that start from the enamel and move to the DEJ are more likely to be found in thinner enamel (eg, the cervical region of the tooth), whereas margin cracks that start in the DEJ and move toward the surface are more common in thick enamel (Fig 2-8). These cracks are usually promoted by internal flaws in enamel due to concentrated tensile stress.[22]

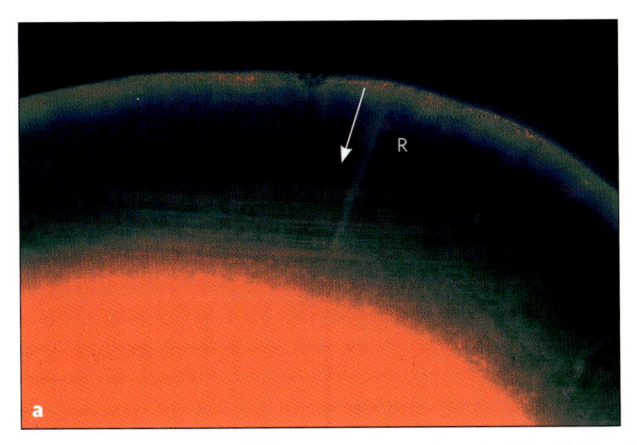

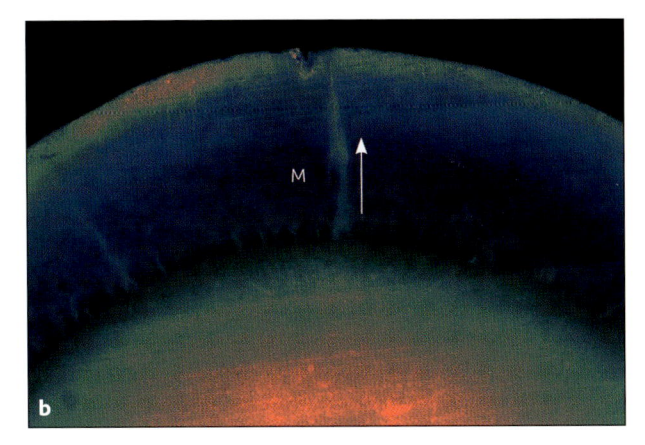

Fig 2-8 *(a)* Radial crack (R) from outer enamel to the DEJ. *(b)* Margin crack (M) from the DEJ to outer enamel.

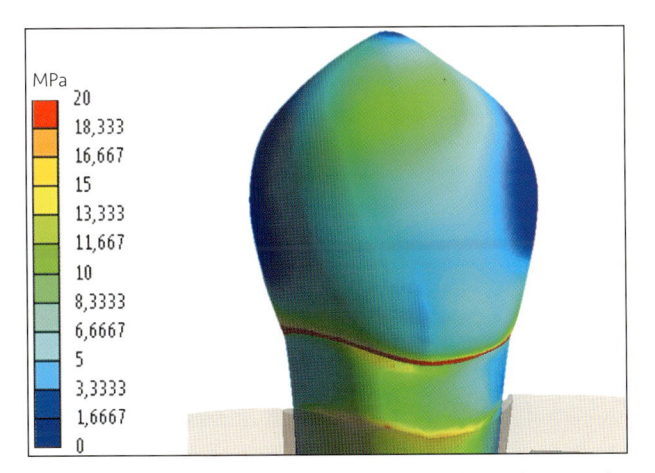

Fig 2-9 Three-dimensional finite element analysis showing the mechanical stress concentration at the cementoenamel junction upon oblique load simulation.

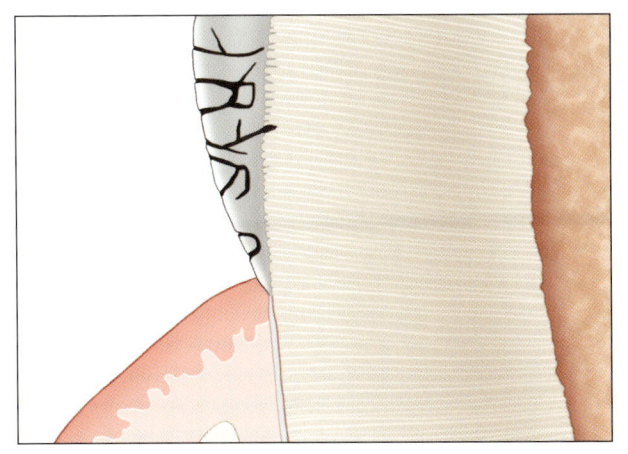

Fig 2-10 Illustration of cracks in the enamel that can lead to the development of NCCLs.

Damage control

The influence of microstructure is not limited to the initial stage of fracture. Conversely, periodic reorientation of the fiber bundles in regions of high decussation tends to disrupt crack propagation by causing cracks to deflect and bifurcate.[24] After that, to continue growing, these cracks have to break up and reform continuously along their front and, in the process, pull out any unruptured enamel rods that bridge the crack walls behind the advancing front.[25] Crack-interface bridging resembles fiber-reinforced composites and is capable of dissipating the stress, with a consequent progressive increase in toughness.[26]

Enamel has innate structural protection to resist fractures.[25] The large dimension of enamel increases the load-bearing capacity by redistributing the stress over a greater base area. With respect to the enamel microstructure, the fill of the gaps with flow proteins within a fluid-rich suspension can arrest crack propagation. Excessive shear displacements can cause stress concentrations leading to crack initiation, but the deformable sheaths decrease the brittleness of the enamel. Such large gaps show a capacity to self-heal by continual replenishment of protein-rich fluids, coupled with stress shielding between toughness and decussation of rod bundles that gives enamel its long-term damage control.[25]

Clinical relevance

Premature occlusal contacts

An etiologic factor of noncarious cervical lesions (NCCLs) is premature eccentric contact during interocclusal activity, which causes flexure of the crowns. Because the enamel is very thin and rodless in the cervical region of the tooth,[27] it is more susceptible to splitting of the rods under tensile and shear stress provoked by flexure, which initiates crack formation and the propagation of NCCLs. Furthermore, the difference between the elastic moduli of enamel and dentin creates large stress concentrations at the cervical area during this flexure (Fig 2-9), supporting the development of NCCLs. Crack initiation from premature eccentric occlusal contacts, coupled with biocorrosion and toothbrush/dentifrice abrasion, promote the growth of these lesions (Fig 2-10).

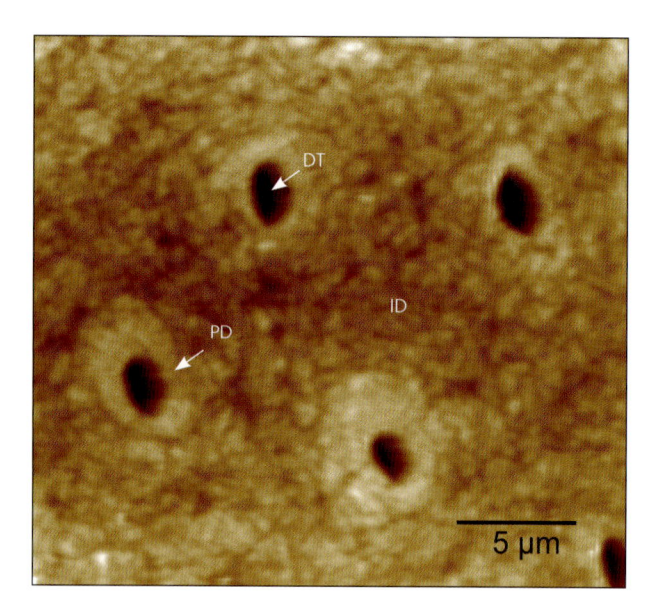

Fig 2-11 Scanning probe microscopy of midcoronal dentin showing dentinal tubules (DT), peritubular dentin (PD), and intertubular dentin (ID).

Demineralization-remineralization process

When exposed to plaque acids, the carbonated components of the crystal are the most susceptible to demineralization and the first to be solubilized. Following the cycles of acid dissolution, the therapeutic substitution of fluoride into the enamel apatite crystal is the key to remineralization. In the presence of fluorides, the enamel crystals affected by incipient caries are replaced or repaired by fluoroapatite and/or fluorohydroxyapatite. This makes the enamel more caries resistant.[28,29] Control of acidic diet and gastroesophageal reflux disease as well as plaque control, especially in the cervical region, are very important to prevent demineralization, which weakens the enamel that is very thin in this region.

Dentin-Pulp Complex

Understanding the dynamic nature of the dentin-pulp complex has meaningful clinical implications for continued advances in novel dental therapies. Structural and developmental interactions between dentin and pulp reflect the biologic regulatory mechanism necessary to maintain tooth vitality and function. While dental pulp has essential sensory, protective, and reparative functions, dentin provides support for the enamel and cementum and acts as a protective barrier against chemical, thermal, and mechanical stimuli. Together, these tissues are referred to as the *dentin-pulp complex*.

Structural composition

Despite the differences in structure and composition, the close relationship between dentin and pulp and the dynamic nature of these structures reflect their anatomical arrangement, structure, and functional organization.[30,31] Dentin provides the main architecture of the tooth and consists of approximately 70 wt% mineral, 20 wt% organic matrix, and 10 wt% water.[32] While the organic matrix is predominantly comprised of type I collagen (~ 90%), the mineral phase is mainly apatite crystallites located either in the spaces between the collagen fibrils or in the gap regions between the collagen molecules within the fibrils. The remainder of the organic matrix is represented by noncollagenous proteins.

Dentin micromorphology is comprised of tubules approximately 1 to 2 µm in diameter surrounded by peritubular dentin and intertubular dentin (Fig 2-11). The tubular structure of dentin provides pathways for the permeation of fluids, solvents, or bacteria (Fig 2-12). As these tubules approach the pulp, both their density and diameter increase. Each individual dentinal tubule is described as an inverted cone surrounded by a collagen-poor, hypermineralized cuff—the peritubular dentin—which forms the wall of the dentinal tubule. The most dominant part of the circumpulpal dentin is formed by intertubular dentin, which is essentially a rich mineral-impregnated network of collagen fibrils (Fig 2-13). These collagen fibrils provide a three-dimensional scaffold for the deposition of apatite crystals.

Dentin-Pulp Complex

Fig 2-12 Dentin components with great significance for the dentin-pulp complex in regard to its mechanical properties and permeability.

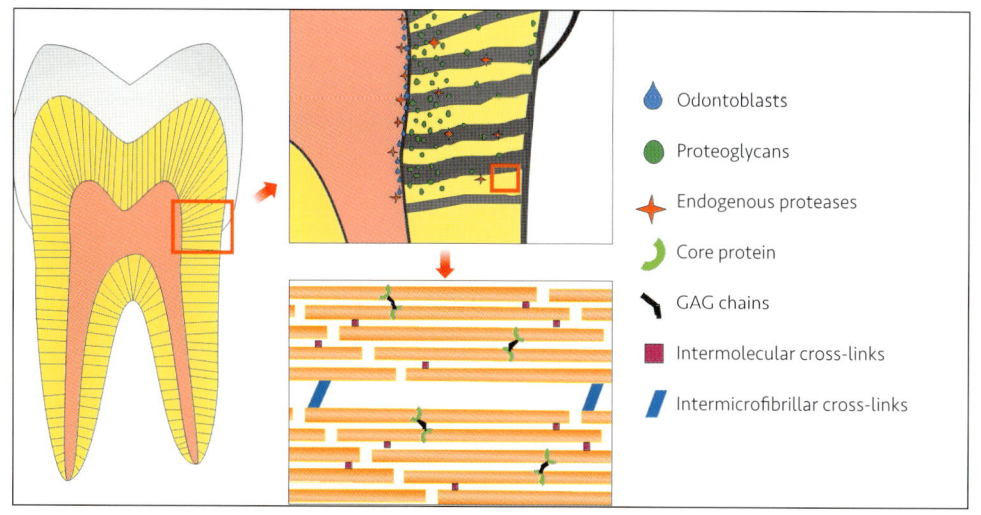

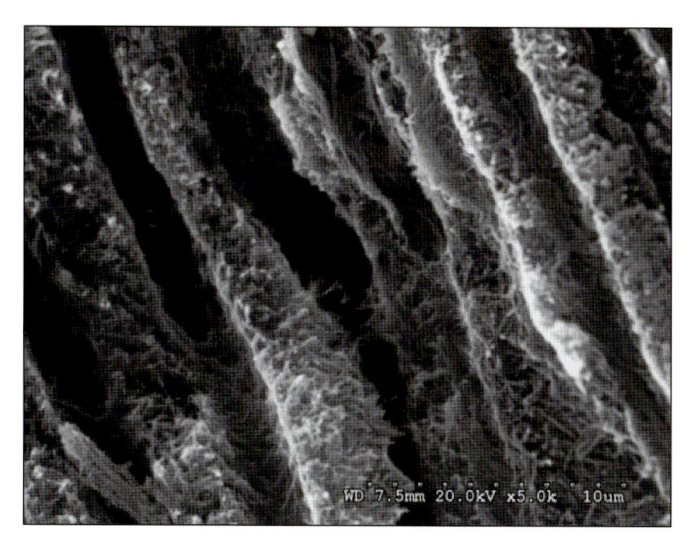

Fig 2-13 Scanning electron microscopic image of the cryofractured dentin matrix depicting the collagen architecture and dentinal tubule orientation.

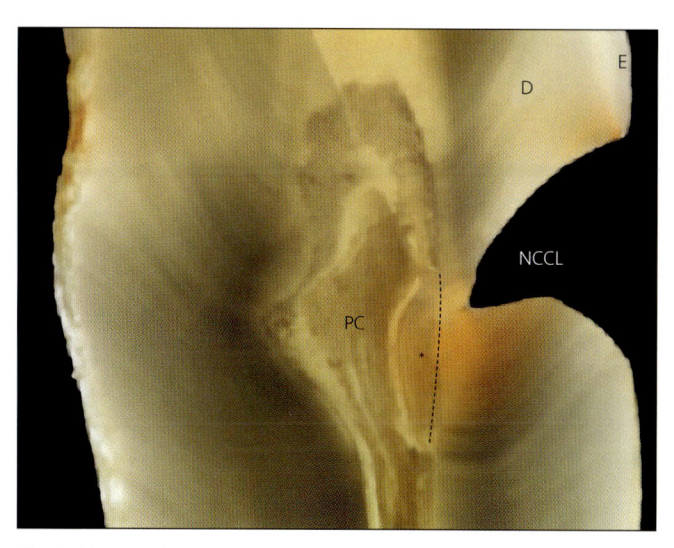

Fig 2-14 An advanced NCCL with reduction of the pulp chamber *(dashed line)* due to the deposition of reactionary dentin *(asterisk)*. D, dentin; E, enamel; PC, pulp chamber.

The pulp comprises an outer layer of odontoblasts and connective tissue made up of undifferentiated cells, blood, lymph vessels, nerves, and interstitial fluid. Two distinguished processes involving dentin deposition should be highlighted: reactionary and reparative tertiary dentin formation.[31] Reactionary dentin shows anatomical, biochemical, and functional similarities to physiologic dentin[33] (Fig 2-14). Reparative tertiary dentin is associated with severe dentinal pathology (eg, the rapid progression of root caries lesions, trauma, dental wear, or exposed hypersensitive cervical dentin), causing severe hard tissue damage that results in the formation of a bonelike structure or a structureless, diffusely mineralized pulp as well as pulp stones.[34]

Differences in the structure of dentin have been described with aging. The gradual enlargement of the peritubular dentin and formation of secondary dentin represent the main structural changes. The deposition of peritubular dentin leads to continuous narrowing of the lumen of the tubules, referred to as *dentin sclerosis*, which results in more transparent dentin.[35] Small changes in the diameter of dentinal tubules can greatly modify permeability.[36,37]

Biomechanical behavior

The organizational level and hierarchy of dentin mineral and organic matrix influence the elastic properties of dentin.[32] Site-specific evaluation of the modulus of elasticity of dentin showed differences in mechanical properties between the intertubular and peritubular dentin, namely the large presence of collagen in the intertubular dentin. These differences result in a protective mechanism against fracture by fatigue or repeated stress.

Because of its viscoelastic nature, dentin acts as a stress-breaker for the overlying enamel. Dentin viscoelasticity is determined by the composition of its organic matrix. The presence of water within the staggered arrangement of the collagen molecules may influence the load absorption. Proteoglycans have also been shown to make a significant contribution to the biomechanical and bioelectric effects of dentin: The negatively charged glycosaminoglycans chains attract water/fluids facilitating the sliding between collagen fibrils,[38] which is believed to aid in bearing compressive loads.[39] The efficiency of load absorption by dentin is impaired by cyclic stress concentration, mainly in the cervical areas[40] of overloaded teeth, which, together with biocorrosion and abrasion, can lead to the development and progression of NCCLs.

Fracture strength of human dentin is affected by cycle-dependent stresses like chewing[41]; lower fatigue strength is observed in older teeth. In addition, the stress orientation seems to play a significant role in resistance to fracture. In the cervical area of the tooth, the mineral deposition in the tubule lumen results in transparent or sclerotic dentin, with lower toughness than normal dentin.[42] Lower fatigue strength was observed when dentinal tubules were oriented parallel to the loading direction, which demonstrates the anisotropic microstructure of the dentin.

Resistance to wear is an important property for the development of NCCLs, and it is directly related to the hardness of dentin. Dentin hardness is mainly affected by its mineral phase, and studies have found a significant decrease in dentin hardness after exposure to low-pH solutions.[43] Biocorrosion produced by an acidic pH, along with proteolytic enzymes and to a lesser degree toothbrush/dentifrice abrasion, facilitates the wear of the dentin surface. Furthermore, the physiologic wear of enamel from mastication can affect the deposition of apatite crystals in the underlying dentin. An increase in hardness of the DEJ was observed as a result of wear of the enamel with aging.[44] However, areas of reactionary dentin exhibited lower hardness, likely due to smaller or poor crystal organization, and may be more susceptible to wear.

Clinical relevance

The permeability of dentin regulates the rate of diffusion of irritants and hence may induce pulpal inflammation. A short and sharp pain in response to chemical, thermal, tactile, or osmotic stimulus has been described as *hypersensitive dentin*.[45] This is related to exposure of dentinal tubules from either the loss of enamel or denudation of root surface by loss of the thin cementum layer (20 to 50 μm).[46] The thin enamel overlying the cervical margin of the coronal dentin makes the cervical region susceptible to hypersensitivity, which is a precursor to NCCLs.

A better understanding of how an appropriate stimulus initiates an instantaneous painful response in cervical dentin has been extensively investigated. Although the exact mechanism is still unknown, the hydrodynamic theory proposed by Brännstrom et al[47–49] is the most accepted theory. This theory explains dentinal hypersensitivity based on mechanical stimulation of nerves in the dentin-pulp interface (see chapter 7).

Periodontium

The tissues supporting and covering the tooth constitute the periodontium. They include the alveolar bone, cementum, gingiva, and periodontal ligament.

Alveolar bone

The architecture of the alveolar process is similar to that of long bone. The thickened ridge of bone in the maxilla and mandible are responsible for supporting the teeth with both cortical bone and trabecular bone. The cortical bone consists of plates of compact bone on the facial and lingual surfaces of the alveolar process. These cortical plates are usually about 1.5 to 3.0 mm thick over posterior teeth, but the thickness is highly variable around anterior teeth. The trabecular bone consists of spongy bone that is located between the alveolar bone that faces the periodontal ligament and the plates of cortical bone.[50] The alveolar bone between two neighboring teeth is called the *interdental septum* (or *interdental bone*).

Bone contains between 10% and 20% water in vivo. Of its dry mass, approximately 60% to 70% is mineral, composed of calcium and phosphate in the form of hydroxyapatite crystals. Most of the organic matrix is composed of type I collagen, but it also contains a small amount of other constituents such as proteoglycans and noncollagenous proteins and some inorganic salts.[30]

Cementum

The cementum is a thin layer of calcified tissue covering the root dentin that, through the periodontal ligament, promotes the insertion of the root into the alveolar bone, thus retaining the position of the tooth. The cementum has dynamic and responsive characteristics that also ensure somewhat reparative and adaptive functions crucial to maintaining the occlusal relationship and the integrity of the root surface. Cementum can be divided into cellular and acellular cementum. Cementum plays a role in inserting the collagen fibers of the periodontal ligament. Although it is similar in chemical composition and physical properties to bone, ce-

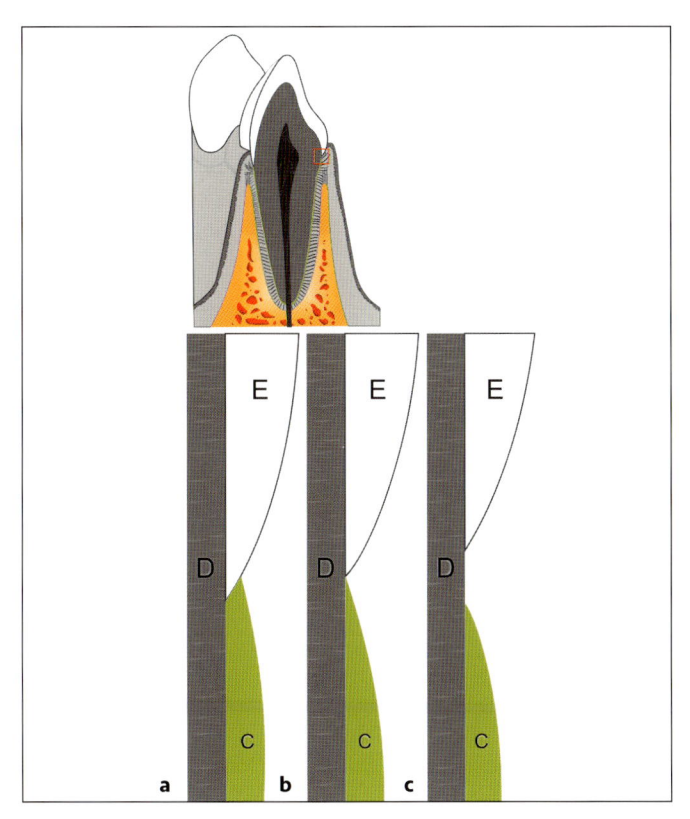

Fig 2-15 Types of relationships between enamel and cementum. *(a)* The cementum overlaps the enamel in 60% of teeth. *(b)* The cementum and enamel meet end to end in 30% of teeth. *(c)* There is no contact between enamel and cementum in 10% of teeth.

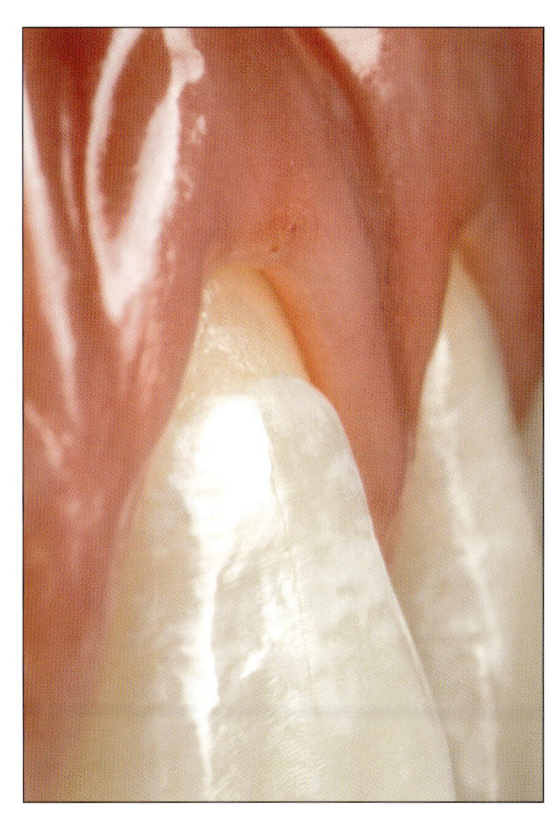

Fig 2-16 Gingival recession with root dentin exposed. (Courtesy of Dr Carlos Ayala, Lima, Peru.)

mentum is avascular; its nutrition depends on the adjacent periodontal ligament.

At the cementoenamel junction (CEJ), three types of mineralized tissues are present—enamel, dentin, and cementum—and three types of relationships between enamel and cementum may occur, even in the same tooth (Fig 2-15). In 60% of all teeth, the cementum overlaps the enamel for a short distance, where connective tissue consisting of cementoblasts that produce a type of cementum called *afibrillar cementum* contacts the enamel directly (see Fig 2-15a). Another 30% of teeth present a pattern with cementum and enamel meeting at a butt joint, or an end-to-end relationship (see Fig 2-15b). Finally, in 10% of teeth there is no contact between enamel and cementum, and the dentin is exposed as an external part of the root surface; in this situation, the CEJ is absent[51] (see Fig 2-15c).

Gingiva

Gingiva, the mucosa immediately surrounding an erupted tooth, has a particular purpose—to provide a seal around the teeth via the junctional epithelium and the epithelial attachment against foreign invaders such as microorganisms. Gingiva is the only periodontal tissue clinically visible upon inspection of the healthy oral cavity. Attached gingiva is most often widest on the vestibular aspect of maxillary anterior teeth and the lingual aspect of mandibular molars; in mandibular premolars, it is narrowest on the vestibular aspect.[52,53] Figure 2-16 shows gingival recession.

Periodontal ligament

The periodontal ligament connects the tooth to the jaw and is capable of absorbing the considerable forces of mastication and receiving sensory stimuli. It is a specialized connective tissue composed of fiber bundles; one end is embedded in bone, and the other end is embedded in cementum at the surface of the root.[54,55] The collagen bundles are capable of being continually remodeled without losing their architecture and function, adapting to the stresses placed on them.[56]

Clinical relevance

Buccal gingival recession continues to be a prevalent problem in populations with a high standard of oral hygiene and is often associated with NCCLs, leading to the need for a combined periodontal-restorative approach for better esthetic and functional results.[57]

The clinical location of the CEJ serves as an important anatomical site for measurement of probing pocket depth and clinical attachment level and is of paramount importance for measuring recession depth and evaluating treatment outcomes.[57-59]

Some clinical cases present gingival recession associated with NCCLs. In these cases, the authors recommend the combination of restorative and periodontal surgery procedures.[45,57-59] More details on these procedures can be found in chapters 9 and 10.

Conclusion

Let's review what we have covered in this chapter:
- Enamel protects the dentin and pulp against mechanical wear and biocorrosion. Because the enamel is thin at the cervical region of the tooth, this area is more susceptible to NCCLs.
- The permeability of dentin makes it susceptible to CDH.
- A healthy periodontium is essential to protect the cervical region of the tooth from biocorrosion.

References

1. Chun K, Choi H, Lee J. Comparison of mechanical property and role between enamel and dentin in the human teeth. J Dent Biomech 2014;5:1-7.
2. Tillberg A, Järvholm B, Berglund A. Risks with dental materials. Dent Mater 2008;24:940-943.
3. Vaderhobli RM. Advances in dental materials. Dent Clin North Am 2011;55:619-625.
4. Cuy JL, Mann AB, Livi KJ, Teaford MF, Weihs TP. Nanoindentation mapping of the mechanical properties of human molar tooth enamel. Arch Oral Biol 2002;47:281-291.
5. Lynch CD, O'Sullivan VR, McGillycuddy CT, Dockery P, Sloan AJ. Hunter-Schreger band patterns in human tooth enamel. J Anat 2010;217:106-115.
6. Nanci A. Ten Cate's Oral Histology: Development, Structure and Function, ed 8. St Louis: Mosby, 2013.
7. Spears IR, van Noort R, Crompton RH, Cardew GE, Howard IC. The effects of enamel anisotropy on the distribution of stress in a tooth. J Dent Res 1993;72:1526-1531.
8. Gwinnett AJ. Structure and composition of enamel. Oper Dent 1992;(suppl 5):10-17.
9. Gašperšič D. Micromorphometric analysis of cervical enamel structure of human upper third molars. Arch Oral Biol 1995;40:453-457.
10. Summitt JB, Robbins JW, Hilton TJ, Schwartz RS. Fundamentals of Operative Dentistry, ed 3. Chicago: Quintessence, 2006.
11. Muller CJ, van Wyk CW. The amelo-cemental junction. J Dent Assoc S Afr 1984;39:799-803.
12. Giannini M, Soares CJ, de Carvalho RM. Ultimate tensile strength of tooth structures. Dent Mater 2004;20:322-329.
13. Craig RG, Peyton FA. Elastic and mechanical properties of human dentin. J Dent Res 1958;37:1072-1078.
14. Craig RG, Sakaguchi RL, Powers JM. Craig's Restorative Dental Materials, ed 13. Philadelphia: Mosby, 2012.
15. Christensen RP, Palmer TM, Ploeger BJ, Yost MP. Resin polymerization problems—Are they caused by resin curing lights, resin formulations, or both? Compend Contin Educ Dent Suppl 1999;(25):S42-S54.
16. Anusavice KJ, Shen C, Rawls HR. Phillips's Science of Dental Materials, ed 12. St Louis: Saunders, 2013.
17. He LH, Yin ZH, van Vuuren LJ, Carter EA, Liang XW. A natural functionally graded biocomposite coating—Human enamel. Acta Biomater 2013;9:6330-6337.
18. Park S, Wang DH, Zhang D, Romberg E, Arola D. Mechanical properties of human enamel as a function of age and location in the tooth. J Mater Sci Mater Med 2008;19:2317-2324.
19. Bajaj D, Arola DD. Role of prism decussation on fatigue crack growth and fracture of human enamel. Acta Biomater 2009;5:3045-3056.
20. Palamara J, Phakey PP, Rachinger WA, Orams HJ. Ultrastructure of spindles and tufts in human dental enamel. Adv Dent Res 1989;3:249-257.
21. Chai H, Lee JJ, Constantino PJ, Lucas PW, Lawn BR. Remarkable resilience of teeth. Proc Natl Acad Sci U S A 2009;106:7289-7293.
22. Lee JJ, Constantino PJ, Lucas PW, Lawn BR. Fracture in teeth: A diagnostic for inferring bite force and tooth function. Biol Rev Camb Philos Soc 2011;86:959-974.
23. Griffith AA. The phenomena of rupture and flow in solids. Phil Trans Roy Soc London A 1921;221:163-198.
24. Koenigswald WV, Rensberger JM, Pretzschner HU. Changes in the tooth enamel of early Paleocene mammals allowing increased diet diversity. Nature 1987;328:159-162.
25. Lee JJ, Constantino PJ, Lucas PW, Lawn BR. Fracture in teeth—A diagnostic for inferring bite force and tooth function. Biol Rev 2011;86:959-974.
26. Marshall DB, Cox BN, Evans AG. The mechanics of matrix cracking in brittle-matrix fibre composites. Acta Metallurgica 1985;23:2013-2021.
27. Fava M, Watanabe I, Moraes FF, Costa LRRS. Prismless enamel in human non-erupted deciduous molar teeth: A scanning electron microscopic study. Rev Odontol Univ São Paulo 1997;11:239-243.
28. Robinson C, Shore RC, Brookes SJ, Strafford S, Wood SR, Kirkham J. The chemistry of enamel caries. Crit Rev Oral Biol Med 2000;11:481-495.
29. Featherstone JD. Prevention and reversal of dental caries: Role of low level fluoride. Community Dent Oral Epidemiol 1999;27:31-40.
30. Pashley DH. Dynamic of the pulpo-dentin complex. Crit Rev Oral Biol Med 1996;72:104-133.
31. Mjör IA, Ferrari M. Pulp-dentin biology in restorative dentistry. Part 6: Reactions to restorative materials, tooth-restoration interfaces, and adhesive techniques. Quintessence Int 2002;33:35-63.
32. Kinney JH, Marshall SJ, Marshall GW. The mechanical properties of human dentin: A critical review and re-evaluation of the dental literature. Crit Rev Oral Biol Med 2003;14:13-29.
33. Smith AJ. Pulpal responses to caries and dental repair. Caries Res 2002;36:223-232.
34. Aguiar MC, Arana-Chavez VE. Ultrastructural and immunocytochemical analyses of osteopontin in reactionary and reparative dentine formed after extrusion of upper rat incisors. J Anat 2007;2010:418-427.
35. Kvaal SI, Koppang HS, Solheim T. Relationship between age and deposit of peritubular dentine. Gerodontology 1994;112:93-98.
36. Prati C. What is the clinical relevance of in vitro dentine permeability test? J Dent 1992;222:83-88.
37. Thaler A, Ebert J, Petschelt A, Pelka M. Influence of tooth age and root section on root dentine dye penetration. Int Endod J 2008;41:1115-1122.
38. Fessel G, Snedeker JG. Evidence against proteoglycan mediated collagen fibril load transmission and dynamic viscoelasticity in tendon. Matrix Biol 2009;28:503-510.
39. Elliott DM, Robinson PS, Gimbel JA, et al. Effect of altered matrix proteins on quasilinear viscoelastic properties in transgenic mouse tail tendons. Ann Biomed Eng 2003;31:599-605.
40. Jakupovic S, Cerjakovic E, Topcic A, Ajanovic M, Prcic AK, Vukovic A. Analysis of the abfraction lesions formation mechanism by the finite element method. Acta Inform Med 2014;22:241-245.
41. Kruzic JJ, Nalla RK, Kinney JH, Ritchie RO. Mechanistic aspects of in vitro fatigue-crack growth in dentin. Biomaterials 2005;26:1195-1204.
42. Kinney JH, Nalla RK, Pople JA, Breunig TM, Ritchie RO. Age-related transparent root dentin: mineral concentration, crystallite size, and mechanical properties. Biomaterials 2005;26:3363-3376.
43. Habelitz S, Balooch M, Marshall GW, Breunig TM, Marshall SJ. AFM-based nanomechanical properties and storage of dentin and enamel. Mater Res Soc Symp Proc 2001;676:Y3.271-Y3.275.

References

44. Senawongse P, Otsuki M, Tagami J, Mjör I. Age-related changes in hardness and modulus of elasticity of dentine. Arch Oral Biol 2006;51:457–463.
45. West NX, Lussi A, Seong J, Hellwig E. Dentin hypersensitivity: Pain mechanisms and aetiology of exposed cervical dentin. Clin Oral Investig 2013;17(suppl 1):S9–S19.
46. Krauser JT. Hypersensitive teeth. Part I: Etiology. J Prosthet Dent 1986;56:153–156.
47. Brännström M, Aström A. The hydrodynamics of the dentine; its possible relationship to dentinal pain. Int Dent J 1972;22:219–227.
48. Brännström M, Lindén LA, Aström A. The hydrodynamics of the dental tubule and of pulp fluid. A discussion of its significance in relation to dentinal sensitivity. Caries Res 1967;1:310–317.
49. Brännström M. The hydrodynamics of the dental tubule and pulp fluid: Its significance in relation to dentinal sensitivity. Annu Meet Am Inst Oral Biol 1966;23:219.
50. Katchburian E, Arana-Chavez VE. Histologia e Embriologia Oral, ed 3. Rio de Janeiro: Guanabara Koogan-Panamericana, 2012.
51. Jeffcoat MK, Jeffcoat RL, Captain K. A periodontal probe with automated cementoenamel junction detection—Design and clinical trials. IEEE Trans Biomed Eng 1991;38:330–333.
52. Ciano J, Beatty BL. Regional quantitative histological variations in human oral mucosa. Anat Rec (Hoboken) 2015;298:562–578.
53. Kolte R, Kolte A, Mahajan A. Assessment of gingival thickness with regards to age, gender and arch location. J Indian Soc Periodontol 2014;18:478–481.
54. Bosshardt DD, Stadlinger B, Terheyden H. Cell-to-cell communication—Periodontal regeneration. Clin Oral Implants Res 2015;26:229–239.
55. Chen FM, Jin Y. Periodontal tissue engineering and regeneration: Current approaches and expanding opportunities. Tissue Eng Part B Rev 2010;16:219–255.
56. Kaku M, Yamauchi M. Mechano-regulation of collagen biosynthesis in periodontal ligament. J Prosthodont Res 2014;58:193–207.
57. Pradeep K, Rajababu P, Satyanarayana D, Sagar V. Gingival recession: Review and strategies in treatment of recession. Case Rep Dent 2012;2012:563421.
58. Moharamzadeh K, Colley H, Murdoch C, et al. Tissue-engineered oral mucosa. J Dent Res 2012;91:642–650.
59. Zucchelli G, Gori G, Mele M, et al. Non-carious cervical lesions associated with gingival recessions: A decision-making process. J Periodontol 2011;82:1713-1724.

Section II

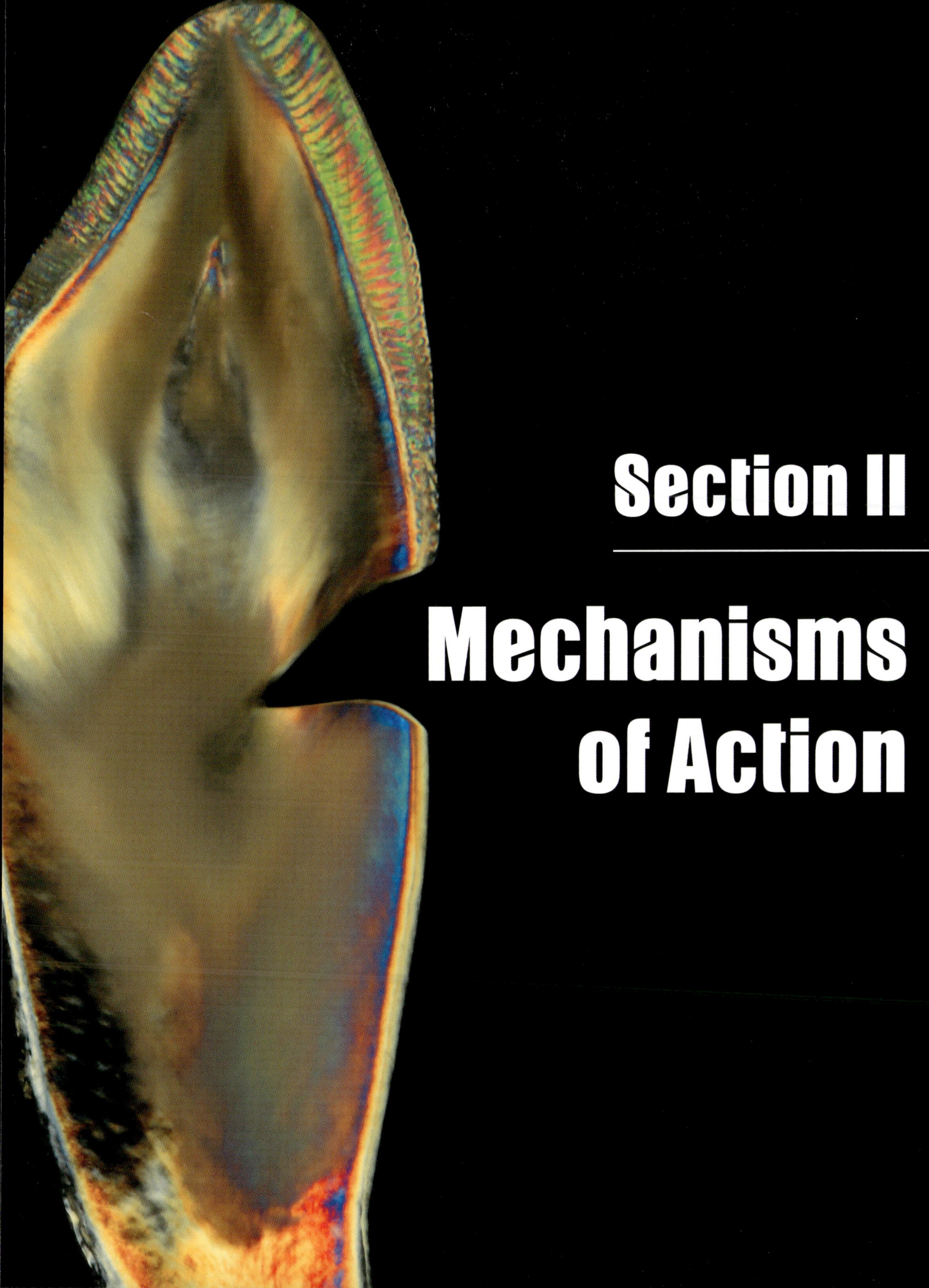

Mechanisms of Action

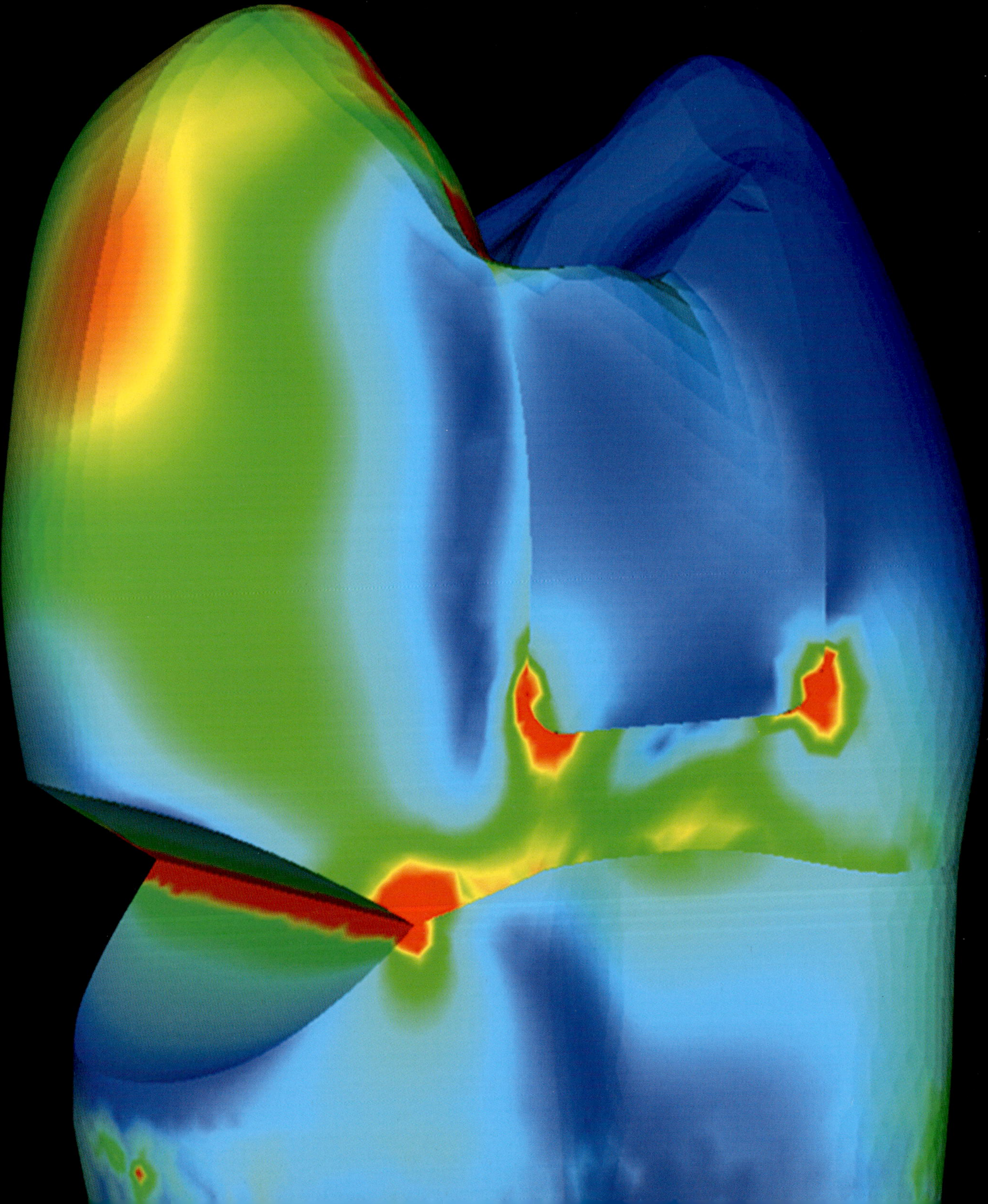

3

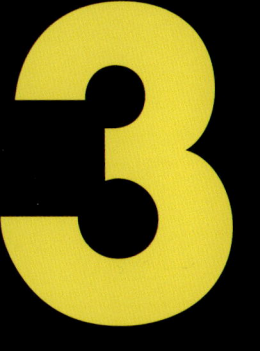

Stress

The loss of dental tissue in the cervical region of the tooth is an increasingly common finding in clinical practice,[1-3] with prevalence rates of up to 85% in some populations.[4] As discussed in chapter 1, noncarious cervical lesions (NCCLs) are related to three distinct and fundamental etiologic mechanisms: stress (Fig 3-1), friction, and biocorrosion[5,6] (see Fig 1-9). This chapter aims to deepen the theoretical knowledge of the etiology of the stress-strain mechanism, explaining how this process influences the origin and development of NCCLs. We will also discuss the significance of stress acting in concert with friction and biocorrosion as a cofactor in the etiology of NCCLs.

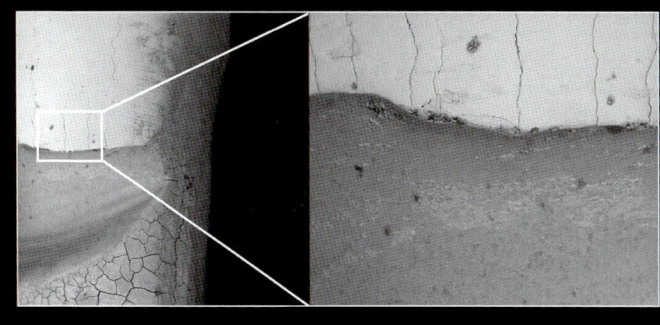

Fig 3-1 Hairline enamel cracks related to excessive loading causing stress to the enamel. The action of a biocorrodent is required to accelerate degradation of the flexible dentin. Toothbrush abrasion can also remove softened dentin.

Stress-Strain

Static or cyclic loading is an action that changes the state of rest or movement of a body. The load applied on a material has internal consequences on the object, understood as mechanical stress[7] (Fig 3-2). The physical and engineering formula for dealing with mechanical stress is designated as force per unit area ($\sigma = F / A$) through a physical point on the surface of a body. Simply stated, stress is the energy from force that propagates in the interior of the material that constitutes its object.[7] Stress can be further classified into tensile stress, compressive stress, and shear stress (Fig 3-3).

The strain of a solid body is considered to be any change in the geometric configuration that leads to a change in shape or dimensions after application of an external action (force). The strain as a consequence of stress can be classified increasingly as transient or elastic, permanent or plastic, and breakage.[7] In elastic strain, the body returns to its original state after the re-

3 Stress

Fig 3-2 Stress dissipation. The load applied dissipates within the material as stress energy, which causes deformation and eventual abfraction from eccentric loading forces. Stress distribution analysis was performed using maximum principal stress, identifying areas with tensile stress (positive) and/or compressive stress (negative).

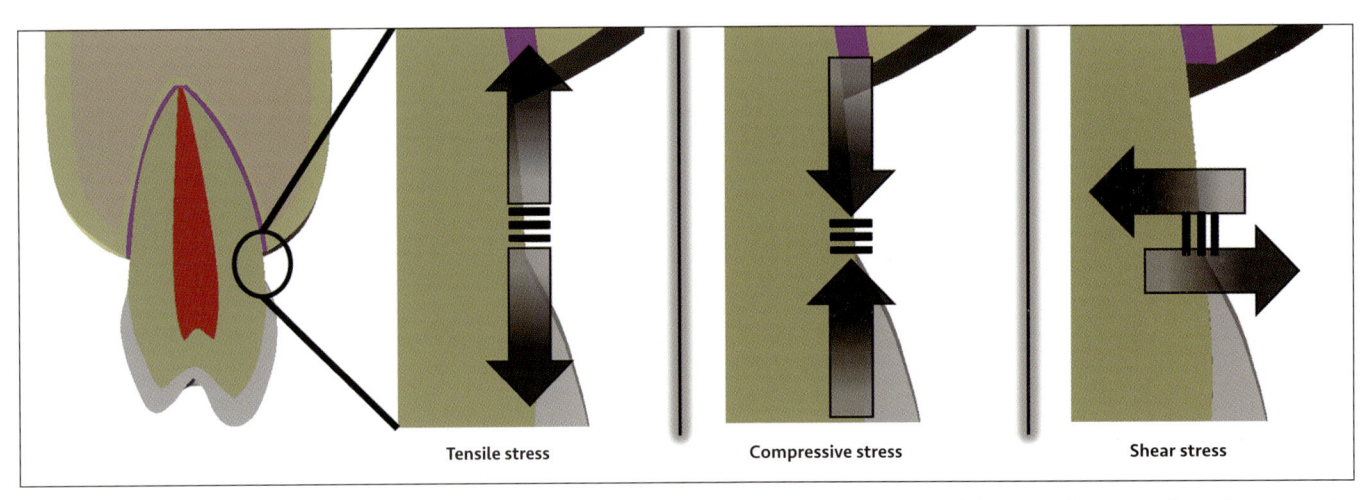

Fig 3-3 Stress classification: tensile, compressive, and shear stress. Tensile stress acts in opposite and diverging directions along the same axis, tending to lengthen the structure on which it operates. Compressive stress acts in opposite and converging directions along the same axis, tending to compress or reduce the structure on which it operates. Shear stress acts in opposite and parallel directions in different planes, tending to slide a portion of the structure along the adjacent part, often leading to dilacerations.

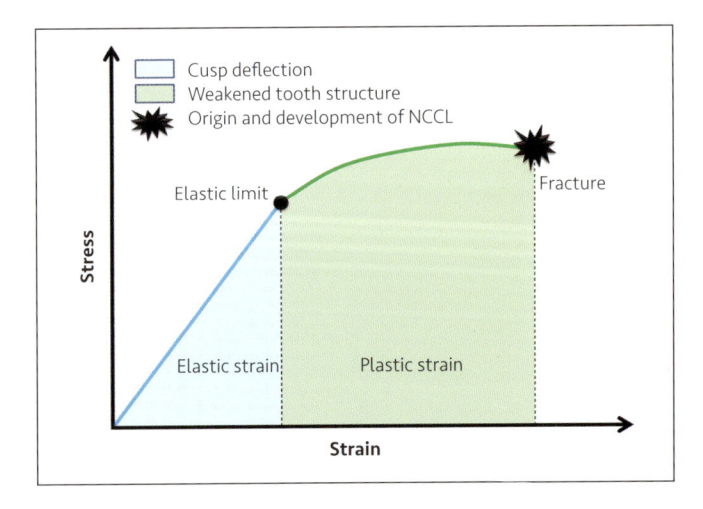

Fig 3-4 Material elastic and plastic strain. In elastic strain, the deformation is reversible and does not promote damage to the dental structure, resulting in only cusp deflection. Plastic strain from higher stress concentration results in permanent deformation, and the dental structure does not return to its original form, promoting the weakening of tooth substance. Should the stress continue to increase, the strain will overcome the plastic limit, resulting in breakage of the structure into two or more parts.

Fig 3-5 Stress-strain pattern by finite element analysis. *(a)* Stress distribution was performed using maximum principal stress, identifying areas with tensile stress (positive) and/or compressive stress (negative). *(b)* Strain analysis was performed by equivalent strain. The areas closer to red have greater strain, and the areas closer to dark blue have lower strain. *(c)* The cervical region has higher stress and strain concentrations, and enamel cracks occur due to plastic strain.

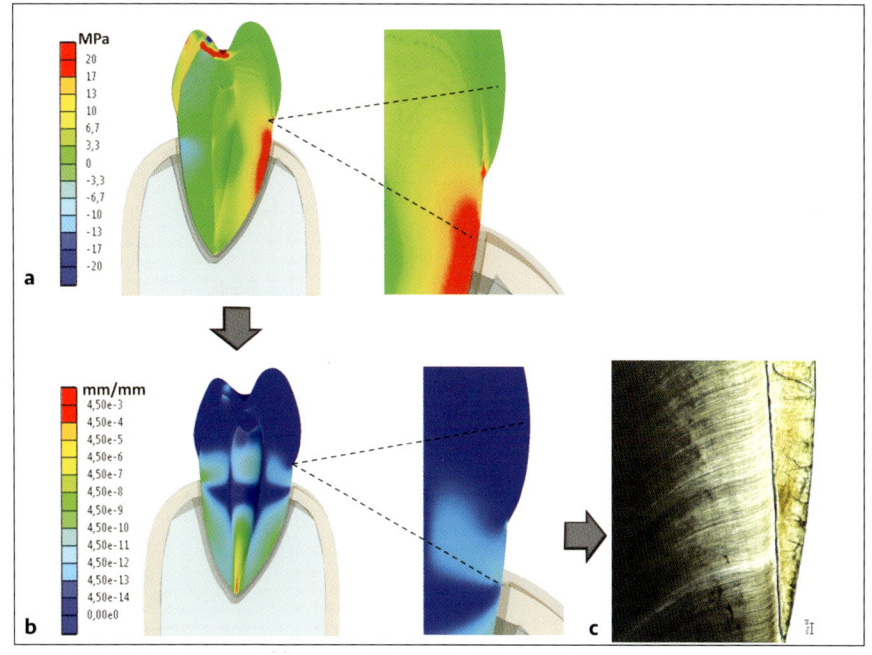

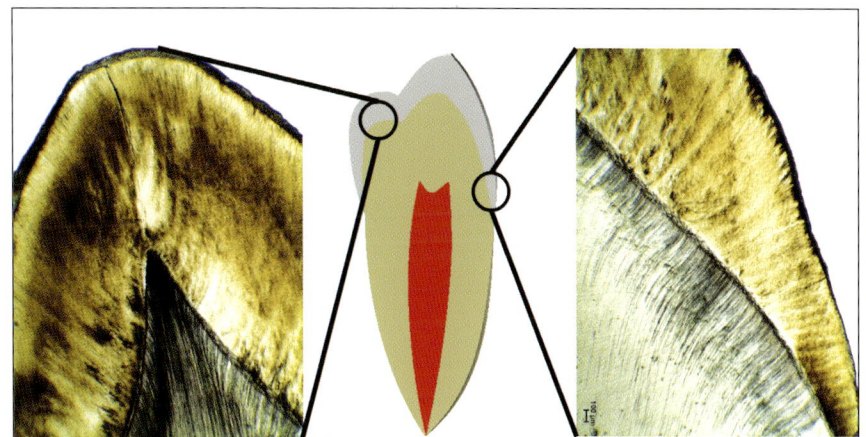

Fig 3-6 Enamel prisms and orientation of dentinal tubules. The cervical region depicts parallel prisms and tubules, which result in less resistant dental tissue than in the occlusal/incisal regions.

moval of the load. In plastic strain, the body does not return to its original state after removal of the load. In breakage strain, the body ruptures into two or more parts[7] (Figs 3-4 and 3-5).

Anatomical Considerations in the Cervical Region

The micromorphology of the tooth structure directly influences the origin and progression of NCCLs (Fig 3-6). In the cervical region, the enamel prisms and dentinal tubules are located transversely to the long axis of the tooth, whereas they are parallel to the long axis in the occlusal/incisal third.[8] The enamel is also thinner and therefore more brittle in the cervical region.[6,8–11] The characteristics of dentin (ie, the amount of peritubular and intertubular dentin) and the direction of the dentinal tubules are significantly altered by localization,[12] which can have profound effects on the maximum tensile strength of the material.[13] This direction together with the higher density and diameter of these tubules[14] result in a more deformable and brittle dentin and consequently promote a major chance of failure.[15–17]

3 Stress

Table 3-1 Ultimate tensile strengths (MPa) of dentin and enamel, according to area and histologic feature[17,18]

Enamel		DEJ	Dentin						
Parallel orientation	Perpendicular orientation		Parallel orientation		Perpendicular orientation		Superficial dentin	Middle dentin	Deep dentin
			Crown	Root	Crown	Root			
40.1–42.2	11.5–17.6	46.9	54.2	49.8	86.5	64.7	61.6	48.7	33.9

DEJ, dentinoenamel junction.

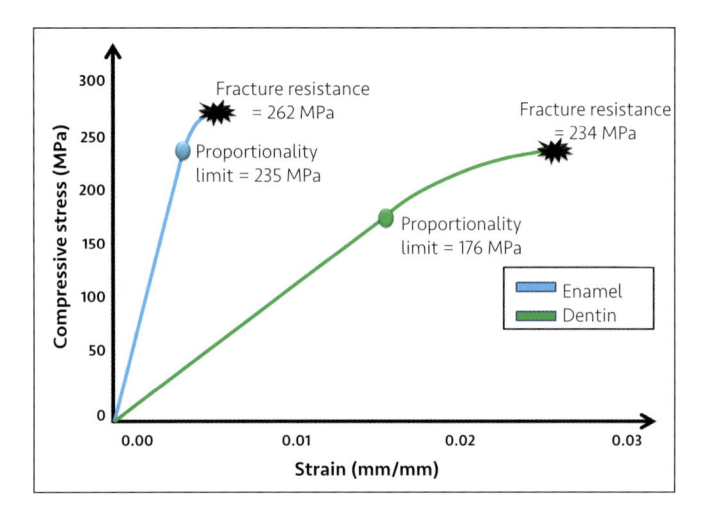

Fig 3-7 Ultimate compressive strengths of enamel and dentin.

These specific characteristics of enamel and dentin (see also chapter 2) result in a less resistant tooth tissue in the cervical area, which can result in micro- and macrofractures caused by stress concentration that exceeds the elastic strain limit of the dental tissue. The ultimate tensile strength value for enamel perpendicular to the prisms is between 40.1 and 42.1 MPa.[17,18] As previously mentioned, in the cervical region the enamel orientation is parallel to the prisms,[8] which results in a less rigid dental structure[16] and lower ultimate tensile strength (11.5 to 17.6 MPa).[17,18] The ultimate tensile strength of dentin depends on the region and the direction of the tubules; the deeper the dentin, the lower the ultimate tensile strength[17,18] (Table 3-1). The ultimate compressive strengths of enamel and dentin are 262 MPa and 234 MPa, respectively[7] (Fig 3-7).

Abfractive Lesions and Occlusal Factors

When stress in the cervical region arising from repeated occlusal loading to the enamel and dentin exceeds their ultimate tensile or compression strength, the resulting strain is greater than the elastic limit of these structures, which manifests as fracture and the development of abfractive lesions.[5,19] These lesions often occur at the cementoenamel junction (CEJ), where flexure can lead to a disruption of the extremely thin layer of enamel prisms and cause microfracture of the cementum and dentin.[5,19,20] *Abfraction* refers to the pathologic loss of hard tissue tooth structure in areas of stress concentration caused by eccentric occlusal loading forces. The size and the development of abfractive lesions are proportional to the direction, magnitude, frequency, duration, and location of the static and cyclic loading forces causing the stress.[5]

The most potentially damaging forces are generally the output of intercuspation of the teeth during lateral excursion or anterior slide from centric relation to maximal intercuspal position in normal function or parafunction. Therefore, there is strong evidence of an association between wear facets on the occlusal surface and NCCLs.[21,22] Nevertheless, not every tooth with wear facets will exhibit NCCLs, and not every tooth with NCCLs will exhibit wear facets.

Abnormal occlusion frequently creates nonaxial loads, which are associated with the presence of NCCLs. There is evidence that up to 100% of teeth with wedge-shaped NCCLs and premature contacts resulted from nonaxial loading.[23] However, this analysis has some limitations and raises some questions. For example, the effects of bruxism and clenching are enhanced by mastication. Clenching does not re-

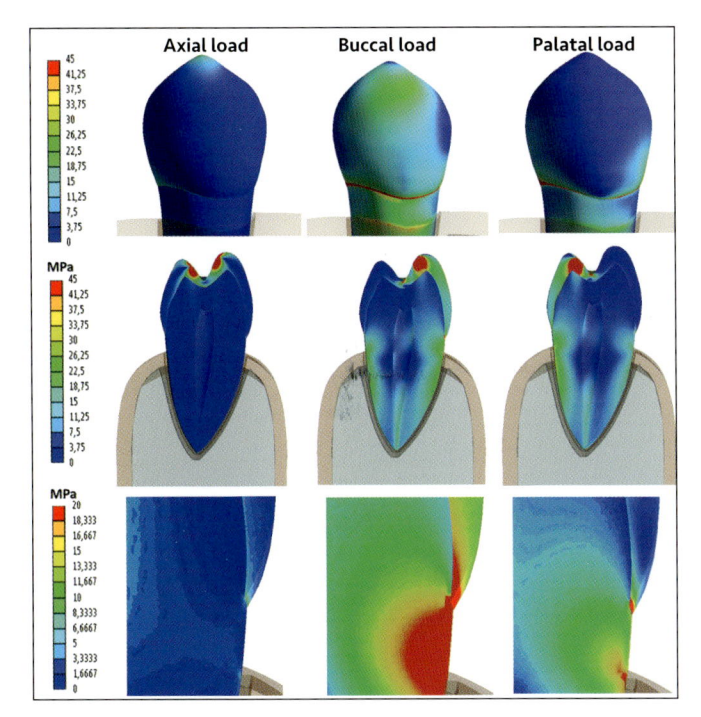

Fig 3-8 Variations of stress concentration according to the direction of the occlusal loading force on the cusps analyzed by the von Mises criterion. The areas closer to red have greater stress concentration, and the areas closer to dark blue have lower stress concentration. The stress concentration varies according to the region where the force is applied, or clinically, where occlusal contact occurs. Simulation of the contact on one cusp (buccal or lingual) promotes higher stress concentration in the cervical region, which will result in greater deformation of the tooth structure.

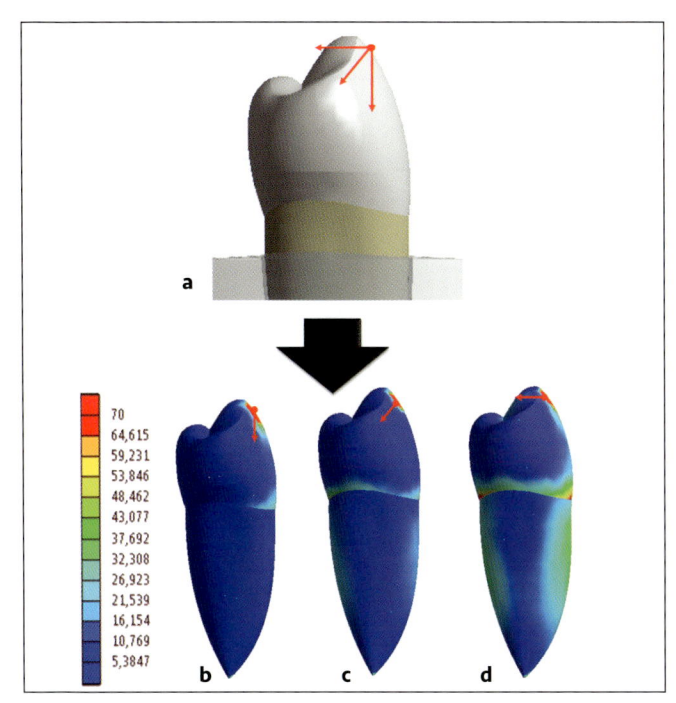

Fig 3-9 Oblique loads result in higher stress concentration in the cervical areas. The areas closer to red have greater stress concentration, and the areas closer to dark blue have lower stress concentration. *(a)* Computer-aided design model exported to finite element analysis software. The models were fixed to resist displacement. The occlusal load (100 N) was simulated to be applied at the same point but with differently directed resultants: *(b)* 0 degrees, *(c)* 45 degrees, and *(d)* 90 degrees.

sult in wear of the broad occlusal facets as does bruxism, yet it can still form Class VI lesions and cause tooth flexure. Furthermore, there is no simple or accurate method for quantifying the effects of bruxism or clenching; bruxism, for example, is underestimated because the wear facets are the only way of measuring its activity.[19] Therefore, both bruxing and clenching become modifying factors in the formation of NCCLs.

In addition to occlusal instability, the dental crown's morphology and geometry may influence the occlusal stress pattern of the tooth. The morphogeometry of the dental crown is primarily based on genetic factors, but environmental factors such as diet and habits may affect their anatomy.[24] Occlusal and incisal wear as well as loss of enamel in the cervical area can alter the anatomy of the tooth; this varying occlusal morphology may affect the chewing efficiency and result in lowered stress concentration in the cervical region due to a decrease in the height and inclination of the cusps.[25]

Despite the availability of studies purporting to show associations between occlusal factors and NCCLs, the literature shows no *clear* association between the two.[20,26] This may be due to the great heterogeneity among methodologies, the lack of standardization, and differences in the diagnosis of NCCLs (wedge-shaped versus rounded). In addition, NCCLs will not always appear in the tooth in which the premature contact is identified; this tooth is more likely the culprit for the interfering movement from centric relation to maximal intercuspal position.

Occlusal Load Direction

Stress concentration in the cervical region due to nonaxial loading has a physical/mechanical relationship with the failure of tooth structure, and the direction of occlusal loading affects this stress concentration (Fig 3-8). When the same magnitude of load is applied to the same position on a tooth but results in a different direction of force, it will create different stress concentrations and strain patterns in the cervical region (Fig 3-9). The same will happen when the location of occlusal contact changes.[27-30] On the other hand, the same load delivered axially tends to have a pattern of uniform stress distribution throughout the tooth.[27-29]

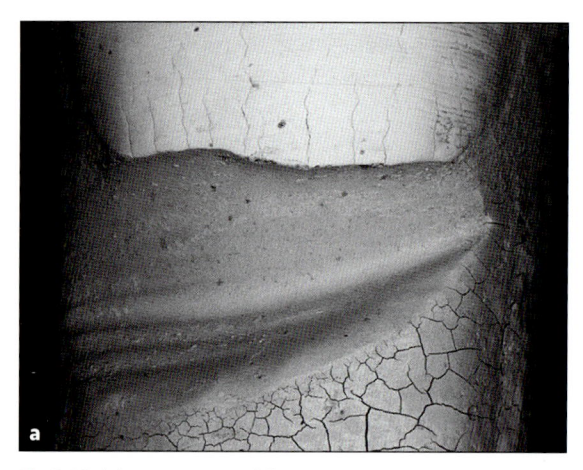

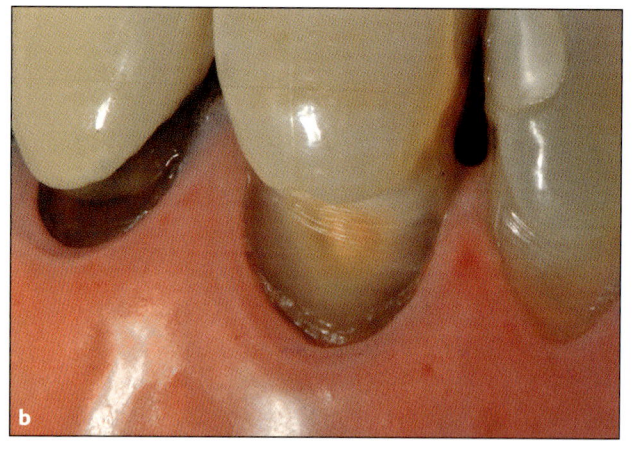

Fig 3-10 *(a)* Biocorrosive abfraction ridges within the wedge-shaped NCCL resulting from variation in the location of the tensile stress concentration over time combined with a biocorrodent, resulting in a lesion with irregular morphology attributed to a changing fulcrum toward the apex of the tooth. *(b)* Clinical aspects of biocorrosive abfraction ridges, or "progression lines," within the wedge-shaped NCCL.

When there is eccentric loading, increased accumulation of stress occurs as well as consequent higher levels of strain.[27–29,31] The contact region is closely related to the flexure of the tooth and its effects on stress to the cervical area.[9,28] In the case of the contacting side, when the loading is applied to the palatal cusp, the tooth will flex toward the lingual region, which then results in tensile stress concentration in the buccal cervical region and corresponding compressive stress to the lingual cervical region. When the load is applied to the contacting part of the buccal cusp, the opposite occurs, wherein tensile stress concentration is at the cervical lingual area and the compressive stress is at the buccal cervical region.[27,29]

Levers

To better understand that fulcrum areas and biomechanical concepts are fundamental, one must consider that the lever is most relevant in biologic systems. While the principles of the lever are well known, their biologic implications are often underestimated or ignored. Yet every living organism has some part or projection, particularly a rigid extension such as a leg or arm, that, when subject to forces acting on it, would act as a simple lever.

The lever is one of the simplest and most primitive mechanisms used by man for the expansion of muscle strength. It consists of a rigid bar that is free to rotate around a fixed point called a *fulcrum* (F) under the action of two or more forces often referred to as *effort* (E) (or applied force) and *resistance* (R) (or force resistance). The purpose of this principle is to multiply the force and motion.[32] In the case of teeth, they may be considered vertical cantilevers and would react accordingly to loads in various directions.

The lever is classified according to the position of the fulcrum and the applied resistance forces. When it comes to teeth in alveolar bone, the class I lever is the one that best represents the situation: the fulcrum (F) is between the effort (E) and resistance (R). The abfractive lesions are located close to the fulcrum point of teeth, which is precisely in the area of highest stress concentration.[9,19] This theory then states that the direction of occlusal forces acting on the tooth will determine the site of NCCLs.[9,19]

Lesion morphology

Changes of the fulcrum point in areas of stress concentration affect the development of NCCLs and result in various morphologies.[9,19,33] The wedge-shaped lesion, for example, is a common pattern for NCCLs caused by changes in the occlusal or incisal contact areas at different times due to various mandibular movements. Changes in the tensile stress concentration within the lesion result in irregular morphology beyond a well-defined internal angle and flat walls.[33] Some lesions appear to have ridges within the notch, or "progression lines" (Fig 3-10). These lines signify high activity of mechanical etiologic factors in developing the NCCL.

The stress-strain concentration at the bottom and along the walls of the lesion has a proximity to the pulp chamber and promotes a stimulus to the pulp cells due to the possibility of damage to dentin and pulp (Fig 3-11). In this case, the deposition of dentin by odontoblasts results in sclerotic dentin. The reactive dentin is the result of an inflammatory stimulus and is deposited close to the offending biocorrodents, also resulting in more mineralized dentin that is less permeable due to obliteration of dentinal tubules. The dentin can also be deposited on the pulp wall chamber to main-

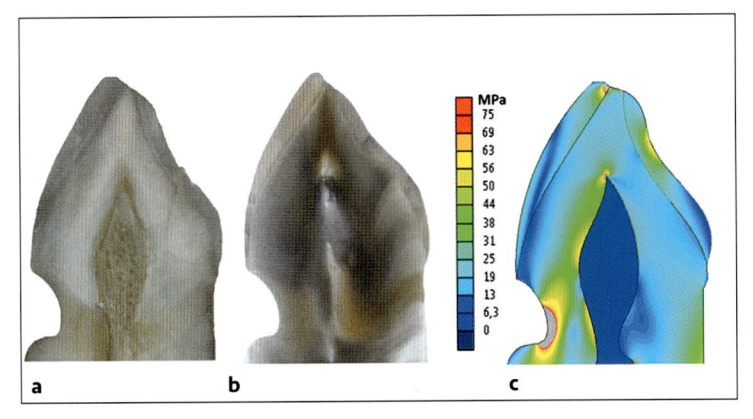

Fig 3-11 *(a)* Longitudinal section of a canine. *(b)* The stress concentration (MPa) at the depth of the lesion results in more mineralized dentin deposition in the pulp chamber. *(c)* Stress pattern by finite element analysis (von Mises criterion). Areas in red have the highest stress concentration, while areas in dark blue have the lowest stress concentration.

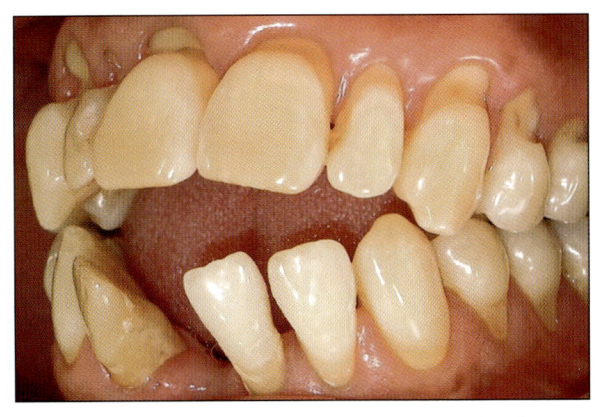

Fig 3-12 Biocorrosive abfractive lesions associated with stress resulting from tongue-thrusting forces and biocorrodents. The patient presented with an anterior open bite and the related parafunctional habit of applying tongue pressure to the teeth. (Courtesy of Dr Alvaro Junqueira, Ribeirão Preto, Brazil.)

tain the vascular and nervous tissue farthest from the stimulus, consequently reducing the volume of the pulp chamber. Because of these depositions, it is common to clinically observe darker dentin at the bottom of the NCCLs and also in teeth with pulp necrosis due to calcification of the pulp tissue and root canals as a consequence of the effects of stress-strain (see Fig 3-11). In these cases, the patient rarely complains of dentin hypersensitivity.

Other considerations

In some cases, it is observed that stress concentration is not caused by opposing contacts but instead by the tongue pressing against the teeth, a parafunctional habit seen especially in patients with open bite. For its small size, the tongue is considered one of the strongest muscles in the body and is capable of producing forces strong enough to exceed the elastic limit of tooth structures when it performs repetitive movements. It exerts a load force along an oblique axis of the tooth, which, combined with biocorrosive agents, can lead to the development and progression of NCCLs, or caries when plaque is present in patients who have poor hygiene (Fig 3-12).

Stress-Biocorrosion

The mechanism of stress is recurring and unavoidable in oral activity, and other modifying etiologic factors also act to define the origin and progression of NCCLs, which may result in different morphologies.[5] *Stress-biocorrosion* refers to the synergistic action of both etiologic mechanisms and serves an important role in the initiation and progression of

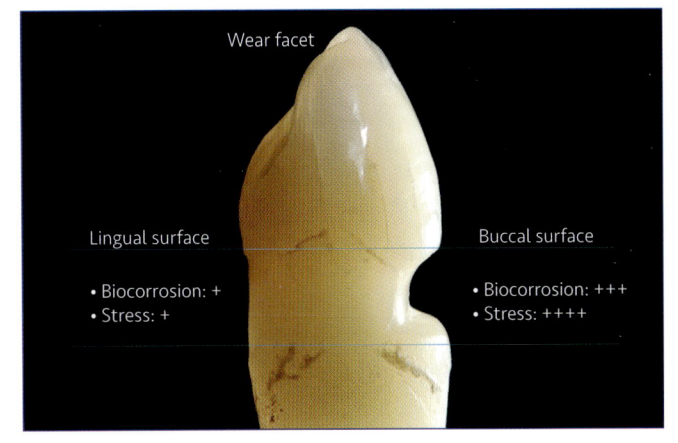

Fig 3-13 Biocorrosive abfraction is greater on the facial than on the lingual due to the lack of serous saliva on the facial.

NCCLs as well as caries in regions of stress concentration.[6] The combination of stress and biocorrosion can cause more damage than either acting alone[5,34] (see chapter 1).

The prevalence of NCCLs on buccal surfaces is influenced by the lack of saliva on these surfaces, causing the increased action of biocorrosive abfraction,[6] even though the magnitude of the stress can be similar in both regions.[27,29] The biocorrosive potential of acidic diets (eg, eating citrus fruits, drinking soda) as well as occupational and recreational habits (eg, pipe smoking) acts together with the stress and strain in the cervical region. Furthermore, the palatal and lingual areas have six times more serous saliva than the vestibule area; this saliva neutralizes the various acidic and proteolytic biocorrosives.[6,34] Dentin can be attacked by exogenous or endogenous acids as well as by proteolytic agents, which degrade the softened dentin and make it susceptible to abfraction. The combined effects of stress and biocorrosion further degrade the dentin on the facial side of the tooth (Fig 3-13).

Fig 3-14 NCCL restorations promote a biomechanical behavior similar to that of a healthy tooth, due to their similar moduli of elasticity.

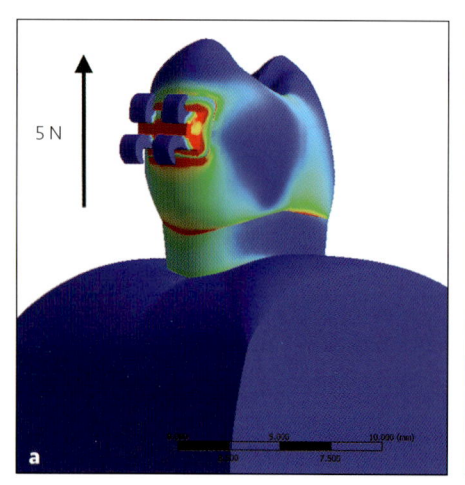

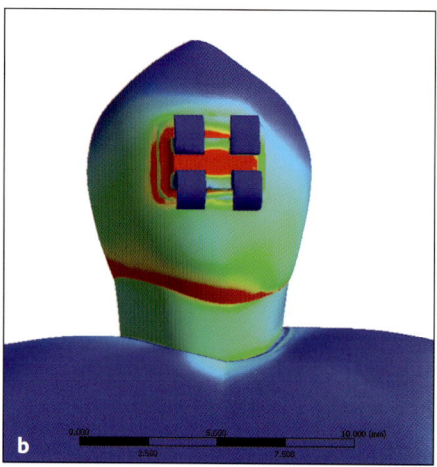

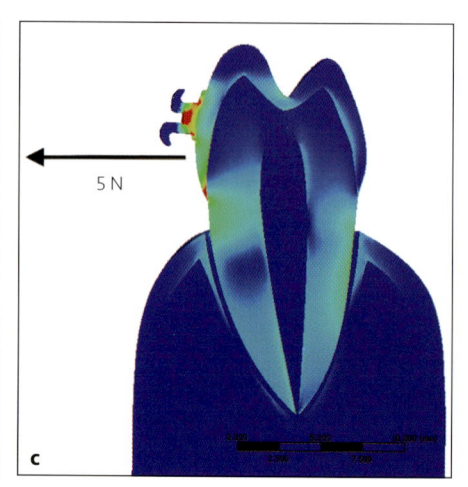

Fig 3-15 Effect of orthodontic movement on mechanical stress concentration in the cervical region of a maxillary premolar (*red* is 10 MPa, *green* is 5 MPa, and *blue* is 0 MPa). *(a)* 3D view of extrusive tooth movement. *(b)* Frontal view of the buccal aspect after buccal tooth movement (load of 5 N). *(c)* Longitudinal cut of a premolar after buccal tooth movement. Observe the stress concentration in the cervical enamel.

Biomechanical Behavior of Abfractive Lesions

Tooth substance loss is a major modifying factor in the biomechanical behavior of a tooth.[12,27,28] This loss results in a less rigid tooth remnant that is now more susceptible to further degradation and eventual failure. Therefore, in the case of loss of tooth structure within the NCCL, the remainder will be changed in its distribution pattern of stress and strain.[27,28,35] In this instance, stress will focus on the walls of the cavity of the lesion. In NCCLs, the accumulation of stress is greater at the depth of the lesions because the stress increases in regions of higher modulus of elasticity with acute angles.[27,28,35] The greater the loss of tooth substance, the greater the stress concentration and progression of the lesion.

Restoration

Restoration of NCCLs is advised to protect the areas from biocorrodents and add strength to the weakened tooth. Restorative materials should have an elastic modulus similar to that of tooth structure to restore the biomechanical behavior of the lost tooth structure.[20,30,35] Restorative procedures result in lower stress magnitude at the depth and walls of the lesion as well as reduced strain on the tooth structure (Fig 3-14).

Orthodontic Treatment

Postorthodontic patients have been proposed as a group at risk for NCCLs and CDH,[36] but studies in the literature conclude that there is a lack of scientific evidence to effectively prove this correlation.[37] Nonetheless, it is important to study the distribution of stress in the cervical region of teeth resulting from excessive eccentric loading forces during orthodontic treatment. Orthodontic movements promote stress concentration at the cervical region of teeth, for example, extrusive and buccal tooth movement (Fig 3-15). In teeth with NCCLs, the stress is most significant in the interior of

Fig 3-16 Variations of stress concentration (finite element analysis) according to status of the cervical region (sound tooth, unrestored NCCL, or NCCL restored with composite resin). All models were submitted to extrusive orthodontic movement and the results plotted by the von Mises criterion. The areas in red have the highest stress concentration, and the areas in dark blue have the lowest stress concentration. For all three teeth, the orthodontic load promotes stress concentration at the cervical region, but the stress value is greater in the presence of an unrestored NCCL.

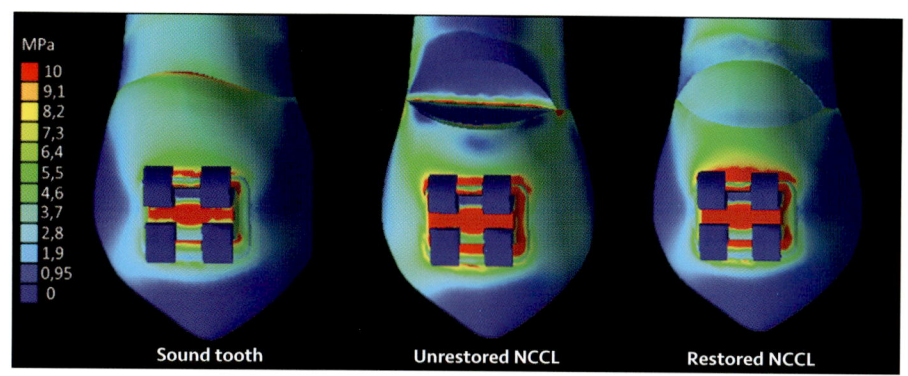

Fig 3-17 *(a to c)* Frontal and lateral views of a patient with multiple NCCLs and a high level of cervical dentin hypersensitivity associated with orthodontic treatment.

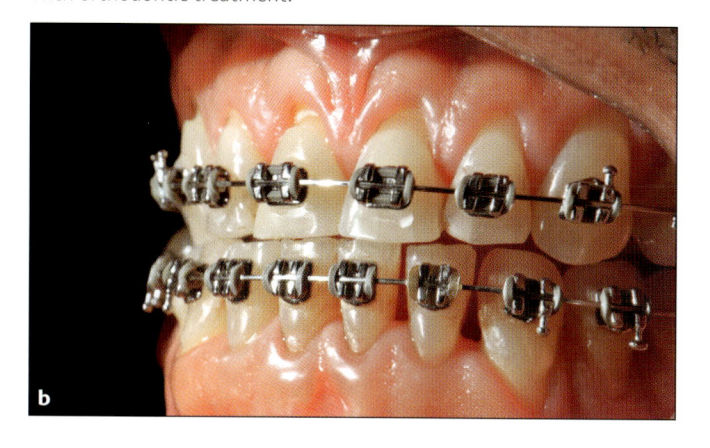

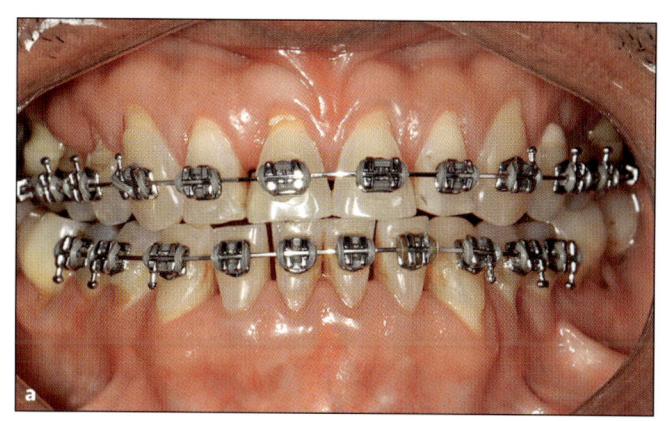

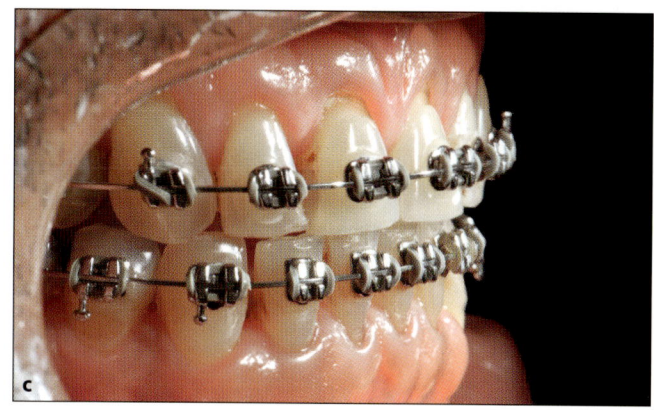

the lesions. Moreover, when the NCCL is restored with composite resin, the stress is more homogenously distributed than in an unrestored NCCL (Fig 3-16). Thus, restorations are indicated to avoid the higher concentration of stress in the NCCL depth and walls during occlusal load application. Figure 3-17 illustrates a patient with multiple NCCLs associated with orthodontic movement therapy. Chapter 9 describes the restoration of NCCLs with adhesive materials.

Periodontal Considerations

Occlusal loading forces applied to the teeth are transmitted to the periodontal supporting structures, which cushion and dissipate the resultant stresses when receiving an axial load. When the periodontal ligament is subjected to compressive stress beyond its elastic limit, cellular mediators are released in the region to induce resorption of the compressive side of the alveolar bone.[38,39] Also known as *bone deflection*, this mechanism absorbs, reduces, and distributes the amount of stress so that it is not restricted to or concentrated in the periodontal tissues. As the teeth lose their bone level, the fulcrum point moves apically, and applied forces will result in less stress concentration at the CEJ (Fig 3-18). However, because of the bone and gingival attachment loss, the cervical region will have a greater amount of cementum and dentin exposed to other etiologic factors for NCCLs such as toothbrush/dentifrice abrasion and especially biocorrosion (Fig 3-19).

Fig 3-18 Periodontal support and the influence of the fulcrum point: The lower the bone and attachment levels, the greater the dental mobility. Stress concentration then becomes located more apically and distant from the CEJ. *(a)* Normal bone level. *(b)* Buccal gingival recession and consequent bone loss. *(c)* Horizontal bone loss.

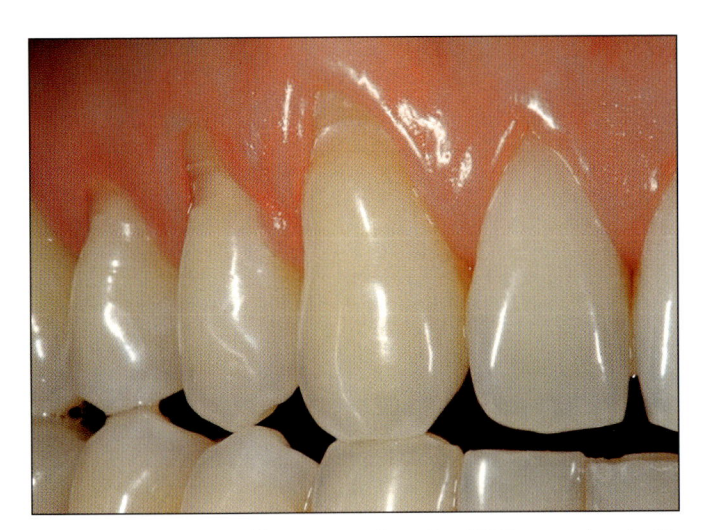

Fig 3-19 Biocorrosive abfractions and varying NCCLs associated with gingival recession resulting from stress concentration.

Conclusion

Let's review what we have covered in this chapter:
- Stress from nonaxial occlusal loading is a major etiologic stress factor in the development and progression of NCCLs.
- The direction of eccentric occlusal loading will affect the stress concentration and strain pattern.
- Loss of tooth structure changes the biomechanical behavior of the tooth, so NCCLs may have irregular morphology as the tensile stress concentration changes with progression.
- The restoration of NCCLs promotes a more homogenous stress concentration on the depth and walls of the cavity.
- The combination of stress and biocorrosion can cause more damage than either acting alone.
- Loss of periodontal attachment may reduce the stress concentration at the CEJ, but it makes the exposed tooth structure more susceptible to biocorrodents and toothbrush/dentifrice abrasion.
- Patients with bruxism or clenching habits as well as patients who have undergone orthodontic treatment are considered at risk for NCCLs and cervical dentin hypersensitivity due to stress factors.

References

1. Levitch LC, Bader JD, Shugars DA, Heymann HO. Non-carious cervical lesions. J Dent 1994;22:195–207.
2. Faye B, Kane AW, Sarr M, Lo C, Ritter AV, Grippo JO. Noncarious cervical lesions among a non-toothbrushing population with Hansen's disease (leprosy): Initial findings. Quintessence Int 2006;37:613–619.
3. Afolabi AO, Shaba OP, Adegbulugbe IC. Distribution and characteristics of non carious cervical lesions in an adult Nigerian population. Nig Q J Hosp Med 2012;22(1):1–6.
4. Que K, Guo B, Jia Z, Chen Z, Yang J, Gao P. A cross-sectional study: Non-carious cervical lesions, cervical dentine hypersensitivity and related risk factors. J Oral Rehabil 2013;40:24–32.
5. Grippo JO, Simring M, Schreiner S. Attrition, abrasion, corrosion and abfraction revisited: A new perspective on tooth surface lesions. J Am Dent Assoc 2004;135:1109–1118.
6. Grippo JO, Simring M, Coleman TA. Abfraction, abrasion, biocorrosion, and the enigma of noncarious cervical lesions: A 20-year perspective. J Esthet Restor Dent 2012;24:10–23.
7. Anusavice KJ, Shen C, Rawls HR. Phillips's Science of Dental Materials, ed 12. St Louis: Saunders, 2013.
8. Hariri I, Sadr A, Shimada Y, Tagami J, Sumi Y. Effects of structural orientation of enamel and dentine on light attenuation and local refractive index: An optical coherence tomography study. J Dent 2012;40:387–396.
9. Lee WC, Eakle WS. Possible role of tensile stress in the etiology of cervical erosive lesions of teeth. J Prosthet Dent 1984;52:374–380.
10. Craig RG, Peyton FA. Elastic and mechanical properties of human dentin. J Dent Res 1958;37:710–718.
11. Atsu SS, Aka PS, Kucukesmen HC, Kilicarslan MA, Atakan C. Age-related changes in tooth enamel as measured by electron microscopy: Implications for porcelain laminate veneers. J Prosthet Dent 2005;94:336–341.
12. Marshall GW Jr, Marshall SJ, Kinney JH, Balooch M. The dentin substrate: Structure and properties related to bonding. J Dent 1997;25:441–458.
13. Carvalho RM, Fernandes CA, Villanueva R, Wang L, Pashley DH. Tensile strength of human dentin as a function of tubule orientation and density. J Adhes Dent 2001;3:309–314.

References

14. Harrán Ponce E, Canalda Sahli C, Vilar Fernandez JA. Study of dentinal tubule architecture of permanent upper premolars: Evaluation by SEM. Aust Endod J 2001;27:66–72.
15. Arola DD, Reprogel RK. Tubule orientation and the fatigue strength of human dentin. Biomaterials 2006;27:2131–2140.
16. Miura J, Maeda Y, Nakai H, Zako M. Multiscale analysis of stress distribution in teeth under applied forces. Dent Mater 2009;25:67–73.
17. Soares CJ, Castro CG, Neiva NA, et al. Effect of gamma irradiation on ultimate tensile strength of enamel and dentin. J Dent Res 2010;89:159–164.
18. Giannini M, Soares CJ, de Carvalho RM. Ultimate tensile strength of tooth structures. Dent Mater 2004;20:322–329.
19. Michael JA, Townsend GC, Greenwood LF, Kaidonis JA. Abfraction: Separating fact from fiction. Aust Dent J 2009;54:2–8.
20. Senna P, Del Bel Cury A, Rösing C. Non-carious cervical lesions and occlusion: A systematic review of clinical studies. J Oral Rehabil 2012;39:450–462.
21. Telles D, Pegoraro LF, Pereira JC. Prevalence of noncarious cervical lesions and their relation to occlusal aspects: A clinical study. J Esthet Dent 2000;12:10–15.
22. Pegoraro LF, Scolaro JM, Conti PC, Telles D, Pegoraro TA. Noncarious cervical lesions in adults: Prevalence and occlusal aspects. J Am Dent Assoc 2005;136:1694–1700.
23. Piotrowski BT, Gillette WB, Hancock EB. Examining the prevalence and characteristics of abfractionlike cervical lesions in a population of US veterans. J Am Dent Assoc 2001;132:1694–1701.
24. Kono RT. Molar enamel thickness and distribution patterns in extant great apes and humans: New insights based on a 3-dimensional whole crown perspective. Anthropol Sci 2004;112:121–146.
25. Benazzi S, Nguyen HN, Kullmer O, Hublin JJ. Unravelling the functional biomechanics of dental features and tooth wear. PLoS One 2013;8(7):e69990.
26. Silva AG, Martins CC, Zina LG, et al. The association between occlusal factors and noncarious cervical lesions: A systematic review. J Dent 2013;41:9–16.
27. Soares PV, Machado AC, Zeola LF, et al. Loading and composite restoration assessment of various non-carious cervical lesions morphologies - 3D finite element analysis. Aust Dent J 2015;60:309–316.
28. Soares PV, Souza LV, Verissimo C, et al. Effect of root morphology on biomechanical behaviour of premolars associated with abfraction lesions and different loading types. J Oral Rehabil 2014;41:108–114.
29. Rees JS. The effect of variation in occlusal loading on the development of abfraction lesions: A finite element study. J Oral Rehabil 2002;29:188–193.
30. Ichim I, Schmidlin PR, Kieser JA, Swain MV. Mechanical evaluation of cervical glass-ionomer restorations: 3D finite element study. J Dent 2007;35:28–35.
31. Benazzi S, Grosse IR, Gruppioni G, Weber GW, Kullmer O. Comparison of occlusal loading conditions in a lower second premolar using three-dimensional finite element analysis. Clin Oral Investig 2014;18:369–375.
32. Fernandes-Neto AJ, Neves FD, Simamoto Junior PC. Oclusão. São Paulo: Medicas Arts, 2013.
33. Michael JA, Kaidonis JA, Townsend GC. Non-carious cervical lesions on permanent anterior teeth: A new morphological classification. Aust Dent J 2010;55:134–137.
34. Grippo JO, Masi JV. Role of biodental engineering factors (BEF) in the etiology of root caries. J Esthet Dent 1991;3:71–76.
35. Soares PV, Santos-Filho PC, Soares CJ, et al. Non-carious cervical lesions: Influence of morphology and load type on biomechanical behaviour of maxillary incisors. Aust Dent J 2013;58:306–314.
36. Spini PH, Machado AC, Lelis E, Raposo LH, Soares PV. Influence of orthodontic loads on premolars with non-carious cervical lesions [abstract]. Presented at the 93rd General Session of the IADR/AADR/CADR, Boston, 11-14 March 2015.
37. Lee WC, Eakle WS. Stress-induced cervical lesions: Review of advances in the past 10 years. J Prosthet Dent 1996;75:487–494.
38. Baumrind S. A reconsideration of the propriety of the "pressure-tension" hypothesis. Am J Orthod 1969;55:12–22.
39. Heller IJ, Nanda R. Effect of metabolic alteration of periodontal fibers on orthodontic tooth movement. An experimental study. Am J Orthod 1979;75:239–258.

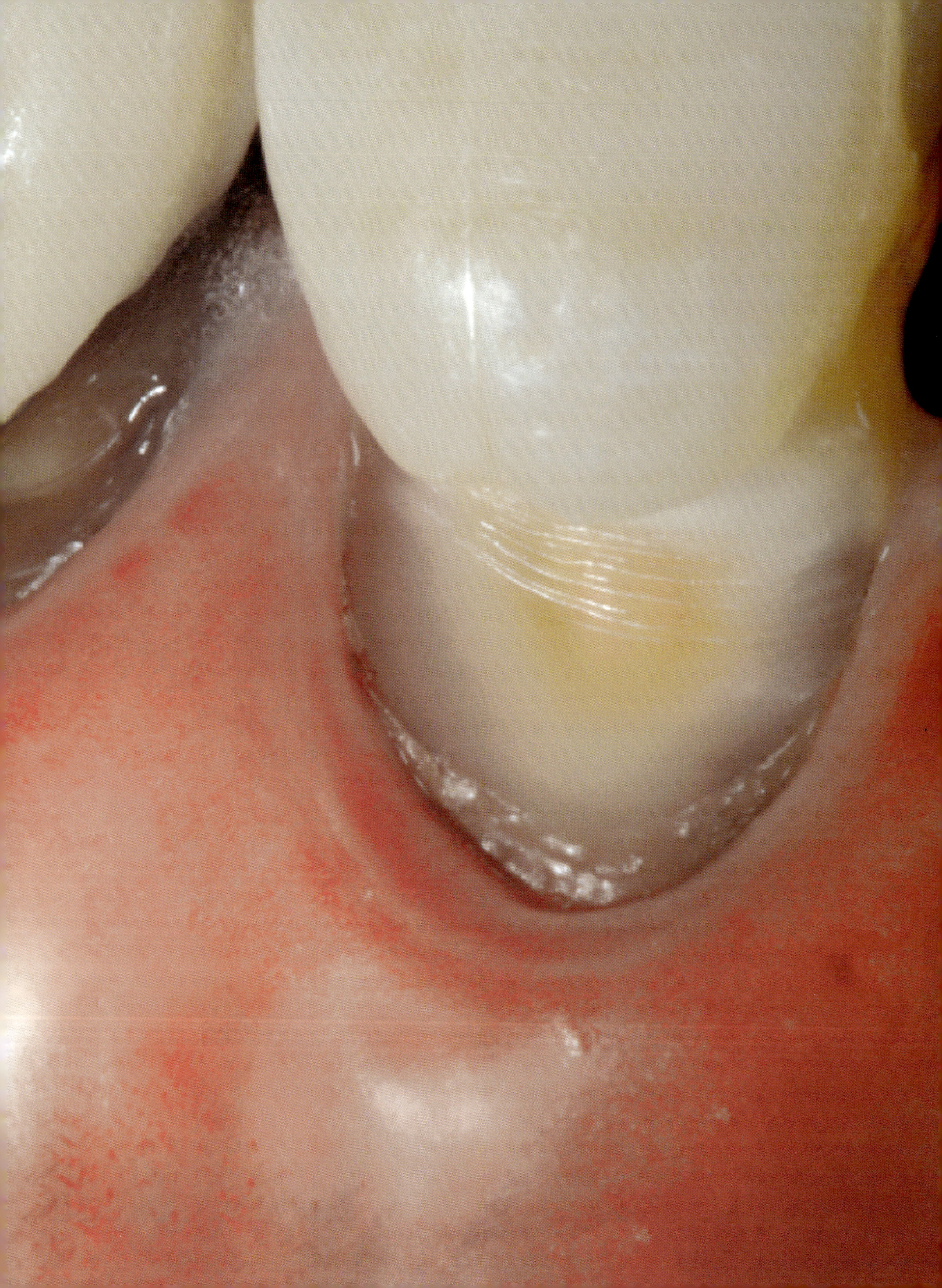

4

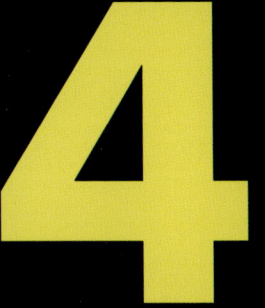

Friction

As a mechanism for noncarious cervical lesions (NCCLs), friction can be classified as endogenous (attrition) or exogenous (abrasion).[1] Attrition occurs as a result of tooth-to-tooth contact (eg, during mastication), whereas abrasion is caused by external objects or substances that are constantly introduced to the mouth (eg, dentifrice).[1,2] This chapter details the mechanism of friction from toothbrush/dentifrice abrasion and its role as a cofactor in the etiology of NCCLs.

The main factors that impact dental abrasion from toothbrushing are the particular brushing technique, the type of toothbrush, the dentifrice used during brushing, and the duration and intensity of brushing.[3]

Brushing Technique

Toothbrushing is the most efficient method for removing biofilm from dental surfaces. The correct brushing technique permits adequate removal of biofilm, protects the periodontal tissues, and reduces the risk of gingival recession.[4] However, incorrect application of the toothbrush can act as a cofactor for NCCLs and increases the loss of softened enamel, particularly at the cervical third of the tooth where stress concentration is the greatest. In severe cases, this can lead to the exposure of dentin to the oral environment[5] (Fig 4-1).

Several methods of manual toothbrushing are recommended by dentists and dental associations to cater to specific age and patient groups. The toothbrushing technique that is most commonly suggested to patients by dentists and hygienists is the modified Stillman technique.[6] This technique emphasizes the removal of biofilm located above and just below the gingival margin. The bristles of the toothbrush are positioned 45 degrees coronal to the gingival margin, and horizontal and vertical brush strokes are applied. Vibratory and slight rotary movements are then applied before moving to the next group of teeth.[6]

Incorrect brushing techniques involve the use of excessive force (which can reach 1.96 N) during the brushing movements. Excessive brushing force increases the friction between the brush bristles and dental enamel or dentin, which can lead to increased wear on these hard tissues.[4] But brush contact does not cause significant wear by itself. A soft-bristle brush promotes dentin wear of less than 0.5 μm per month, which is clinically insignificant.[7] Wear upon enamel from toothbrush abrasion is even more negligible.

4 Friction

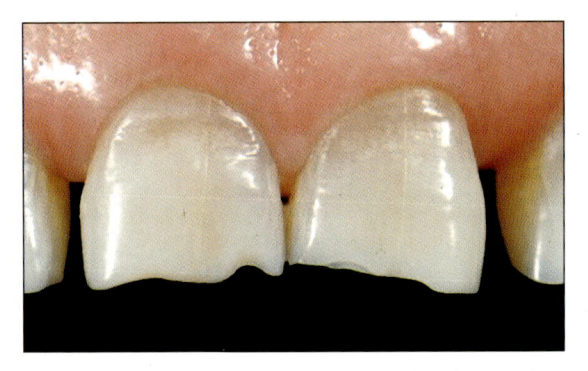

Fig 4-1 Note the smooth NCCLs and tooth substance loss on the facial surfaces of the central incisors associated with incorrect brushing technique.

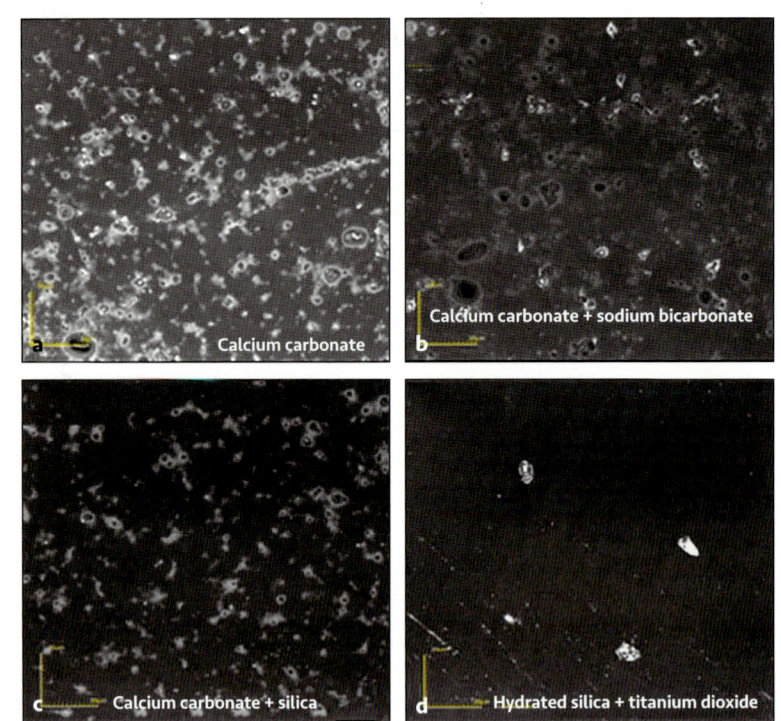

Fig 4-2 *(a to d)* Presence of different abrasive agents in commercial dentifrices. Note that in *d*, some large abrasive particles are used either in isolation or in combination with microabrasive particles.

Generally, brushing with a manual toothbrush results in greater brushing forces than brushing with a sonic toothbrush, and brushing speed has not been shown to influence enamel or dentin abrasion.[8] Studies have suggested that there is no difference in hard tissue abrasion between electric and manual brushing with toothpaste,[9,10] despite the finding that the head and/or filament actions of electric toothbrushes may quickly dislocate the toothpaste from the brush head.[11,12]

Another aspect that should be considered is the type of bristle in the brush. It has been shown that soft-bristle brushes exhibit the best bristle tip morphologies, which result in improved quality control. In contrast, hard-bristle toothbrushes exhibit the worst bristle tip morphologies and may injure the hard and soft tissues, thus leading to gingival recession.[13] Nevertheless, soft- and hard-bristle toothbrushes were not found to produce significant differences in the abrasion of enamel.[14]

Toothbrushes

The toothbrush influences the wear process in combination with the dentifrice because soft bristles are able to retain more toothpaste and create a larger contact surface with the substrate. Moreover, increased filament diameter promotes more abrasion. It has been found that dentifrices in combination with toothbrushes with 0.20-mm filament diameters induce enamel losses greater than 0.15 to 0.25 mm.[13] In contrast, an increase in the number of filaments can decrease the average roughness and volume loss values and increase the surface contact, which improves the cleaning ability. Indeed, the toothbrush-dentifrice combination can simultaneously cause increased volume loss but fewer deep scratches, promoting a smoother surface.[13]

Dentifrices

Dentifrices are composed of an abrasive, an aqueous humectant, and an active therapeutic. Therapeutic agents may include dentin desensitizers, whitening agents, or substances that promote bacteriostatic/bactericidal activity. The abrasive content promotes the removal of stains because the particles are harder than the stain but softer than sound enamel. Wear is dependent on the particle hardness, shape, size, distribution, concentration, and load applied during brushing.[13]

Dentifrices of different abrasiveness are available on the market, depending on the solid contents and the type(s) of abrasive present (Fig 4-2). The amount of abrasive in the formulation and the degree of abrasiveness are not correlated,

Table 4-1 Average roughness, volume loss, and RDA of the different dentifrices after a brushing time of 6 hours according to abrasive composition[17]

Abrasive	Average roughness (μm)	Volume loss (mm³)	RDA
Hydrated silicon dioxide	0.97 ± 0.56	1.82 ± 1.41	44
Silica	1.30 ± 0.53	10.61 ± 6.60	70
Calcium phosphate, calcium carbonate, and aluminum silicate	1.15 ± 0.24	1.76 ± 0.76	130
Natriummeta phosphate	0.50 ± 0.19	1.10 ± 0.25	45–60
Silicon dioxide	2.37 ± 1.30	5.25 ± 3.56	142
Hydrated silica	1.46 ± 0.46	2.72 ± 0.90	65–96
Pumice	7.83 ± 5.89	14.79 ± 11.76	250
Pumice	8.99 ± 1.55	20.20 ± 2.41	170
Hydrated silica	1.70 ± 0.56	3.42 ± 1.63	120
Hydrated silica	0.65 ± 0.34	1.42 ± 1.06	40

and the physical characteristics of the minerals that compose dentifrices should be considered. Calcium carbonate in the rhombohedral or ovoid shape is more regular and exhibits an abrasiveness that is lower than that of aragonitic particles, which are more irregular.[15] However, when thin particles of carbonate or silica are used, the dentifrice exhibits reduced abrasiveness. Manufacturers indicate only the main type of abrasive used in the formulation; fundamental data such as the shapes and sizes of the particles are not disclosed.[16]

Abrasivity

The abrasivity of toothpastes varies, and wear depends on the interaction of the toothpaste and toothbrush.[13] The abrasive potential of any toothpaste is determined according to the radioactive enamel abrasion (REA) and radioactive dentin abrasion (RDA) values (Table 4-1). These values are set based on the International Organization for Standardization (ISO) 11609 standards, and dentifrices are classified according to their abrasiveness into low, medium, high, and harmful categories.[18] The primary abrasive substances that are used in toothpastes to remove tooth stains are sodium bicarbonate, hydrated silica, aluminum oxide, calcium carbonate, dicalcium phosphate, pumice powder, and mixes involving other powders such as metal oxides, phosphates, plant extracts, and active components with preventive actions; thus, each dentifrice may contain more than one abrasive.[15]

According to the ISO, there is a degree of abrasivity that must be tolerated by a dentifrice.[19] The RDA standard indicates that the maximum dentin abrasivity must not exceed 250. Whitening toothpastes typically exhibit RDAs between 60 and 100 or over 100, which represent medium and high abrasiveness, respectively.[20–22] It is important to emphasize that it is not RDA alone that defines abrasivity of a dentifrice but rather its association with roughness value.

Dentifrice abrasivity is normally described via the use of a radiotracer technique to calculate the RDA value. This quantitative technique is based on the irradiation of the tooth substance in the test material with neutrons that convert the phosphorous of the hydroxyapatite of the dentin into its radioactive isotope.[23] However, this technique needs to be complemented by other quantitative and qualitative measurements.

Despite the importance of abrasivity, it is necessary to evaluate a dentifrice's cleaning efficacy on the dentin (ie, the pellicle cleaning ratio [PCR]) in relation to the abrasivity. In general, toothpastes with silica exhibit good PCR/RDA values that are lower than those of some toothpastes with calcium carbonate and alumina trihydrate,[24] and the addition of abrasives can improve the cleaning power and PCR/RDA ratio[17] (Fig 4-3).

Other considerations

Another important factor that should be considered is the pH of the dentifrice, because a hallmark of a more alkaline pH is a reduced degree of abrasion. Some dentifrices with lower pH exhibit higher abrasiveness that can potentially be indicative of the combination of biocorrosive and abrasive effects.[16] Moreover, the interaction of detergents and abrasives in toothpaste formulations may increase the net effect of abrasion.[23] Lesions with sharply defined margins may be related to abrasive factors, whereas biocorrosion produces broader, dish-shaped, and shallower lesions.[25]

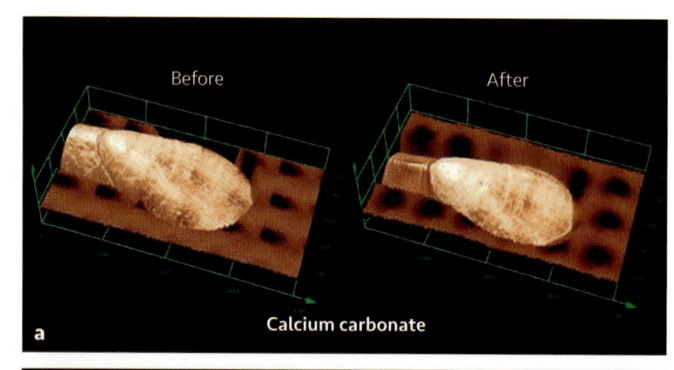

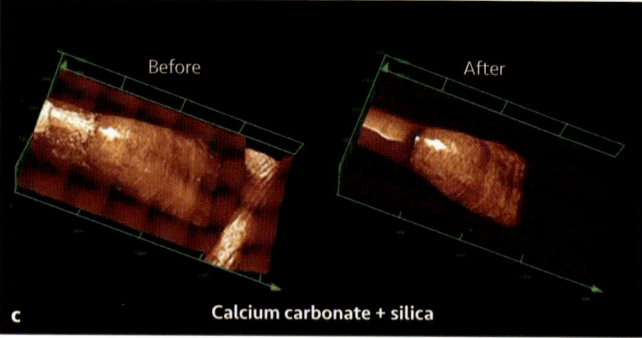

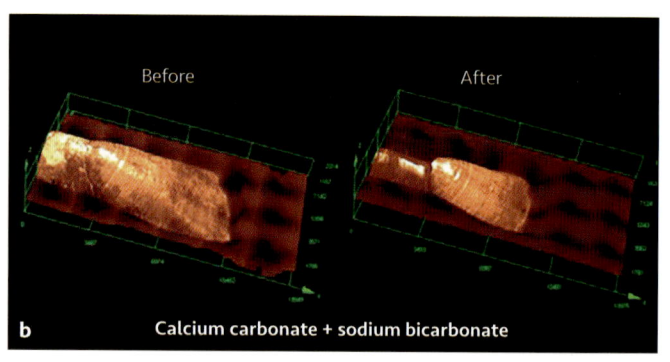

Fig 4-3 *(a)* Tested wear on a tooth using a dentifrice with calcium carbonate as the abrasive component. Observations after toothbrushing revealed that the root and enamel surfaces exhibited smoother, polished appearances, while the dentin exhibited wear. *(b)* Tested wear of a tooth using a dentifrice with calcium carbonate plus sodium bicarbonate as the abrasive components. After toothbrushing, the root and enamel surfaces showed more wear than in *a*. *(c)* Tested wear of a tooth using a dentifrice with calcium carbonate plus silica as the abrasive components. After toothbrushing, the root and enamel surfaces were smooth and polished, whereas the radicular dentin showed pronounced wear.

Whitening Toothpastes

Due to an increased demand for whiter teeth, new toothpastes specifically designed for dental bleaching have been released. As a general rule, whitening toothpastes contain greater amounts of abrasives and detergents than typical toothpastes to remove tougher stains.[26] The basic components of abrasive whitening dentifrices are hydrated silica, calcium carbonate, perlite, dicalcium phosphate dihydrate, and sodium bicarbonate.[27,28] Perlite is an abrasive considered to be more effective in stain removal than silica and results in enamel wear at less than clinically relevant values.[29] As previously mentioned, the extent of dental wear by abrasion is dependent on the hardness, size, shape, and concentration of the abrasive particles in addition to the pressure (ie, force) used during brushing. The thin particles of perlite are effective at tooth cleaning with minimal tooth abrasion. The optimized particle size and geometry are responsible for the improved performance of perlite toothpastes compared to whitening toothpastes with high-cleaning silica.[30]

Bleaching agents such as hydrogen peroxide and carbamide can also be incorporated into dentifrices at low concentrations (0.5% to 1.5%)[26] and act as mild antibacterial agents.[24] These agents oxidize the dental pigments to promote chemical removal and thus dental bleaching. The presence of hydrogen peroxide in toothpaste does not promote significant changes in the soft tissues and has no adverse oral manifestation.[24]

Typically, whitening toothpastes can lighten tooth color by one or two shades. However, these dentifrices can contain abrasives with potential side effects on tooth structure and should therefore be used with caution.[31] Bleaching toothpastes are not associated with increased abrasion,[17] but studies have shown that whitening dentifrices promote more deleterious effects on enamel and dentin than regular toothpastes[32] (Fig 4-4), and the combined use of a dentifrice and mouthwash for bleaching can cause intensive dentin wear.[33]

Nevertheless, the abrasivity of whitening dentifrices is the main actuation factor and exhibited evident correlations with RDA (Table 4-2) and color alteration.[27] These findings suggest that the whitening effect of the dentifrice is primarily related to its ability to mechanically remove stains from enamel surfaces and that abrasive toothpaste can cause some degree of dental wear. However, abrasive dentifrices containing sodium bicarbonate produce more severe lesions, while dentifrices containing carbamide peroxide produced less severe lesions,[21] when associated with other etiologic factors.

Alternative whitening toothpastes contain natural enzymes. These enzymes break down the organic components of biofilm and remove stains. For example, the bleaching effects of whitening dentifrices that contain papain and bromelain have been found to be superior to those of abrasive and control toothpastes without affecting enamel or dentin wear.[34-36]

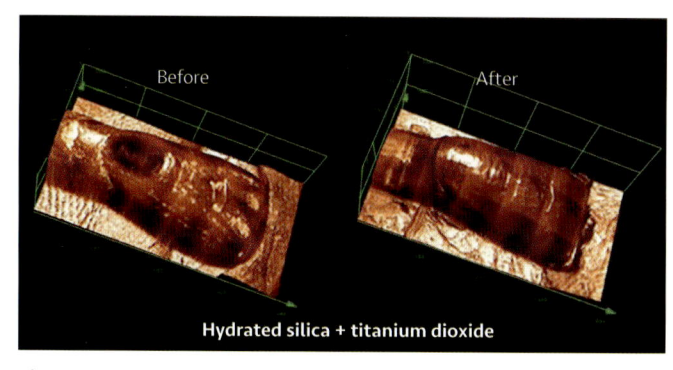

Fig 4-4 Tested wear on a tooth using a whitening dentifrice with hydrated silica plus titanium dioxide as abrasive components. The root and enamel surfaces were smooth and polished, while the radicular dentin showed intense wear.

Table 4-2 RDA of the abrasives employed in different dentifrices indicated for dental bleaching[27]

Abrasive ingredients	RDA
Silica + disodium pyrophosphate	189.2
Calcium pyrophosphate + silica + tetrasodium pyrophosphate + hydrogen peroxide	98.0
Hydrated silica + sodium bicarbonate + tetrasodium pyrophosphate	188.2
Hydrated silica + pentasodium triphosphate	123.7
Hydrated silica in nonwhitening dentifrice	98.6
Hydrated silica + sodium hexametaphosphate	220.0
Hydrated silica in whitening dentifrice	101.2

Fig 4-5 Radicular dentin submitted to an abrasion test and the observed open tubules and wear profiles compared with the control area. The open dentinal tubules from biocorrosion were maintained after toothbrushing with dentifrice. *(a)* Open dentinal tubules resulting from biocorrosion. *(b)* Open dentinal tubules after toothbrushing. Note the very little, if any, difference in numbers of open tubules or their diameter following toothbrushing.

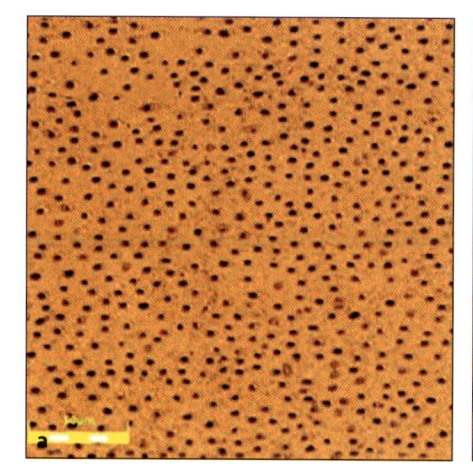

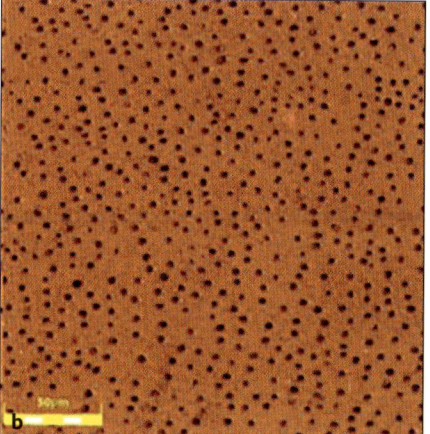

Cervical dentin hypersensitivity

Cervical dentin hypersensitivity (CDH) represents one of the first clinical signs during the formation of an NCCL. The loss of tooth structure in the cervical area of a tooth may be responsible for tooth sensitivity, but dental whitening may also promote CDH. The mechanisms of action of bleaching agents are based on their oxidizing powers, which cause the decomposition of pigmented organic material through the release of free radicals and oxygen. Once these bleaching agents infiltrate the dental tissue, they might be able to elicit morphologic changes in the molecular structure or composition of the tooth.[30] Although the mineral loss from toothbrushing with whitening dentifrices is due to the frictional effects of the brushing itself and not the bleaching agents,[19,37] when exposed to the oral environment, dentin is more susceptible to chemical degradation, and the bleaching agents may permeate the open dentinal tubules and result in CDH[21,22,38] (Fig 4-5).

Interaction Between Etiologic Factors of NCCLs

The genesis of NCCLs has been described as a multifactorial process that involves the mechanisms of stress, biocorrosion, and friction. While some clinicians still view toothbrush/dentifrice abrasion as a major cofactor during NCCL development, the authors aver that biocorrosion and cervical stress concentration are the primary etiologic factors in the formation and progression of NCCLs.

However, abrasion of the hard tissues increases if the tooth has been affected by a biocorrosive challenge, such as acidic foods or drinks or stomach acid from regurgitation.[1,3,39] In such situations, the acidic attack leads to an irreversible loss of dental hard tissue that is accompanied by a progressive softening of the surface; consequently, this softened zone becomes more susceptible to mechanical forces such as toothbrush/dentifrice abrasion.[40,41] Therefore, brushing after meals should be delayed for at least several minutes to allow for remineralization and glycoprotein redeposition.[42]

There is evidence that toothbrushing of a biocorroded tooth with a dentifrice causes tooth wear and can result in pathology as the dentin becomes exposed.[43,44] The main consequence of this situation is CDH, which arises due to the movement of fluids into the exposed dentinal tubules and manifests as pain. If a patient is using an effective desensitizing agent such as fluoridated dentifrice or Sensodyne (GlaxoSmithKline), then CDH may not precede or be present during the progression of an NCCL.

It is important to remember that the mineral composition of dentin is less than that of enamel; consequently, dentin is more susceptible to abrasion. These findings suggest that the use of low or moderate RDA pastes should be advised for safety and the prevention of tooth substance loss. Another concept that must be considered is that the detergent that is present in a dentifrice partially removes the smear layer but can also chemically attack the organic material of the dentin, primarily collagen. Thus, the abrasion caused by a dentifrice in situations in which the dentin has been continuously exposed due to chemical degradation and stress is more intense.[45]

Friction during toothbrushing acts to influence the speed of the progression of NCCLs and is dependent on the abrasive type, vehicle, shape, and applied force of the toothbrush. It is paramount that professionals understand these interactions so as to advise patients on the methods and materials used to maintain proper oral hygiene.

Conclusion

Let's review what we have covered in this chapter:
- Friction causes toothbrush/dentifrice abrasion, which is a minor cofactor in the etiology of NCCLs.
- Using excessive force during toothbrushing can lead to increased hard tissue loss, but this wear is negligible.
- The abrasiveness of dentifrices vary, and more abrasive toothpastes lead to increased wear.
- Whitening toothpastes have greater numbers of abrasives than normal toothpastes and can lead to increased wear as well as CDH.
- Biocorrosion makes teeth more susceptible to abrasion.
- Friction during toothbrushing influences the speed of progression of NCCLs.

References

1. Grippo JO, Simring M, Schreiner S. Attrition, abrasion, corrosion and abfraction revisited: A new perspective on tooth surface lesions. J Am Dent Assoc 2004;135:1109–1118.
2. Shellis RP, Addy M. The interactions between attrition, abrasion and erosion in tooth wear. Monogr Oral Sci 2014;25:32–45.
3. Grippo JO, Simring M, Coleman TA. Abfraction, abrasion, biocorrosion, and the enigma of noncarious cervical lesions: A 20-year perspective. J Esthet Restor Dent 2012;24:10–23.
4. Wiegand A, Schlueter N. The role of oral hygiene: Does toothbrushing harm? Monogr Oral Sci 2014;25:215–219.
5. Hooper S, West NX, Pickles MJ, Joiner A, Newcombe RG, Addy M. Investigation of erosion and abrasion on enamel and dentine: a model in situ using toothpastes of different abrasivity. J Clin Periodontol 2003;30:802–808.
6. Wainwright J, Sheiham A. An analysis of methods of toothbrushing recommended by dental associations, toothpaste and toothbrush companies and in dental texts. Br Dent J 2014;217(3):E5.
7. Joiner A, Pickles MJ, Lynch S, Cox TF. The measurement of enamel wear by four toothpastes. Int Dent J 2008;58:23–28.
8. Wiegand A, Burkhard JP, Eggmann F, Attin T. Brushing force of manual and sonic toothbrushes affects dental hard tissue abrasion. Clin Oral Investig 2013;17:815–822.
9. Comar LP, Gomes MF, Ito N, Salomão PA, Grizzo LT, Magalhães AC. Effect of NaF, SnF(2), and TiF(4) toothpastes on bovine enamel and dentin erosion-abrasion in vitro. Int J Dent 2012;2012:134350.
10. Sorensen JA, Pham MM, Mcinnes C. In vitro safety evaluation of a new ultrasound power toothbrush. J Clin Dent 2008;19(1):28–32.
11. Addy M. Oral hygiene products: Potential for harm to oral and systemic health? Periodontol 2000 2008;48:54–65.
12. Van Der Weijden GA, Timmerman MF, Reijerse E, Snoek CM, Van Der Velden U. Toothbrushing force in relation to plaque removal. J Clin Periodontol 1996;23:724–729.
13. Tellefsen G, Liljeborg A, Johannsen A, Johannsen G. The role of the toothbrush in the abrasion process. Int J Dent Hyg 2011;9:284–290.
14. Voronets J, Jaeggi T, Buergin W, Lussi A. Controlled toothbrush abrasion of softened human enamel. Caries Res 2008;42:286–290.
15. Pascaretti-Grizon F, Mabilleau G, Chappard D. Abrasion of 6 dentifrices measured by vertical scanning interference microscopy. J Appl Oral Sci 2013;21:475–481.
16. Andrade ACC, Andrade MRTC, Machado WAS, Fischer RG. In vitro study of dentifrice abrasivity. Rev Odontol Univ São Paulo 1998;12:231–236.
17. Johannsen G, Tellefsen G, Johannsen A, Liljeborg A. The importance of measuring toothpaste abrasivity in both a quantitative and qualitative way. Acta Odontol Scand 2013;71:508–517.
18. González-Cabezas C, Hara AT, Hefferren J, Lippert F. Abrasivity testing of dentifrices—Challenges and current state of the art. Monogr Oral Sci 2013;23:100–107.
19. Ren YF, Amin A, Malmstrom H. Effects of tooth whitening and orange juice on surface properties of dental enamel. J Dent 2009;37:424–431.
20. Kuroiwa M, Kodaka T, Abe M. Dentin hypersensitivity. Occlusion of dentinal tubules by brushing with and without an abrasive dentifrice. J Periodontol 1994;65:291–296.
21. Pinto SC, Batitucci RG, Pinheiro MC, Zandim DL, Spin-Neto R, Sampaio JE. Effect of an acid diet allied to sonic toothbrushing on root dentin permeability: An in vitro study. Braz Dent J 2010;21:390–395.
22. Sauro S, Watson TF, Thompson I. Dentine desensitization induced by prophylactic and air-polishing procedures: An in vitro dentine permeability and confocal microscopy study. J Dent 2010;38:411–422.
23. Liljeborg A, Tellefsen G, Johannsen G. The use of a profilometer for both quantitative and qualitative measurements of toothpaste abrasivity. Int J Dent Hyg 2010;8:237–243.
24. Meyers IA, McQueen MJ, Harbrow D, Seymour GJ. The surface effect of dentifrices. Aust Dent J 2000;45:118–124.
25. Bartlett DW, Shah P. A critical review of non-carious cervical (wear) lesions and the role of abfraction, erosion, and abrasion. J Dent Res 2006;85:306–312.

26. Carey CM. Tooth whitening: What we now know. J Evid Based Dent Pract 2014;14(suppl):70–76.
27. Alshara S, Lippert F, Eckert GJ, Hara AT. Effectiveness and mode of action of whitening dentifrices on enamel extrinsic stains. Clin Oral Investig 2014;18:563–569.
28. Hattab FN, Qudeimat MA, al-Rimawi HS. Dental discoloration: An overview. J Esthet Dent 1999;11:291–310.
29. Joiner A. Whitening toothpastes: A review of the literature. J Dent 2010;38(suppl 2):e17–e24.
30. Wang B. Cleaning, abrasion, and polishing effect of novel perlite toothpaste abrasive. J Clin Dent 2013;24(3):88–93.
31. Majeed A, Farooq I, Grobler SR, Moola MH. In vitro evaluation of variances between real and declared concentration of hydrogen peroxide in various tooth-whitening products. Acta Odontol Scand 2015;73:387–390.
32. Turssi CP, Faraoni JJ, Rodrigues Jr AL, Serra MC. An in situ investigation into the abrasion of eroded dental hard tissues by a whitening dentifrice. Caries Res 2004;38:473–477.
33. Lima JP, Melo MA, Passos VF, Braga CL, Rodrigues LK, Santiago SL. Dentin erosion by whitening mouthwash associated to toothbrushing abrasion: A focus variation 3D scanning microscopy study. Microsc Res Tech 2013;76:904–908.
34. Kalyana P, Shashidhar A, Meghashyam B, Sreevidya KR, Sweta S. Stain removal efficacy of a novel dentifrice containing papain and bromelain extracts—An in vitro study. Int J Dent Hyg 2011;9:229–233.
35. Lima DA, Silva AL, Aguiar FH, et al. In vitro assessment of the effectiveness of whitening dentifrices for the removal of extrinsic tooth stains. Braz Oral Res 2008;22:106–111.
36. Patil PA, Ankola AV, Hebbal MI, Patil AC. Comparison of effectiveness of abrasive and enzymatic action of whitening toothpastes in removal of extrinsic stains—A clinical trial. Int J Dent Hyg 2015;13:25–29.
37. Worschech CC, Rodrigues JA, Martins LR, Ambrosano GM. In vitro evaluation of human dental enamel surface roughness bleached with 35% carbamide peroxide and submitted to abrasive dentifrice brushing. Pesqui Odontol Bras 2003;17:342–348.
38. Erdemir U, Yildiz E, Kilic I, Yucel T, Ozel S. The efficacy of three desensitizing agents used to treat dentin hypersensitivity. J Am Dent Assoc 2010;141:285–296.
39. Grippo JO, Simring M. Dental 'erosion' revisited. J Am Dent Assoc 1995;126:619–620,623–624,627–630.
40. Attin T, Knöfel S, Buchalla W, Tütüncü R. In situ evaluation of different remineralization periods to decrease brushing abrasion of demineralized enamel. Caries Res 2001;35:216–222.
41. Moretto MJ, Magalhães AC, Sassaki KT, Delbem AC, Martinhon CC. Effect of different fluoride concentrations of experimental dentifrices on enamel erosion and abrasion. Caries Res 2010;44:135–140.
42. Addy M. Tooth brushing, tooth wear and dentine hypersensitivity—Are they associated? Int Dent J 2005;55:261–267.
43. Lussi A, Lussi J, Carvalho TS, Cvikl B. Toothbrushing after an erosive attack: Will waiting avoid tooth wear? Eur J Oral Sci 2014;122:353–359.
44. West NX, Lussi A, Seong J, Hellwig E. Dentin hypersensitivity: Pain mechanisms and aetiology of exposed cervical dentin. Clin Oral Investig 2013;17(suppl 1):S9–S19.
45. Moore C, Addy M. Wear of dentine in vitro by toothpaste abrasives and detergents alone and combined. J Clin Periodontol 2005;32:1242–1246.

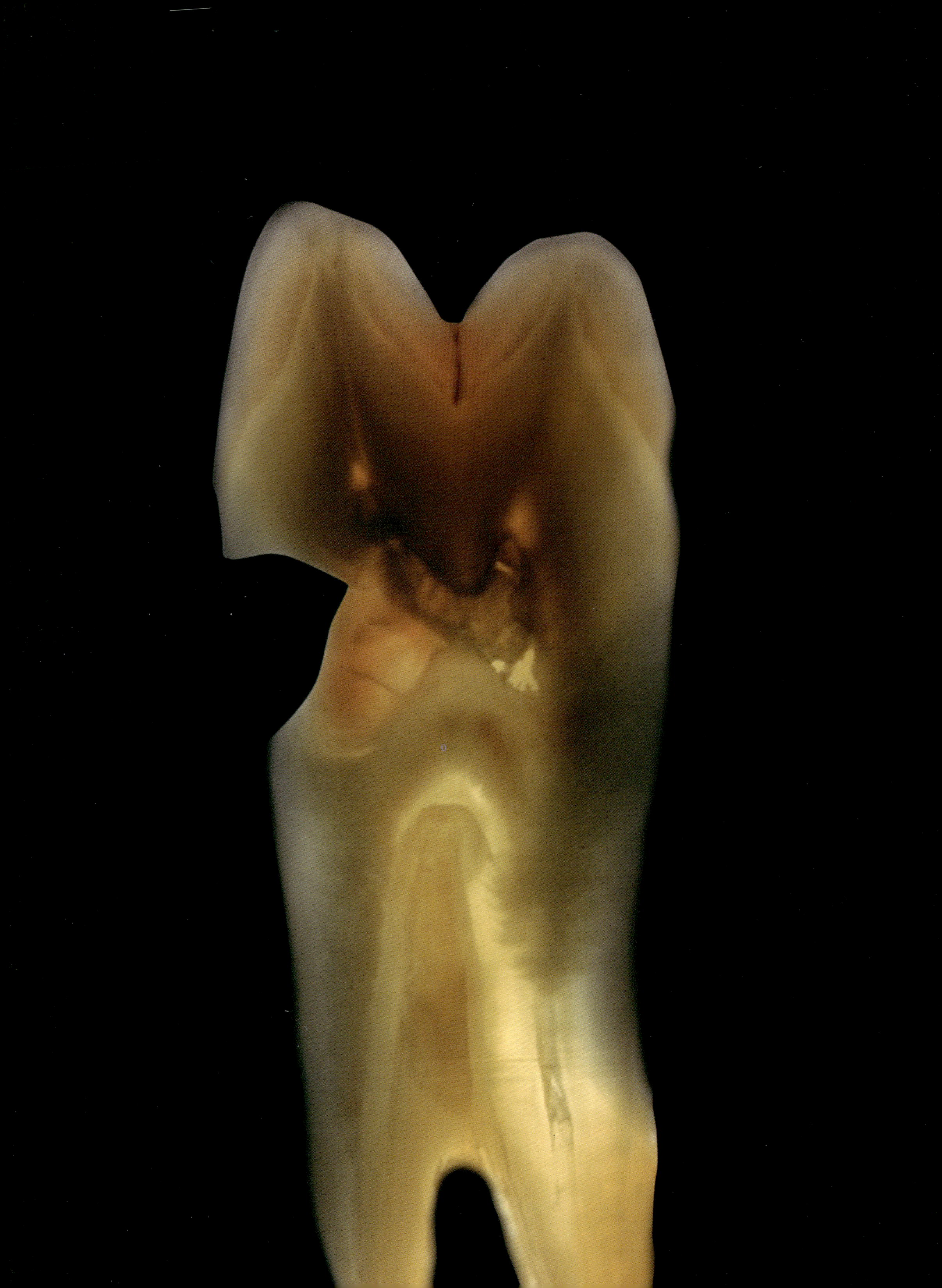

5 Biocorrosion

The biocorrosion mechanism occurs by means of exogenous chemicals, biochemical endogenous acids,[1-3] biochemical proteolytic enzymes,[4,5] and piezoelectric effects[6-8] that cause molecular degradation of the essential properties of the living tooth tissue. There is evidence that the prevalence of dental acidic degradation is growing steadily.[9] Studies in Greece, Turkey, and Australia showed prevalence rates of 51.6%, 52.6%, and 68%, respectively, among adolescents.[10-12] Prevalence rates in Brazil range from 1.8% to 34.1%.[13-16] This chapter describes the exogenous and endogenous etiologic factors involved in the degradation of tooth substance and the development of cervical dentin hypersensitivity (CDH) and noncarious cervical lesions (NCCLs).

Chemical Degradation Mechanism in Dental Structures

The biocorrosion mechanism is a complex process that involves chemical reactions between acids derived from different sources and components of dental structures. This process was described by Featherstone and Lussi[17] and is based on degradation of the hydroxyapatite of the dental hard tissue due to long and frequent effects from acids. Chemical degradation of the teeth occurs either by the H^+ derived from acids or by the chelating action of anions (capable of binding or complexing calcium).[17]

During a biocorrosive challenge, protons of the acidic agent attack the components of hydroxyapatite such as carbonate, phosphate, and hydroxyl ions. This attack results in degradation of the hydroxyapatite crystals with the release of calcium ions.[18] The acids dissociate in water and release hydrogen ions (H^+). The H^+ contacts the mineral crystals and degrades them by combining with either the carbonate or the phosphate ions. This chemical degradation process promotes the releasing of all ions from that region of the crystals, leading to etching[17] (Fig 5-1), and it occurs when any acid contacts the tooth structure. However, according to the characteristics of the acidic agent, the degradation may be slower or more aggressive. No matter the rate of degradation, the continuous action of acids removes the smear layer, which opens dentinal tubules to the oral environment and increases the risk of CDH development.

The strength of an acid is defined by its acid dissociation constant value (Ka). Thus, it is necessary to determine the

5 Biocorrosion

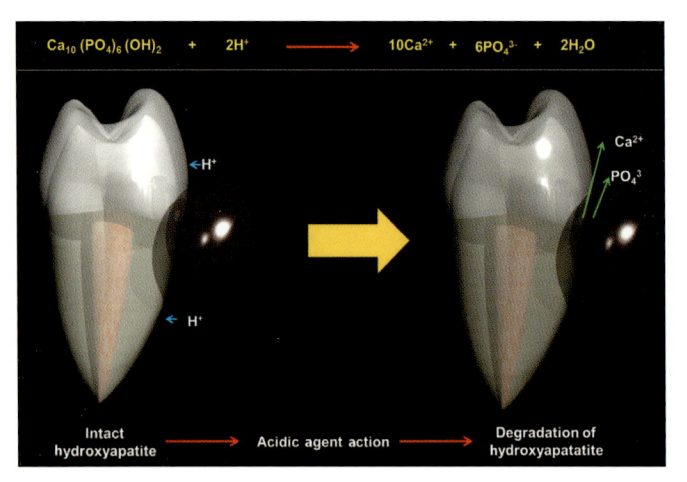

Fig 5-1 Illustration of the biocorrosive effects of acids on dental structures.

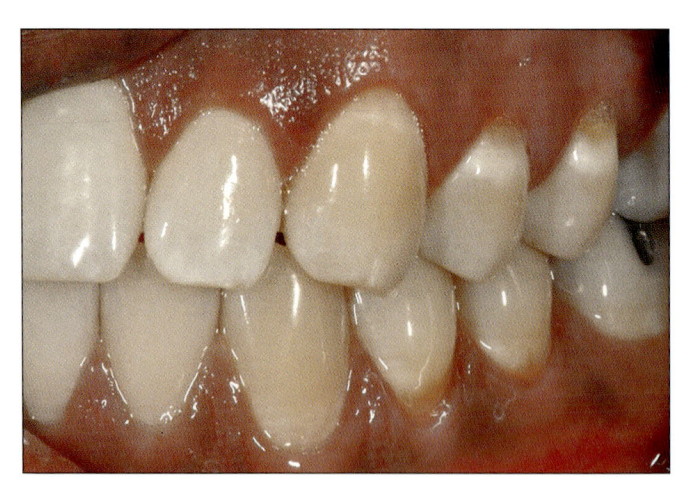

Fig 5-2 Note the initial areas of enamel demineralization in the maxillary teeth of this 30-year-old woman with gastroesophageal reflux disease. (Courtesy of the NCCL Research Group, Uberlândia, Brazil.)

pKa value, or negative logarithm of the Ka value, for a given acid. In this context, when the pH value is equal to the pKa of a weak acid, the acid exists as a half anion and half undissociated acid molecule, releasing H^+ to the solution.[17]

Acids such as citric acid, present in many foods and beverages, have a more complex action with tooth substance. In water they exist as a mixture of H^+, acidic anions (citrate), and undissociated acidic molecules.[19] In contact with the teeth, H^+ attacks their mineral crystals. In addition, the citrate anion binds to the calcium, forming a complex, and removes it from the crystal surface.[18] The stronger the bond between the anion and calcium, the greater the amount of calcium removed from the dental structure, promoting more chemical degradation.[17] Because of this dual action, acids such as citric are more deleterious to the dental structures than, say, acetic acid, which uses up all the H^+ in its interaction with the apatite and makes little association with calcium.[17]

Action of acids on enamel and dentin

Dentin and enamel have similar mineral compositions, but the carbonate content is much higher in dentin (5% to 6%) than in enamel (3%). Moreover, the crystals in enamel are much bigger than those in dentin, making the surface area per gram much higher in dentin and thus providing more surface availability for acid action.[17] In addition, enamel is porous, which leads to the diffusion of H^+ into enamel and the escape of dissolved mineral ions.[20]

The mineral content and, correspondingly, the calcium concentration and density of enamel decrease toward the cementoenamel junction (CEJ), but the concentrations of carbonate and magnesium increase, promoting a greater susceptibility of degradation at the CEJ.[21] Because dentin is made up of tubules with low surface area at the dentinoenamel junction,[22] the presence of tubular deposits affects the demineralization response, and acidic agents lead to increased dentinal permeability by removing and dissolving the smear layer in this region.[22]

Stages of dental biocorrosion

Chemical degradation of enamel

The initial phase of chemical degradation involves mainly the demineralization of the ultrastructural components of the tooth enamel (Fig 5-2). In general, at this stage the condition is reversed by saliva remineralization.[23,24] The acid contact with enamel promotes the degradation of its mineral content from a layer extending a few micrometers below the surface, a process called *softening*.[25] With time, as softening progresses further into the enamel, degradation in the most superficial enamel will reach the point where this layer of enamel is lost completely.[26,27] When the frequency and strength of the acid challenge are greater than the neutralization process (by saliva), dental chemical degradation will be clinically manifested. Therefore, chemical degradation can involve two types of enamel loss: *(1)* the direct removal of hard tissue by complete dissolution or *(2)* the creation of a thin softened layer that is vulnerable to subsequent mechanical wear, mainly from toothbrush/dentifrice abrasion.[28]

Initially, exposure to an acid leads to removal of the smear layer,[29] thereby exposing the natural enamel surface. In contact with the enamel, the H^+ component of the acid will start to degrade the enamel crystal. The first attacked area is the prism sheath, followed by the prism core[29]; this creates a honeycomb appearance.[30] In addition, the free un-ionized acid will eventually diffuse into the interprismatic areas of

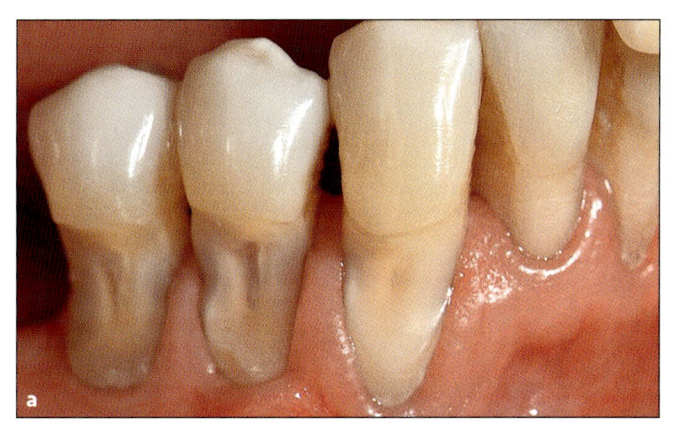

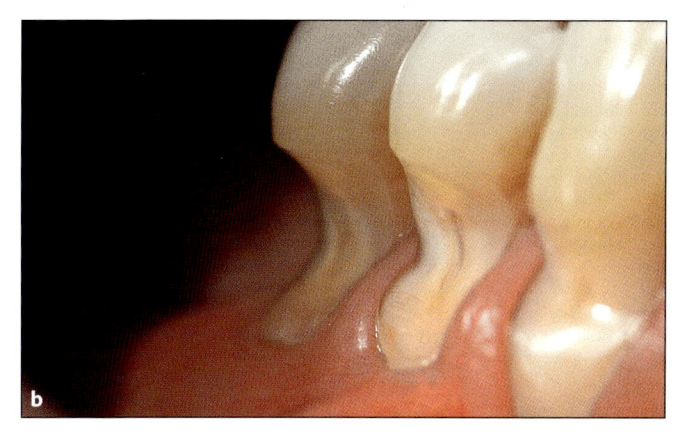

Fig 5-3 *(a and b)* Note the severe NCCLs resulting from dentin degradation in this 50-year-old woman with a highly acidic diet. (Courtesy of the NCCL Research Group, Uberlândia, Brazil.)

the enamel and further dissolve minerals in the region beneath the surface.[31,32] Acid degradation could compromise the crystals, decrease their amount, or enlarge their size,[33] resulting in an uneven reduction of the surface structure volume and therefore increased surface roughness.[34] Thus, the acidic agents could enter enamel through internal pore channels to weaken cervical enamel, thereby contributing to the development of NCCLs.[35]

Chemical degradation of dentin

The frequent and constant contact of tooth structure with acidic agents leads to the degradation of the enamel and thereby the exposure of dentin. Chemical degradation of the dentin is in principle the same as in the enamel but even more complex. Due to its high content of organic material, the diffusion of the acidic agent into deeper regions is hindered by the dentin matrix, and so is the outward flux of dissolved tooth mineral.[4] However, once this matrix is chemically or mechanically degraded, demineralization will follow.[36] The process in dentin begins at the junction of the peritubular and intertubular dentin.[37] Next, the peritubular dentin is lost, and as a consequence the dentinal tubules are wider,[38] resulting in the formation of a superficial layer of demineralized collagenous matrix that is vulnerable to mechanical and enzymatic action.[28,39] The degradation of dentin not only exposes dentinal tubules, resulting in CDH, but also leads to rapid progression of NCCLs (Fig 5-3).

The Role of Saliva

Saliva consists of approximately 98% water and a large organic content of proteins, hormones, and electrolytes, as well as mucosal, antimicrobial, enzyme, and immune agents[40,41] (Fig 5-4). This fluid is present throughout the oral cavity and provides the only inherent protection against potentially biocorrosive effects of acidic challenges to hard dental structures. The main protective mechanisms of saliva against the biocorrosion action are described in Box 5-1. The contact of saliva with dental surfaces promotes the formation of salivary acquired pellicle.[44] This pellicle is characterized as a bacteria-free biofilm composed of mucins, glycoproteins, and proteins, including several enzymes.[31] The acquired pellicle may protect against chemical degradation by acting as a diffusion barrier or a perm-selective membrane that prevents direct contact between the acids and the tooth surface, thereby reducing the chemical degradation rate of tooth substance.[45]

The presence of acid in the oral cavity stimulates an increase in salivary flow. In normal conditions, when an acid comes in contact with enamel, it must first diffuse through the acquired pellicle, and only thereafter can it interact with the enamel.[45]

The buffering capacity of saliva is another important factor and has the ability to neutralize acids.[44] After an acidic challenge, it is possible to remineralize the softened enamel by the deposition of calcium and phosphate from the saliva, thus reducing the vulnerability of dental hard tissues to mechanical wear. In this context, remineralization of some of the softened enamel will take place through salivary calcium, fluoride,[46] and phosphate deposition.[23]

The protective capacity of saliva against degradation was shown to be limited to weak acidic challenge on enamel that does not involve the dentin. The neutralization is related to the balance between the frequency and severity of the acid challenge and the protective effects of saliva.[44]

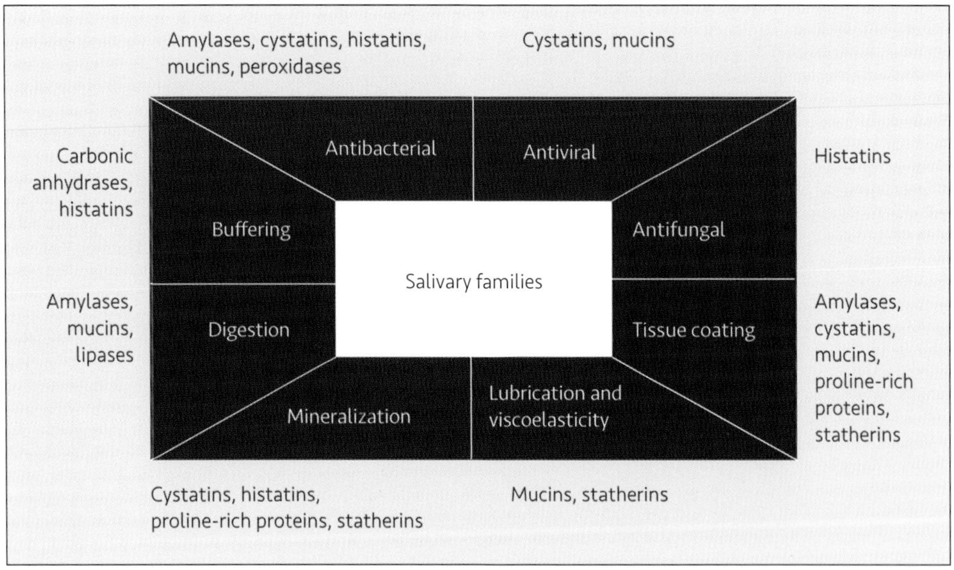

Fig 5-4 Functions of salivary components. (Adapted from Levine.[42])

Box 5-1	**Protective functions of saliva against biocorrosive action[43]**

- Dilution and clearance of potentially corrosive agents from the mouth
- Neutralization and buffering of dietary acids
- Maintaining a supersaturated state next to the tooth surface due to the presence of calcium and phosphate in the saliva
- Formation of the acquired pellicle by the adsorption of salivary proteins and glycoproteins, which has the ability to protect the enamel surface from demineralization by dietary acids
- Providing the calcium, phosphate, and possible fluoride necessary for remineralization

Importance of the acquired pellicle thickness and salivary flow

Salivary action varies in different locations in the mouth.[44] These differences affect the saliva's ability to protect teeth from chemical degradation. In sites that have the greatest salivary pellicle thickness (eg, lingual surface of mandibular molars), rarely does dental degradation occur. In general, greater pellicle thickness correlates with lower incidence of cervical lesions.[44,47]

Depending on the oral stimuli, different salivary glands may be affected, leading to variations in salivary flow and composition and thus influencing the level of salivary protection.[48] A higher flow rate with higher hydrogen bicarbonate content increases the capacity of saliva in neutralizing and buffering acids as well as the ability to clear acids from tooth surfaces.[24,49] This explains why, in some cases, individuals subjected to similar dietary conditions present with different biocorrosive patterns.[46] Patients taking medications, athletes, those frequently consuming acidic foods and beverages, as well as those who have received radiation therapy for head and neck cancer have a higher potential for a decrease in saliva output.[50,51]

Salivary flow is extremely important in its protective role against gastric acids in the mouth; in fact, the human body's immediate response to vomitus is an increase in salivary flow.[52]

Exogenous Sources of Acid

Diet

The patient's diet—particularly the excessive consumption of various acidic fruits and juices, carbonated beverages, sports drinks, and vinegar-containing salad dressing—are factors

Fig 5-5 A 45-year-old woman with NCCLs on the maxillary premolars and first molar. Severe CDH existed in the first molar. There was no data about gastroesophageal diseases or use of any medicines in her report. She had an acidic diet including frequent consumption of orange juice. In addition, she had an unstable occlusal pattern. (Courtesy of the NCCL Research Group, Uberlândia, Brazil.)

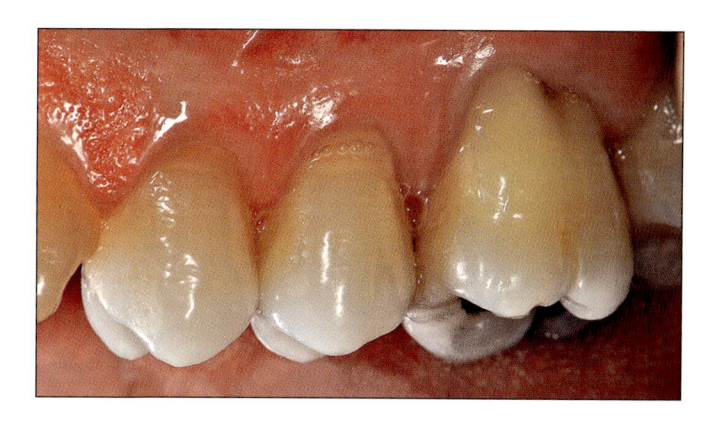

associated with the chemical degradation of dental structures[46,53] (Fig 5-5). Industrialization, urbanization, economic development, and the globalization of markets have reverberated in the health and nutritional status of the population. The frequency of consumption of acidic foods (acidic candies and citric fruits) and drinks (soft drinks and fruit juices) have increased over the last several decades.[23,45,54,55]

Fruits and fruit juices

Rapid transportation has facilitated the availability of citrus fruits and fruit juices year round instead of seasonally.[56] Among the most consumed fruits in the United States are oranges, apples, grapes, apricots, and kiwi,[57] all of which contribute to acidity. If frequently consumed, the various organic acids in theses fruits increase the risk of dental chemical degradation.[23,46] The consumption of citric fruits more than twice daily poses a 37-fold higher risk for the development of lesions by enamel chemical degradation and a 5- to 8-fold higher risk than other fruits.[58,59] Orange juice has been the target of much attention because of its high consumption rate and proven record for causing dental demineralization in children.[60]

Because of their high fiber content, fruits may have abrasive particles that, when combined with acidic degradation, result in the acceleration of friction to the teeth and thus increase the chance of damage. Studies have shown that vegetarians (who presumably eat more fruits and vegetables than nonvegetarians) have higher rates of biocorrosion than nonvegetarians.[61,62] Linkosalo and Markkanen compared dental biocorrosion in a group of lactovegetarians (who eat no meat or eggs but other dairy products) with their sex- and age-matched controls.[61] None of the controls were found to have chemical degradation, whereas over 75% of the lactovegetarians had acidic degradation.

However, fruits should not be excluded from the diet because they are important sources of fiber, vitamins, and minerals. Instead they should be part of a balanced diet that includes neutralizing and calcium-rich foods (eg, cheese).

Other acidic foods

Tomatoes, yogurt, salad dressings, pickles, and various condiments also have high acidity because of their vinegar content or fermentation byproducts. This acidity is often minimized when combined with other food.

Soft drinks and energy drinks

People are consuming soft drinks (carbonated and noncarbonated) and energy drinks more than ever before.[63] It is estimated that about 26% of American adults consume soft drinks at least once per day,[64] and almost one in every four American adults consumes energy and sports drinks at least once a week.[65] In fact, soft drink consumption in the United States increased by 300% in just 30 years.[66] As of 2005, between 56% and 85% of US schoolchildren consumed at least one soft drink daily, and 20% consumed four or more servings daily.[67] Studies in children and adults have shown that the number of servings per day is associated with the presence and progression of chemical degradation to teeth when other risk factors are present.[49,68] These beverages contain modifying agents such as phosphoric acid (to stimulate taste and counteract sweetness)[55,69] and/or citric (orange), ascorbic (vitamin C), tartaric (grape), maleic (apple), or lactic acid that contribute to the low pH value.[46,55] Citric acid, very likely the most widely used additive in beverages, has a great affinity for attacking the calcium in teeth, causing rapid degradation. Carbonated beverages also contain carbonic acid.[69] Soft drinks therefore have the ability to chelate calcium at higher pHs as well as maintain a pH below the level for dental biocorrosion (pH of 5.5).[37,46,55] The daily intake of cola soft drinks causes significant and irreversible loss of surface structure, in both the enamel and the dentin.[70,71]

Soft drinks	Ice cream	Pasta	Oats
Energy drinks	Popcorn	Bread	Oysters
Alcohol	Meat	Pasteurized fruit juice	Dark chocolate
Sugar	Coffee	Eggs	Peanuts
Carbonated drinks	Yellow cheese	Fish	Nuts
Processed and refined food	Tea	Rice	
Citric juices	Artificial sweeteners	Soy milk	

Fig 5-6 List of acidic foods and drinks from most acidic to least acidic.

Table 5-1 Biocorrodents and pH values of acidic foods and beverages common to Western diets

Food or drink	Biocorrodent(s)	pH
Coca-Cola	Phosphoric acid and flavorings	2.45
Diet Coca-Cola	Phosphoric acid and citric acid	2.60
Sprite	Carbonic acid and citric acid	2.54
Fanta	Orange juice and citric acid	2.67
Pepsi	Phosphoric acid and citric acid	2.39
Diet Pepsi	Phosphoric acid and citric acid	2.77
Regular iced tea	Black tea extract	2.94
Lemon iced tea	Black tea extract and lemon juice	3.03
Peach iced tea	Black tea extract and peach juice	2.94
Red Bull	Taurine and complex B vitamins	3.3
Gatorade	Citric acid and flavorings	3.17
Apricot	NA	3.25
Kiwi	NA	3.25
Orange	NA	3.6
Orange juice	Orange juice	3.56
Apple juice	Apple juice and pear juice	3.41
Carrot juice	Carrot juice, orange juice, agave juice, lemon juice, and ascorbic acid	4.16
Grapefruit juice	Grapefruit juice	3.15
Smirnoff Ice vodka	40% alcohol	3.07
Beer (Carlsberg)	5% alcohol	4.2
Red wine	13% alcohol	3.43
White wine	12.1% alcohol	3.6
Salad dressing (classic)	Vinegar and lemon juice	4.04
Yogurt (forest berries)	Forest berries	3.77
Yogurt (natural)	NA	3.91
Yogurt (slim line)	NA	4.03
Coffee espresso	NA	5.82

Adapted from Lussi et al.[72] NA, not applicable.

Alcohol

In drinks such as champagne, red and white wine, and vodka, the acidity is a result of a substance formed in its fermentation process.

Figure 5-6 lists a range of acidic foods and drinks from most acidic to least acidic, and Table 5-1 shows the biocorrodents and pH values for various acidic foods and drinks related to dental chemical degradation.[72]

Nutritional habits

In addition to the type of diet, nutritional habits such as the frequency and time of consumption and the method of retaining acidic foods and beverages in the mouth affect chem-

| Box 5-2 | Habits that accelerate dental chemical degradation and should be avoided[74] |

- Frequent consumption of acidic drinks
- Swishing the drink before swallowing
- Consuming acidic drinks just before sleep, when the protective benefits of saliva are reduced
- Brushing teeth immediately following the acid challenge, which increases the wear of the enamel due to the abrasive action of the toothpaste on the still-softened tooth surface

| Box 5-3 | Recommendations for patients at high risk of dental biocorrosion |

- Avoid leaving sports drinks, energy drinks, soft drinks, acidic juices, and herbal teas for a long time in the mouth. When possible, use a straw to drink these beverages.
- Avoid brushing your teeth immediately after the intake of acidic foods and drinks, and rinse the mouth with water after the intake.
- End meals with calcium-rich foods like cheese after ingestion of acidic foods.
- Reduce the consumption of acidic foods, sweets, acidic juices, and wine, and only consume them during meal times.
- Avoid acidic foods late in the evening.
- Avoid prolonged fasting to maintain the pH of the saliva and help control gastroesophageal disorders.
- Drink water throughout the day to contribute to the dilution of foods in the oral cavity.
- Avoid the intake of acidic fruits and fiber sources like cereal bars without subsequent water intake.
- Avoid daily ingestion of noncariogenic chewing gum due to its acidic ingredients.
- When eating fruits, choose the least acidic and those with a softer texture (eg, puree).

Adapted from Lussi et al,[80] Amaechi and Higham,[81] and Touger-Decker et al.[82]

ical degradation of tooth structure.[73] Some habits are reported in the literature as accelerators of dental chemical degradation and need to be avoided for proper control[74] (Box 5-2).

Frequency

The frequency of ingestion of acidic foods and drinks is equally important as, if not more important than, the amount consumed.[75] The consumption of citrus fruits two or more times a day, soft drinks once a day, and vinegar and sports drinks more than once a week contributes significantly to the emergence of dental biocorrosion.[60,76]

Method of introduction to and retention in mouth

The mode of introduction of foods and beverages to the mouth (mulling, sipping, use of a straw, or swishing) is very important.[77] The habit defines which teeth come into contact with the acid challenge and can affect the degradation pattern. When an acidic drink is held, swished, swirled, or sluiced in the mouth before swallowing, it will intensify the interaction time between the solution and tooth surface, thereby increasing the risk of dissolution of the hard tissues.[78] High chemical degradation was associated with a method of drinking whereby the drink was kept in the mouth for a longer period.[79] A suggested strategy for reducing the acidic challenge is to use straws and limit consumption of acidic beverages to mealtimes only.[57] This will reduce the amount of time the liquid is in contact with the teeth and thereby limit its destructive potential.[80,81]

Box 5-3 provides dietary and nutritional habit recommendations for patients at high risk of dental biocorrosion.

Lifestyle

Western culture and media currently prizes a slim body,[83] and people wanting this "ideal" body shape often adhere to diets involving greater consumption of fruits and vegetables as well as intense exercise regimens. This increase in exercise frequency promotes loss of body fluids and may lead to decreased salivary flow and greater consumption of sports drinks and carbonated beverages.[45,56] Some individuals may adopt obsessive dieting and/or exercise behaviors, increasing the risk of eating disorders such as anorexia nervosa and bulimia.[84]

Among patients with a "healthy lifestyle," the group that deserves the most attention regarding NCCLs are those with a lactovegetarian diet. This diet, excluding all meat products and eggs, leads to frequent consumption of acidic foods like salads with vinegar and citrus fruits,[85] which makes these patients susceptible to the degradation of their teeth.[46]

Alternatively, unhealthy lifestyle habits can have negative implications and increase the risk of biocorrosion.[46] Mental stress, excessive work, "lack of time," and the rapid intake of meals are all factors that promote the development of diseases such as gastrointestinal problems and acid reflux.[86] In most cases, patients with these diseases require medication that can affect the salivary flow.[86] The combination of acidic agents in the mouth (such as vomitus) and a reduction of salivary secretion increase the risk of dental chemical degradation.

Drug use

The use of illicit drugs is also related to the development of dental biocorrosion. Ecstasy, a widely used party drug, promotes dehydration (dry mouth), thus increasing the desire to consume excessive amounts of low-pH beverages. This increases the susceptibility of teeth to degradation.[87]

Drug addicts are especially prone to the development of CDH and NCCLs. In addition to causing systemic changes such as gastrointestinal disorders and vitamin deficiencies, cocaine and other illicit drugs lead to dry mouth, decreased salivary flow and buffering capacity, dental wear, bone loss, tooth decay, periodontal disease, and parafunction,[88,89] all of which can contribute to the emergence or progression of CDH and NCCLs.

Abusive effects of mouthrinses

The abusive use of some oral hygiene products has been associated with biocorrosive effects on tooth structures.[90,91] However, little attention has been given to the biocorrosive effects of an acidic mouthrinse. The main ingredients of most mouthrinses are chlorhexidine, ethylenediaminetetraacetic acid,[92] and acidified sodium chlorite.[90] Studies report that the chemical degradation of dental structures by mouthrinses would not be clinically significant when used for a short period of time. However, the prolonged use of these products is contraindicated because it would represent another acidic challenge in the mouth.[90] These mouthrinses should be used only for short to medium periods of time as adjuncts to oral hygiene. In addition, these mouthrinses should not be used before brushing.[90]

Medications

Many medications available on the market have the potential to chemically degrade teeth when used frequently or for prolonged periods.[93] The biocorrosive action of these medicines is related to the relatively acidic composition in the form of liquid and effervescent tablets as well as their low pH. Many commonly used medications have the capacity to reduce the salivary flow rate or buffering capacity of saliva, including antihistamines, tranquilizers, antiparkinsonian drugs, and steroids used in inhalers and aerosols (treating asthma).[46]

Acetylsalicylic acid (aspirin) is one of the most widely used medications throughout the world. Reports have stated that as much as 10 tons of the drug are consumed each day. Chronic use of chewable aspirin tablets, as may be used by patients with chronic headache[94] or juvenile rheumatoid arthritis, can also result in increased dental biocorrosion.[95]

Vitamin C (L-ascorbic acid) preparations have also received some attention.[93] Although the pH level varies from manufacturer to manufacturer, the level of acidity in these preparations is always high.[46,93] Chewable vitamin C tablets have been reported to have a pH of 2.3 and are associated with the development of tooth wear.[68] This pH value is lower than the critical point at which enamel degrades (pH 5.5). In comparison with citric and phosphoric acid (present in carbonated drinks), ascorbic acid has been proven to have greater potential for dental chemical degradation, especially when consumed frequently and when in direct contact with teeth.[53] However, when used in moderation and conforming with the manufacturer's instructions, chewable vitamin C tablets pose no obvious risk to the dentition.[96]

Occupational hazards

Occupational chemical degradation to teeth is caused by exposure to different types and applications of acids in the workplace. Among those with the greatest risk of contact with acids are professional athletes (major consumers of energy and sports drinks), swimmers (constantly in contact with treated pool water), professional wine tasters, and factory workers who manufacture acidic products.[46]

Athletes

People involved in vigorous sporting activities may be at higher risk of biocorrosion due to their frequent ingestion of acidic sports drinks.[97] In addition, dehydration occurs during strenuous activity, which results in decreased salivary flow; rehydration and electrolyte replacement are often accomplished with drinks that have a high biocorrosive potential.[98,99] Athletes in contact sports also often wear mouthguards to protect their teeth from trauma, but these appliances harbor any acidic beverages drunk by the athlete close to the teeth, thus causing stress concentration and subsequent enamel demineralization.

Swimmers. Large public and small home swimming pools are chlorinated to reduce bacterial and algal contamination. Chlorine is the most commonly used agent to maintain swimming pool pH balance.[100] When the dissociation of the chlorine compound occurs in water, it generates two substances: hypochlorous acid (HOCl), a weak acid with disinfectant (germicidal) properties, and hydrochloric acid, a highly corrosive acid.[101-103] These compounds require neutralization and buffering to maintain the recommended pH of the pool (7.2 to 8.045),[104] ensuring no harm to the teeth. Soda ash (Na_2CO_3) is most commonly used for this purpose.[104] However, if the water is inadequately buffered, the pH of the pool water may be as low as 3.7.[104] Therefore, young adults and competitive swimmers who spend a lot of time in the pool may be more susceptible to acidic enamel degradation.[105] Moreover, some competitive and recreational swimmers may increase their risk by consuming acidic sport drinks during training. For this population, lesions are clinically observed on the facial surfaces of central and lateral incisors of both arches. Apparently, no effect was observed on premolars and molars.[106]

Winemakers and wine tasters

Wines have a low pH (3.0 to 4.0) and contain acids with high biocorrosive potentials, such as lactic, malic, and tartaric acids.[107] Chemical degradation of teeth is therefore a problem for winemakers and wine tasters because they sip the wine and keep it in the mouth long enough for the wine to damage the enamel.[108]

Factory workers manufacturing acidic products

Acidic fumes at work seem to be associated with chemical degradation of tooth surfaces.[109-112] Individuals working in factories manufacturing batteries, galvanized steel, and fertilizers[18] are constantly exposed to an acid environment and are at risk for dental biocorrosion. In these populations, the chemical degradation first occurs on the facial surfaces of the incisors. The canines are rarely affected, and no degradation of the posterior teeth has been observed.[18,111] Adequate ventilation is crucial to mitigating the acidic atmosphere of these factories.[113]

Radiotherapy

Another group particularly at risk for biocorrosion is patients who have received radiation therapy for head and neck cancer. Radiotherapy forms free radicals of hydrogen and hydro-

Fig 5-7 Characteristic appearance of a tooth after radiotherapy and chemotherapy to control a tumor in the floor of the mouth. Note the radiation caries and darkened dentin. This tooth stands little chance against acidic challenge, favoring NCCL development.

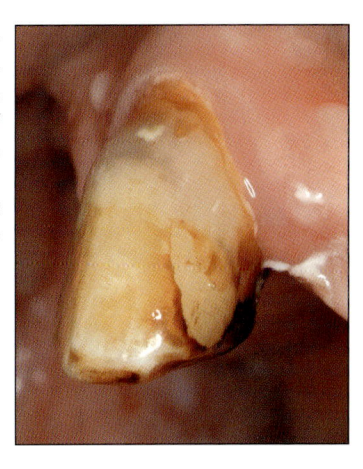

gen peroxide that can cause denaturation of the enamel and dentin organic components,[114] thus promoting changes in their properties.[115-120] In addition, hyposalivation/xerostomia and radiation caries are common side effects of radiotherapy, making the teeth more susceptible to damage. With xerostomia, the neutralizing capacity of saliva is reduced, meaning that acidic challenges may go unchecked. If this occurs in conjunction with radiation caries, the already weakened tooth structure will rapidly degrade when it comes into contact with acids (Fig 5-7).

Chemical Parameters of Exogenous Acids

The biocorrosive potential of an exogenous acid is a measure of its deleterious effects on hard dental structures.[121] It is related to the chemical properties of the acid, not only its pH value. Thus, the pH value, titratable acidity, buffering capacity, degree of saturation, kind of acid, and calcium and phosphate content[19,23,122,123] all must be investigated when determining the biocorrosive potential of a given acid.

Hydrogen potential (pH)

The pH, or actual acidity, is the most commonly used measure for determining the acidity, neutrality, or alkalinity of an aqueous solution. It is the negative logarithm of the H^+ concentration and is measured on a scale of 0 to 14.[69] The pH value 7 indicates a neutral content; anything below 7 indicates an acidic content and above 7 an alkaline content.[69]

The literature reports that the critical pH value for degradation of tooth structure (hydroxyapatite) is 5.5.[124] However, using the pH alone is not sufficient to determine the biocorrosive potential of a food or beverage because it only provides a measure of the initial and dissociated H+ concentration and does not indicate the presence of undissociated acid.[125]

Titratable acidity

The titratable acidity is the quantity of base required to bring a solution to neutral pH and determines the actual H+ availability for interaction with the tooth surface.[125,126] It is therefore a more representative measure than pH for determining the acidic potential of a food or beverage.[46,125]

Buffering capacity

Buffering capacity is generally used in chemistry to define a solution's ability to maintain its pH value.[45] Buffering capacity is associated with the undissociated acid in beverages.[127] Undissociated acid is not charged and can diffuse into the hard tissue of the tooth and act as a buffer to maintain the H+ concentration. Consequently, the driving force for demineralization at the site of dissolution is maintained.[127] Here it is important to distinguish buffering capacity from titratable acidity. The latter measures total available H+ over a wide range of pH values, whereas the former is defined at a certain pH value.[128] Therefore, the greater the buffering capacity of the acid, the longer it will take for saliva to neutralize it[23] and the greater the amount of tooth mineral that may be degraded. For this reason, in some cases, although the pH is similar for different types of acids, the biocorrosion potential can be distinct.[2] For example, the strong acid in grapefruit has a higher biocorrosion potential than that in a cola drink.[2]

Degree of saturation

The degree of saturation (DS) with respect to the tooth mineral content is determined by the concentration of calcium, phosphate, and fluoride ions as well as the pH value of the acidic solution.[129] The concentration gradient of those ions is thought to be the basic thermodynamic driving force for dissolution.[130] A low DS with respect to dental hard structures leads to an initial surface degradation. A local rise in pH then occurs, causing an increased mineral content in the liquid surface layer adjacent to the tooth surface.[129] Solutions oversaturated with respect to dental structures will not degrade them.[125] For this reason, a small increase in DS can generate a reduction in the dissolution rate.[131]

Clinical Aspects of NCCLs from Exogenous Biocorrosion

The final morphology of NCCLs varies according to the predominant etiologic factor (see chapter 6). In cases in which the exogenous acidic degradation is more intense, the lesions present with the following specific features.

Early stages

In early stages, the acidic action produces a smooth and silk-glazed enamel surface[132] that usually lacks developmental ridges and stain lines. In these situations, the lesions are located coronal to the CEJ and present an intact ring of enamel along the gingival margin[133] (Fig 5-8). The preserved enamel band could be explained by the presence of some remaining plaque, which acts as a diffusion barrier for acids, or by an acid-neutralizing effect of the gingival crevicular fluid.[80,132] In addition, it is common to find a loss of surface anatomy, increased incisal translucency, lack of enamel, and chipping of the incisal edges.[68]

Intermediate stages

Further progression of the exogenous biocorrosive effects in the lesion leads to the development of shallow flat concavities with rounded limits, where the width exceeds the depth.[132] In some situations, the enamel is totally removed, leading to exposure of dentin and a polished-looking surface. Clinically, rounding of the cusps, grooves, and incisal edges can occur.[23,132] A common sign of dental biocorrosion in posterior teeth is characteristic "cupping," or concavities in the enamel of cusp tips with or without dentinal involvement[134] (Fig 5-9).

Severe stages

In more severe cases, when the continuing biocorrosive loss of dentin occurs, reactionary and reparative dentin forms, thus obliterating the dentinal tubules as a biologic response to compensate for the loss of tooth substance (see Fig 5-3). Beyond the clinically visible lesions, continuing acid exposure changes the physical properties of the remaining tooth structure and makes the softened surface more susceptible to further biocorrosion and mechanical abrasion.[133] In some situations, the progression of chemical degradation exceeds the reparative capacity of the dentin-pulp complex and can lead to exposures of the pulp or complete destruction or loss of the tooth.[135]

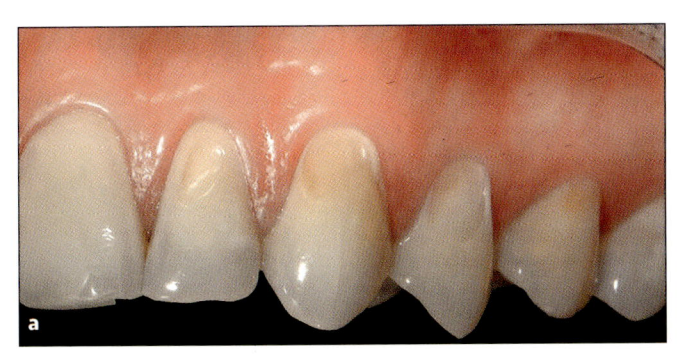

Fig 5-8 *(a to c)* Early-stage NCCLs in a 35-year-old woman with an acidic diet and aggressive brushing habits. Note the signs of biocorrosion, namely a silk-glazed appearance of the teeth and intact enamel along the margins of the NCCLs. (Courtesy of the NCCL Research Group, Uberlândia, Brazil.)

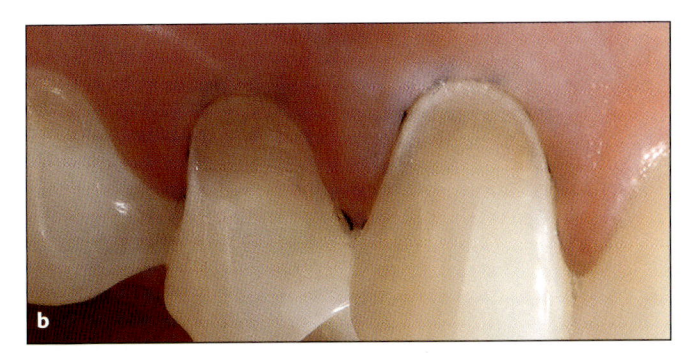

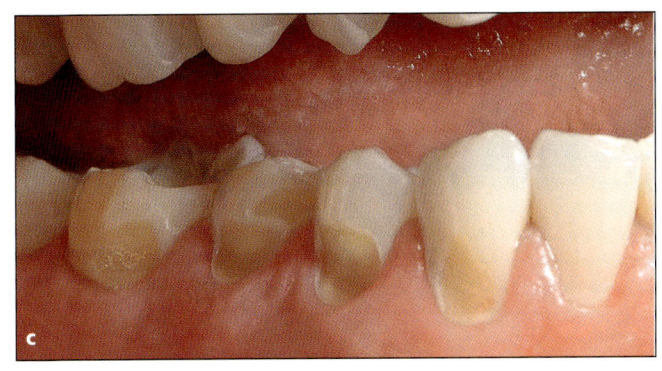

Fig 5-9 The signs of biocorrosion are very evident in the posterior teeth of this 45-year-old man with an acidic diet and unstable occlusal pattern. Note the "cupping" of the cusp tips and rounding of the cusps and grooves. (Courtesy of the NCCL Research Group, Uberlândia, Brazil.)

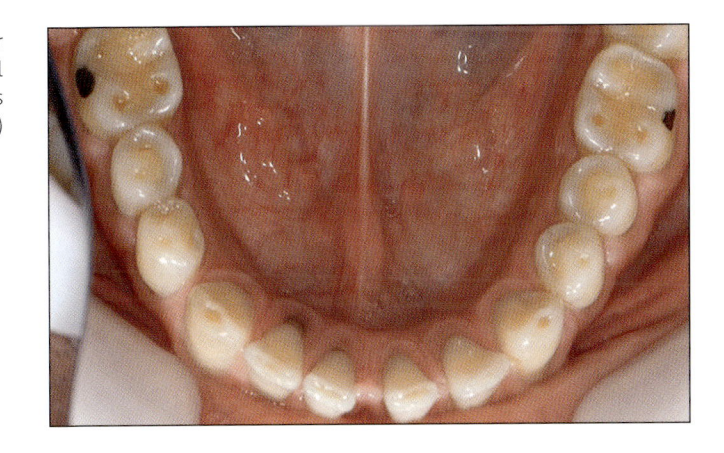

Association of Exogenous Biocorrosion and Other Etiologic Factors

Biocorrosion and abrasion

The association between biocorrosion and abrasion occurs whenever the surfaces of teeth are covered with acids and then abraded by friction from an external source, namely toothbrush/dentifrice.[3,9,136]

Biocorrosion and stress (abfraction)

These combined mechanisms can occur as a result of either sustained or cyclic loading. Static stress-biocorrosion occurs during clenching, deglutition, or active orthodontic treatment. Cyclic stress-biocorrosion occurs during bruxism, parafunctional activities, and mastication. Regardless of stress type, the chemical degradation is accelerated in the presence of stress.[1]

Attrition, stress, and biocorrosion

The association between stress, biocorrosion, and attrition is manifested as the loss of tooth structure due to the action of an acid in areas in which there is interocclusal contact of teeth.[3,9,136,137] This process may lead to a loss of vertical dimension in aggressive cases. When stress, biocorrosion, and attrition are combined, the occlusal surfaces may change in appearance, with rounding or cupping of the cusps. According to G. V. Black's classification, these lesions are classified as Class VI lesions. This type of lesion is not common, but it can be seen on both the occlusal surfaces of posterior teeth as well as the incisal surfaces of anterior teeth. These lesions are occasionally associated with NCCLs.

Endogenous Sources of Acid

The prime endogenous source of acid is the stomach. Biocorrosion occurs when highly acidic gastric contents are brought into the oral cavity via reflux or regurgitation. Biocorrosive episodes are established when the acid vomitus periodically reaches the dental tissue for a prolonged period of time. This generally affects patients with eating disorders or gastroesophageal disorders. The pH of the acidic vomitus is lower than the critical level for dissolution of tooth enamel (pH 5.5) and exceeds the mineralization protective barrier of secreted saliva,[138] hence resulting in biocorrosion of tooth substance.

Gastroesophageal reflux disease

Gastroesophageal reflux disease (GERD) is a severe, chronic form of acid reflux found in otherwise healthy people.[139–141] Whereas gastroesophageal reflux is a normal physiologic process whereby gastric contents retrograde from the stomach to the esophagus without producing symptoms or mucosal damage,[142] GERD involves the reflux of gastric contents into the oral cavity, larynx, or lung and causes troublesome symptoms or complications.[143] This process involves episodes of transient lower esophageal sphincter relaxations or when the sphincter tone improperly adapts to changes in intra-abdominal pressure.[144]

Prevalence

GERD is a widely reported condition and one of the most prevalent diseases of the gastrointestinal tract. The prevalence rates vary substantially depending on whether the analysis is based on symptoms (eg, heartburn and regurgitation) or signs of disease (ie, esophagitis). Given that GERD is defined as at least twice weekly heartburn and/or acid regurgitation, an approximate prevalence of 10% to 20% was identified in the Western world.[145]

Clinical presentation

Heartburn and acid regurgitation are the classic symptoms of GERD. Symptoms such as difficulty swallowing, painful swallowing, the feeling of a lump in the throat, burping, water brash, and cough are other possible presentations of GERD.[146] GERD may also cause a wide spectrum of conditions including noncardiac chest pain, asthma, posterior laryngitis, chronic cough, recurrent pneumonitis, and dental degradation.

Oral manifestations

Oral manifestations due to the presence of gastric acid include biocorrosion to teeth, specifically the palatal surface of maxillary anterior teeth (Fig 5-10), halitosis, nonspecific burns, mucosal ulceration, loss of taste, dry mouth, and/or change in salivary flow. In primary dentitions, the teeth most affected and subject to degradation are the molars. Teeth affected by GERD tend to appear as if they were being prepared for full crown coverage with a chamfered finishing line margin[134] (see Fig 5-10).

In patients with GERD and bruxism, tooth wear becomes more severe as attrition hastens tooth substance loss (Fig 5-11). Although causal factors of NCCLs can act independently, the combination of these mechanisms can also occur during the dynamics of occlusal activity (Fig 5-12).

GERD is also associated with hyposalivation, which causes dry mouth and an oral burning sensation. This hyposalivation reduces the salivary neutralizing capacity and can result in injury to the esophageal mucosa.[147]

Diagnosis and treatment

The diagnosis of and treatment for GERD are beyond the scope of this text and can be found elsewhere. Basic dietary and lifestyle modifications that can be recommended to patients with GERD include elevating the head in bed at night, avoiding meals within 2 to 3 hours of bedtime, sleeping on the left side, and weight loss.[148,149]

Bulimia nervosa

Bulimia nervosa is an eating disorder characterized by episodic binge eating, self-induced vomiting, use of laxatives and diuretics, and excessive exercise.[138] The prevalence of bulimia varies from 1% to 5% depending on the population studied.[150]

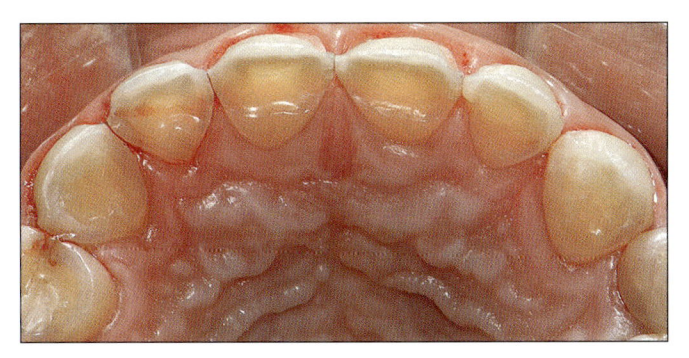

Fig 5-10 Aggressive NCCLs on the palatal surface of the maxillary anterior teeth in this 45-year-old man with diagnosed but untreated GERD. The teeth look as though they have been prepared for a full-coverage restoration with a chamfered margin. (Courtesy of the NCCL Research Group, Uberlândia, Brazil.)

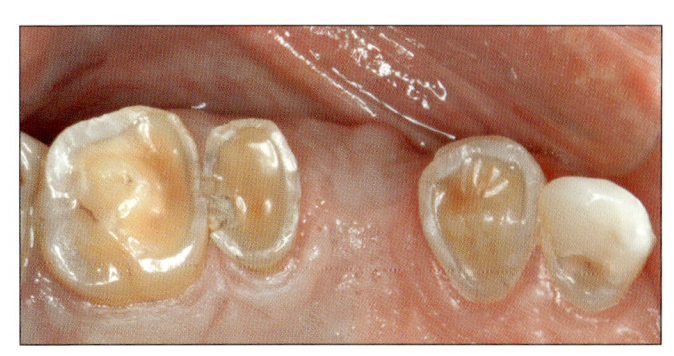

Fig 5-11 Maxillary right quadrant of a patient with GERD and bruxism. Biocorrosion of the teeth has been accelerated by attrition and abrasion.

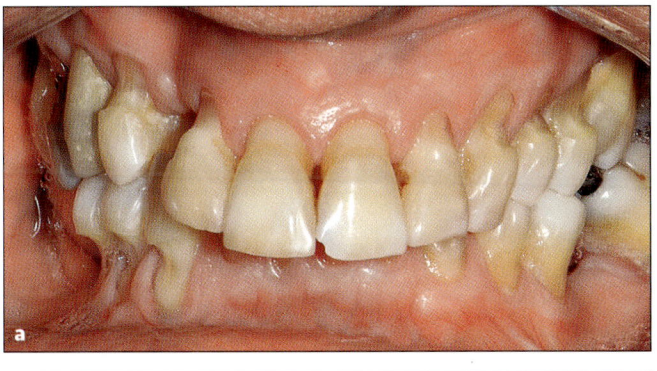

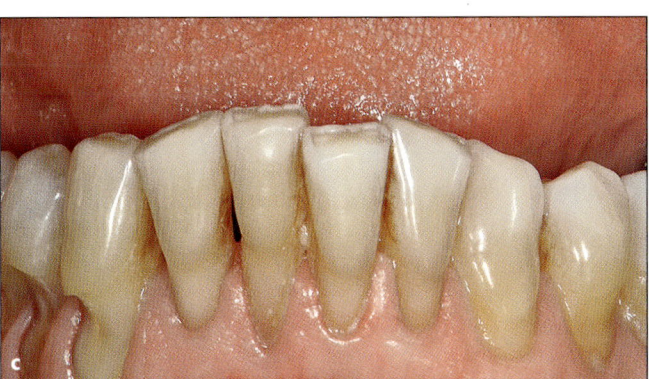

Fig 5-12 *(a to e)* Multiple and very deep NCCLs on the maxillary and mandibular teeth of a 40-year-old woman. She related severe CDH in several teeth and presented with characteristics of bruxism. She also reported having uncontrolled GERD. In addition, she had an unstable occlusal pattern with an anterior open bite. There is no data about acidic diet, use of medicines, or addictions. (Courtesy of the NCCL Research Group, Uberlândia, Brazil.)

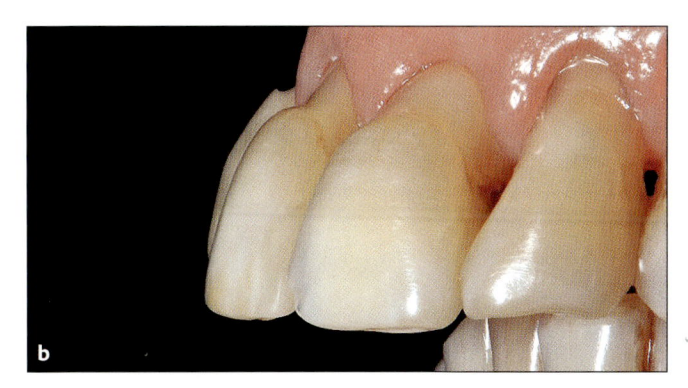

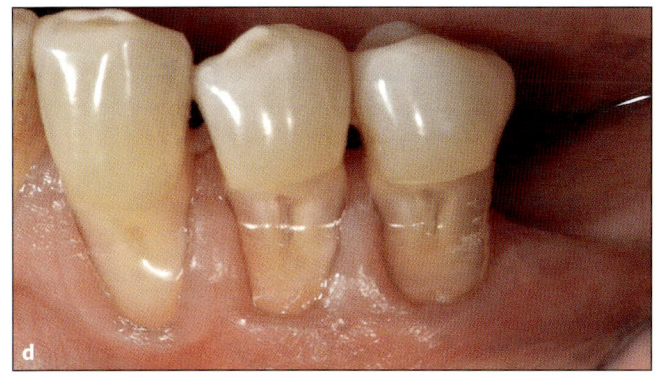

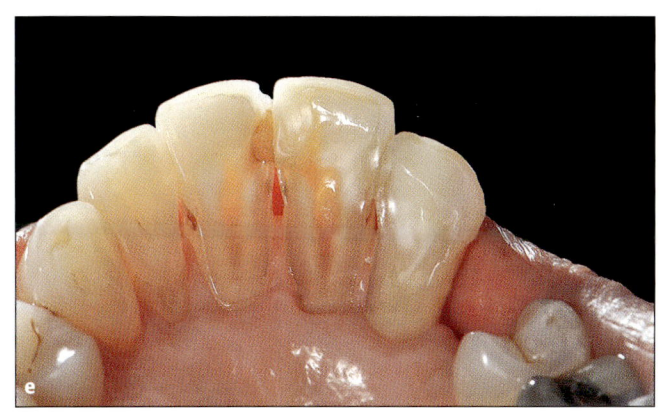

Oral manifestations

The most common oral manifestations of bulimic individuals are tooth degradation, sore throat, and swelling of the parotid glands.[151] During self-induced vomiting, the gastric juice passes through the pharynx and reaches the oral cavity and is retained in the palatal region. The severity of dental chemical degradation depends on the duration and frequency of purging incidents per day, oral hygiene habits, the degree of acid dilution by means of water rinsing or drinking neutralizing liquids such as milk, and timing of tooth cleaning.

The palatal surfaces of the maxillary anterior teeth are the most susceptible to biocorrosion in bulimic patients because of the anatomy of the oral cavity. Mandibular teeth are not affected in the initial stages of biocorrosion because of their relative distance from the vomitus and their protection by the major salivary glands.[141] In general, biocorrosion is most commonly found on the palatal surfaces of teeth in patients who routinely vomit to expel food.[152]

Furthermore, bulimic patients may have decreased function of the parotid gland, resulting in a reduction of serous salivary production and lowered concentration of bicarbonate.[141]

Diagnosis and treatment

The diagnosis of and treatment for bulimia nervosa are beyond the scope of this text and can be found elsewhere. It is important to note, however, that dental treatment should be conservative until the vomiting cycle has been broken and the patient is medically stable.

Other conditions

Rumination syndrome

Rumination syndrome is a rare condition in which patients, usually children, effortlessly regurgitate recently ingested food into the mouth, which is then either rechewed and reswallowed or spat out.[153] This condition is rarely seen in dentistry but can cause severe dental acidic biocorrosion. The pattern of tooth degradation in these patients is similar to that found in patients with bulimia. The first developing signs of biocorrosion appear on the palatal surfaces of the maxillary incisors; if the condition continues, other surfaces of the teeth will be involved.

Hyperthyroidism

Hyperthyroidism has been found to be associated with dental biocorrosion, although the exact cause is unknown; an increase in the thyroid hormone level or the metabolic effects of said increase is likely involved.[154]

Pregnancy

Pregnancy itself does not cause dental biocorrosion, but different eating habits as well as the tendency to vomit during the early months of pregnancy increase the risk of chemical degradation.[155] Bulimic patients especially may have increased effects to their teeth from endogenous acids while pregnant.[156]

Enzymatic Action in the Progression of NCCLs

Recent studies of the progression of dental caries indicate that degradation of the dentin organic matrix is caused by endogenous enzymes present in dentin, saliva, and gingival crevicular fluid (GCF) that minimize the role of bacterial proteases in the process.[157-159] The progression of NCCLs has also been associated with the activity of host-derived enzymes. Hence, in biocorrosive challenges caused by eating disorders and gastric diseases, proteases present in gastric and intestinal fluids can reach the oral cavity and have a role in the degradation of collagen in exposed dentin (Table 5-2).

The hypothesis that host-derived proteolytic enzymes are involved in the progression of NCCLs, mainly due to the activation of matrix metalloproteinases (MMPs) in acidic conditions (Fig 5-13), has been supported by studies showing the in situ reduction of dentin loss when specific inhibitors of enzymes are used under simulated biocorrosive challenges.[160-162] Chlorhexidine (CHX) is widely indicated to control periodontal diseases and, more recently, has been used for MMP inhibition to reduce collagen degradation in dentin adhesive interfaces.[163,164] Dentin tooth substance loss from biocorrosive challenges was significantly reduced when the tissue was treated with CHX.[160,162] Similar effects were observed for epigallocatechin-gallate (EGCG), a monomeric form of proanthocyanidin (PAC).[160] PACs have been shown to be effective natural compounds able to modify the dentin organic matrix by cross-linking collagen, which results in enhanced biomechanical and biochemical properties including greater stability against degradation by collagenases.[165,166] Dentin biocorrosion caused by the flow of acidic beverages was reduced when the tissue was treated with PAC-rich extract (*Camellia sinensis*, green tea)[167] or when drinks were supplemented with it.[168] It is believed that besides enzyme inhibition, both CHX and EGCG gels cause occlusion of dentinal tubules, probably by interacting with metal ions such as calcium from apatite crystals,[160] thereby reducing dentin biocorrosion.

Table 5-2 Endogenous enzymes involved in collagen degradation and progression of NCCLs

Enzyme	Classification	Source	Optimal pH	Mechanism of collagen degradation
Matrix metalloproteinases	Metalloproteinase	Dentin, saliva, GCF	Neutral	Cleavage of native collagen molecule (collagenases); denatured collagen (gelatinases) and nonhelical ends of collagen molecule (telopeptides, telopeptidases)
Cysteine cathepsins	Cysteine protease	Dentin, saliva, GCF	Acid	Cleavage of nonhelical telopeptides and gelatin; cleavage of collagen molecule triple helix (cysteine cathepsin K)
Pepsin	Aspartyl protease	Gastric juice	Acid	Cleavage of nonhelical ends of collagen molecule (telopeptides)
Trypsin	Serine protease	Pancreatic origin to intestinal content, gastric juice	Neutral	Collagen fibril disaggregation

Sodium fluoride (NaF) has also showed a protective effect against biocorrosive attacks, although lower than that of CHX and EGCG.[160,162,169] Concentrations as low as 1.23% of NaF applied for only 1 minute protected dentin from collagenase degradation in vitro. More recently, alternative fluoride compounds including stannous fluoride (SnF_2)[170] and titanium tetrafluoride (TiF_4)[171] have also been assessed as inhibitors of biocorrosion. The use of SnF_2- and TiF_4-containing toothpastes prevented enamel and dentin loss from biocorrosion and wear from abrasion and was even more effective when associated with NaF in enamel.[170] Application of 2.5% TiF_4 for 1 minute on acid-etched smear layer–covered dentin improved its nanomechanical properties and protected the dentin from biocorrosion.[171] It has been shown that TiF_4 forms a coating on dentin,[171,172] composed of organometallic complexes of titanium and dentin organic matrix, which occludes the tubules.

Although the effect of NaF in reducing the progression of biocorrosion by inhibiting MMPs has been reported, the potential of some specific metal fluorides to inhibit such enzymes has yet to be tested. Studies showed that silver diamine fluoride, an agent proposed for the prevention of caries, can inhibit recombinant cysteine cathepsins B and K and MMP-2, -9, and -8 more efficiently than fluoride, so the inhibition potential has been associated with the presence of silver.[173,174] The specific mechanism of inhibition is still unknown, and no studies have tested the effect of silver diamine fluoride on dentin biocorrosion.

Effect of endogenous acids and gastric enzymes on exposed dentin

Besides mineral dissolution caused by exogenous acids, patients with chronic GERD or eating disorders involving chronic vomiting can have demineralization caused by endogenous acids. The biocorrosion in this situation is caused by the very

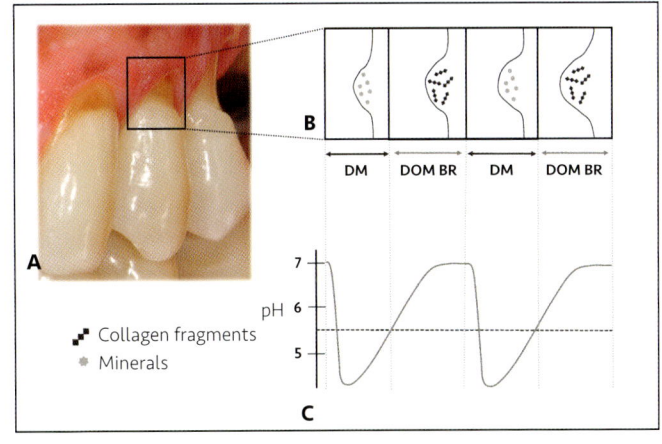

Fig 5-13 Schematic showing the formation and progression of NCCLs in dentin due to demineralization (DM) and dentin organic matrix breakdown (DOM BR) by endogenous enzymes. The mechanism proposed for MMP activation is characterized by an initial decrease in pH (C) caused by acid ingestion or exposure to gastric juice. The acid pH causes dentin demineralization (B) and activates MMPs in dentin and saliva. Because of the buffering capacity of saliva, the pH returns to neutral, when MMPs have proteolytic activity and can cleave demineralized dentin organic matrix. This DM–DOM BR cycle will result in extensive degradation of dentin and progression of the NCCL (A). (Adapted from Tjäderhane et al[159] with permission.)

acidic pH (1 to 3) of gastric juice due to the presence of hydrochloric acid, which has a higher in vitro potency to dissolve enamel than citric acid (pH 1.76). Dentin chemical degradation progression is a diffusion-controlled phenomenon. The thick exposed matrix slows mineral dissolution, regardless of the source of acid content. Similarly to the dentin organic matrix degradation by host-derived proteases from dentin and saliva, when this layer is enzymatically removed, NCCLs progress.

Gastric fluid also contains proteolytic enzymes involved in the progression of NCCLs. Pepsin has been found in the oral environment of patients with GERD,[175] while trypsin from the pancreas, an intestinal enzyme, occurs in the stomach due to its reflux content from the duodenum.[176] Higher enzymatic activity of pepsin and trypsin was found in the oral cavities of bulimic patients with NCCLs than in healthy patients.[177] When there is a combination of biocorrosion and exposure to gastric content, dentin organic matrix degradation by these enzymes occurs.

It has been shown in vitro that when pepsin and trypsin act together, the degradation of collagen in exposed dentin is greater than that when either enzyme acts alone.[177] However, these two enzymes have different mechanisms of degradation. The optimal pH for pepsin activity is an acidity of around 1 to 3, whereas trypsin activity occurs at the neutral conditions of pH 7 to 8. As previously mentioned, saliva neutralizes acid content within a few minutes after vomiting or reflux, which guarantees optimal conditions for both enzymes. Dentin collagen is resistant to degradation by trypsin[178] but becomes more susceptible when denatured, and pepsin alone does not influence tissue loss but compromises remineralization by fluoride.[179] Therefore, trypsin probably makes the collagen matrix more susceptible to degradation by pepsin by opening binding sites to this enzyme, explaining why degradation occurs only when pepsin and trypsin are together.

Prevention and Management of Biocorrosion

The best method to prevent biocorrosive action by exogenous and endogenous sources is to eliminate the etiologic factors, which requires a close collaboration between the patient and the dentist.[9] For this reason, it becomes necessary that a detailed survey of the patient's medical history, behavioral habits, and an inventory of his or her diet be taken. The medical history should consider any medication that may be acidic or may be reducing the salivary protection of the dentition. In addition, the knowledge of the patient's natural salivary condition is also important, due to the intense relationship between decreased salivary flow and susceptibility to biocorrosive tooth substance loss. With this data, the predisposing factors for the biocorrosive process can be determined, and specific instructions can be given to the patient for management and prevention of further dental substance loss. The role of the dentist is to work with patients to identify individual risks and to develop preventive plans that conform with and are agreeable to the individual's dietary and lifestyle requirements.

Conclusion

Let's review what we have covered in this chapter:
- Biocorrosion is based on degradation of the hydroxyapatite of the dental hard tissue from the effects of acid.
- Both exogenous and endogenous acids can cause biocorrosion.
- Saliva neutralizes acid and protects the oral cavity against the biocorrosive effects of acid.
- Exogenous sources of acid include fruits and fruit juices, other acidic foods, soft drinks and sports/energy drinks, alcohol, certain medications, and occupational hazards like unneutralized chlorine in pools.
- Lifestyle choices like excessive exercise as well as medical treatments involving radiotherapy may alter salivary flow and thereby affect biocorrosion.
- The prime source of endogenous acid is the stomach. Biocorrosion occurs when highly acidic gastric contents are brought into the oral cavity via reflux or regurgitation.
- GERD and bulimia are both associated with biocorrosion.
- Endogenous enzymes are responsible for the progression of NCCLs.
- The authors consider patients with GERD and/or a highly acidic diet to be at risk for NCCLs and CDH.

References

1. Grippo JO. Biocorrosion vs erosion: The 21st century and time to change. Compend Contin Educ Dent 2012;33:e33–e37.
2. Grippo JO, Simring M, Coleman TA. Abfraction, abrasion, biocorrosion, and the enigma of noncarious cervical lesions: A 20-year perspective. J Esthet Restor Dent 2012;24:10–23.
3. Grippo JO, Simring M, Schreiner S. Attrition, abrasion, corrosion and abfraction revisited: A new perspective on tooth surface lesions. J Am Dent Assoc 2004;135:1109–1118.
4. Hara AT, Ando M, Cury JA, Serra MC, Gonzalez-Cabezas C, Zero DT. Influence of the organic matrix on root dentine erosion by citric acid. Caries Res 2005;39:134–138.
5. Schlueter N, Hardt M, Klimek J, Ganss C. Influence of the digestive enzymes trypsin and pepsin in vitro on the progression of erosion in dentine. Arch Oral Biol 2010;55:294–299.
6. Braden M, Bairstow AG, Beider I, Ritter BG. Electrical and piezo-electrical properties of dental hard tissues. Nature 1966;212(5070):1565–1566.
7. Grippo JO, Masi JV. Role of biodental engineering factors (BEF) in the etiology of root caries. J Esthet Dent 1991;3:71–76.
8. Marino AA, Gross BD. Piezoelectricity in cementum, dentine and bone. Arch Oral Biol 1989;34:507–509.
9. Bartlett D. Etiology and prevention of acid erosion. Compend Contin Educ Dent 2009;30:616–620.
10. Margaritis V, Mamai-Homata E, Koletsi-Kounari H, Polychronopoulou A. Evaluation of three different scoring systems for dental erosion: A comparative study in adolescents. J Dent 2011;39:88–93.
11. Caglar E, Sandalli N, Panagiotou N, Tonguc K, Kuscu OO. Prevalence of dental erosion in Greek minority school children in Istanbul. Eur Arch Paediatr Dent 2011;12:267–271.

References

12. Taji S, Seow WK. A literature review of dental erosion in children. Aust Dent J 2010;55:358–367.
13. Gurgel CV, Rios D, de Oliveira TM, Tessarolli V, Carvalho FP, Machado MA. Risk factors for dental erosion in a group of 12- and 16-year-old Brazilian schoolchildren. Int J Paediatr Dent 2011;21:50–57.
14. Auad SM, Waterhouse PJ, Nunn JH, Steen N, Moynihan PJ. Dental erosion amongst 13- and 14-year-old Brazilian schoolchildren. Int Dent J 2007;57:161–167.
15. Vargas-Ferreira F, Praetzel JR, Ardenghi TM. Prevalence of tooth erosion and associated factors in 11-14-year-old Brazilian schoolchildren. J Public Health Dent 2011;71:6–12.
16. Mangueira DF, Sampaio FC, Oliveira AF. Association between socioeconomic factors and dental erosion in Brazilian schoolchildren. J Public Health Dent 2009;69:254–259.
17. Featherstone JD, Lussi A. Understanding the chemistry of dental erosion. Monogr Oral Sci 2006;20:66–76.
18. Wiegand A, Attin T. Occupational dental erosion from exposure to acids: A review. Occup Med (Lond) 2007;57:169–176.
19. West NX, Hughes JA, Addy M. Erosion of dentine and enamel in vitro by dietary acids: The effect of temperature, acid character, concentration and exposure time. J Oral Rehabil 2000;27:875–880.
20. Robinson C, Weatherell JA, Hallsworth AS. Variation in composition of dental enamel within thin ground tooth sections. Caries Res 1971;5:44–57.
21. Carvalho TS, Lussi A. Susceptibility of enamel to initial erosion in relation to tooth type, tooth surface and enamel depth. Caries Res 2015;49:109–115.
22. Choi S, Park KH, Cheong Y, Moon SW, Park YG, Park HK. Potential effects of tooth-brushing on human dentin wear following exposure to acidic soft drinks. J Microsc 2012;247:176–185.
23. Lussi A, Jaeggi T, Zero D. The role of diet in the aetiology of dental erosion. Caries Res 2004;38(suppl 1):34–44.
24. Eisenburger M, Addy M, Hughes JA, Shellis RP. Effect of time on the remineralisation of enamel by synthetic saliva after citric acid erosion. Caries Res 2001;35:211–215.
25. Koulourides T. Experimental changes of mineral density. In: Harris RS (ed). Art and Science of Dental Caries Research. New York: Academic Press, 1968:355–378.
26. Schweizer-Hirt CM, Schait A, Schmidt R, Imfeld T, Lutz F, Mühlemann HR. Erosion und Abrasion des Schmelzes: Eine experimentelle Studie. Schweiz Monatsschr Zahnheilkd 1978;88:497–529.
27. Eisenburger M, Hughes J, West NX, Jandt KD, Addy M. Ultrasonication as a method to study enamel demineralisation during acid erosion. Caries Res 2000;34:289–294.
28. Addy M, Shellis RP. Interaction between attrition, abrasion and erosion in tooth wear. Monogr Oral Sci 2006;20:17–31.
29. Parkinson CR, Shahzad A, Rees GD. Initial stages of enamel erosion: An in situ atomic force microscopy study. J Struct Biol 2010;171:298–302.
30. Meurman JH, Frank RM. Scanning electron microscopic study of the effect of salivary pellicle on enamel erosion. Caries Res 1991;25:1–6.
31. Lussi A. Erosive tooth wear—A multifactorial condition of growing concern and increasing knowledge. Monogr Oral Sci 2006;20:1–8.
32. Eisenburger M, Hughes J, West NX, Shellis RP, Addy M. The use of ultrasonication to study remineralisation of eroded enamel. Caries Res 2001;35:61–66.
33. Mahoney EK, Rohanizadeh R, Ismail FS, Kilpatrick NM, Swain MV. Mechanical properties and microstructure of hypomineralised enamel of permanent teeth. Biomaterials 2004;25:5091–5100.
34. Poggio C, Lombardini M, Dagna A, Chiesa M, Bianchi S. Protective effect on enamel demineralization of a CPP-ACP paste: An AFM in vitro study. J Dent 2009;37:949–954.
35. Rees JS. A review of the biomechanics of abfraction. Eur J Prosthodont Restor Dent 2000;8:139–144.
36. Ganss C, Klimek J, Starck C. Quantitative analysis of the impact of the organic matrix on the fluoride effect on erosion progression in human dentine using longitudinal microradiography. Arch Oral Biol 2004;49:931–935.
37. Meurman JH, Ten Cate JM. Pathogenesis and modifying factors of dental erosion. Eur J Oral Sci 1996;104:199–206.
38. Meurman JH, Drysdale T, Frank RM. Experimental erosion of dentin. Scand J Dent Res 1991;99:457–462.
39. Kinney JH, Balooch M, Haupt DL Jr, Marshall SJ, Marshall GW Jr. Mineral distribution and dimensional changes in human dentin during demineralization. J Dent Res 1995;74:1179–1184.
40. Gleeson M, Pyne DB. Special feature for the Olympics: Effects of exercise on the immune system: Exercise effects on mucosal immunity. Immunol Cell Biol 2000;78:536–544.
41. Humphrey SP, Williamson RT. A review of saliva: Normal composition, flow, and function. J Prosthet Dent 2001;85:162–169.
42. Levine MJ. Salivary macromolecules. A structure/function synopsis. Ann N Y Acad Sci 1993;694:11–16.
43. Mandel ID. The functions of saliva. J Dent Res 1987;(66 spec no):623–627.
44. Young WG, Khan F. Sites of dental erosion are saliva-dependent. J Oral Rehabil 2002;29:35–43.
45. Wang X, Lussi A. Functional foods/ingredients on dental erosion. Eur J Nutr 2012;51(suppl 2):S39–S48.
46. Zero DT. Etiology of dental erosion—Extrinsic factors. Eur J Oral Sci 1996;104:162–77.
47. Dawes C. Physiological factors affecting salivary flow rate, oral sugar clearance, and the sensation of dry mouth in man. J Dent Res 1987;66(spec no):648–653.
48. Engelen L, de Wijk RA, Prinz JF, van der Bilt A, Bosman F. The relation between saliva flow after different stimulations and the perception of flavor and texture attributes in custard desserts. Physiol Behav 2003;78:165–169.
49. Lussi A, Schaffner M. Progression of and risk factors for dental erosion and wedge-shaped defects over a 6-year period. Caries Res 2000;34:182–187.
50. Dreizen S, Brown LR, Daly TE, Drane JB. Prevention of xerostomia-related dental caries in irradiated cancer patients. J Dent Res 1977;56:99–104.
51. Wynn RL, Meiller TF. Drugs and dry mouth. Gen Dent 2001;49:10–12,14.
52. Pace F, Pallotta S, Tonini M, Vakil N, Bianchi Porro G. Systematic review: Gastro-oesophageal reflux disease and dental lesions. Aliment Pharmacol Ther 2008;27:1179–1186.
53. Li H, Zou Y, Ding G. Dietary factors associated with dental erosion: A meta-analysis. PLoS One 2012;7(8):e42626.
54. Dugmore CR, Rock WP. A multifactorial analysis of factors associated with dental erosion. Br Dent J 2004;196:283–286.
55. Tahmassebi JF, Duggal MS, Malik-Kotru G, Curzon ME. Soft drinks and dental health: A review of the current literature. J Dent 2006;34:2–11.
56. Gambon DL, Brand HS, Veerman EC. Dental erosion in the 21st century: What is happening to nutritional habits and lifestyle in our society? Br Dent J 2012;213:55–57.
57. United States Department of Agriculture Economic Resarch Service website. http://www.ers.usda.gov/data-products/food-availability-(per-capita)-data-system.aspx. Accessed 21 September 2016.
58. Grobler SR, Senekal PJC, Kotze TJ. The degree of enamel erosion by five different kinds of fruit. Clin Prev Dent 1989;11(5):23–28.
59. Moynihan PJ. The role of diet and nutrition in the etiology and prevention of oral diseases. Bull World Health Organ 2005;83:694–699.
60. Järvinen VK, Rytömaa I, Heinonen OP. Risk factors in dental erosion. J Dent Res 1991;70:942–947.
61. Linkosalo E, Markkanen H. Dental erosive in relation to lactovegetarian diet. Scand J Dent Res 1985;93:436–441.
62. Staufenbiel I, Adam K, Deac A, Geurtsen W, Günay H. Influence of fruit consumption and fluoride application on the prevalence of caries and erosion in vegetarians—A controlled clinical trial. Eur J Clin Nutr 2015;69:1156–1160.
63. Shenkin JD, Heller KE, Warren JJ, Marshall TA. Soft drink consumption and caries risk in children and adolescents. Gen Dent 2003;51:30–36.
64. Kumar GS, Pan L, Park S, et al. Sugar-sweetened beverage consumption among adults - 18 states, 2012. MMWR Morb Mortal Wkly Rep 2014;63(32):686–690.
65. Park S, Onufrak S, Blanck HM, Sherry B. Characteristics associated with consumption of sports and energy drinks among US adults: National Health Interview Survey, 2010. J Acad Nutr Diet 2013;113:112–119.
66. Calvadini C, Siega-Riz AM, Popkin BM. US adolescent food intake trends from 1965 to 1996. Arch Dis Child 2000;83:18–24.
67. Gleason P, Suitor C. Children's Diets in the Mid-1990s: Dietary Intake and Its Relationship with School Meal Participation. Alexandria: US Department of Agriculture, Food and Nutrition Service, Office of Analysis, Nutrition and Evaluation, 2001.

68. O'Sullivan EA, Curzon ME. A comparison of acidic dietary factors in children with and without dental erosion. ASDC J Dent Child 2000;67:186-192, 160.
69. Kitchens M, Owens BM. Effect of carbonated beverages, coffee, sports and high energy drinks, and bottled water on the in vitro erosion characteristics of dental enamel. J Clin Pediatr Dent 2007;31:153-159.
70. Waterhouse PJ, Auad SM, Nunn JH, Steen IN, Moynihan PJ. Diet and dental erosion in young people in south-east Brazil. Int J Paediatr Dent 2008;18:353-360.
71. Fushida CE, Cury JA. Manuscript: Estudo in situ do efeito da frequência de ingestão de Coca-Cola na erosão do esmalte-dentina e reversão pela saliva. Rev Odontol USP 1999;13:127-134.
72. Lussi A, Megert B, Shellis RP, Wang X. Analysis of the erosive effect of different dietary substances and medications. Br J Nutr 2012;107:252-262.
73. Johansson AK, Lingstrom P, Birkhed D. Comparison of factors potentially related to the occurrence of dental erosion in high- and low-erosion groups. Eur J Oral Sci 2002;110:204-211.
74. Holbrook WP. Tooth erosion. In: Limeback H (ed). Comprehensive Preventive Dentistry. Ames, IA: Wiley, 2012.
75. Milward A, Shaw L, Harrington E, Smith AJ. Continuous monitoring of salivary flow rate and pH at the surface of the dentition following consumption of acidic beverages. Caries Res 1997;31:44-49.
76. Järvinen VK, Rytömaa II, Heinonen OP. Risk factors in dental erosion. J Dent Res 1991;70:942-947.
77. Zero DT, Lussi A. Behavioral factors. Monogr Oral Sci 2006;20:100-105.
78. Lussi A, Jaeggi T. Chemical factors. Monogr Oral Sci 2006;20:77-87.
79. Johansson AK, Lingström P, Birkhed D. Comparison of factors potentially related to the occurrence of dental erosion in high- and low-erosion groups. Eur J Oral Sci 2002;110:204-211.
80. Lussi A, Jaeggi T, Zero D. The role of diet in the aetiology of dental erosion Caries Res 2004;38:34-44.
81. Amaechi BT, Higham SM. Dental erosion: Possible approaches to prevent and control. J Dent 2005;33:243-252.
82. Touger-Decker R, Sirois DA, Mobley CC. Nutrition and Oral Medicine. New York: Human Press, 2014.
83. Hawkins N, Richards PS, Granley HM, Stein DM. The impact of exposure to the thin-ideal media image on women. Eat Disord 2004;12:35-50.
84. Lindberg L, Hjern A. Risk factors for anorexia nervosa: A national cohort study. Int J Eat Disord 2003;34:397-408.
85. Linkosalo E, Markkanen H. Dental erosions in relation to lactovegetarian diet. Scand J Dent Res 1985;93:436-441.
86. Meurman JH, Toskala J, Nuutinen P, Klemetti E. Oral and dental manifestations in gastroesophageal reflux disease. Oral Surg Oral Med Oral Pathol 1994;78:583-589.
87. Duxbury AJ. Ecstasy—Dental implications. Br Dent J 1993;175:38.
88. Boghdadi MS, Henning RJ. Cocaine: Pathophysiology and clinical toxicology. Heart Lung 1997;26:466-483.
89. McGrath C, Chan B. Oral health sensations associated with illicit drug abuse. Br Dent J 2005;198:159-162.
90. Pontefract H, Hughes J, Kemp K, Yates R, Newcombe RG, Addy M. The erosive effects of some mouthrinses on enamel. A study in situ. J Clin Periodontol 2001;28:319-324.
91. Sales-Peres SH, Pessan JP, Buzalaf MA. Effect of an iron mouthrinse on enamel and dentine erosion subjected or not to abrasion: An in situ/ex vivo study. Arch Oral Biol 2007;52:128-132.
92. Rytömaa I, Meurman JH, Franssila S, Torkko H. Oral hygiene products may cause dental erosion. Proc Finn Dent Soc 1989;85:161-166.
93. Hellwig E, Lussi A. Oral hygiene products and acidic medicines. Monogr Oral Sci 2006;20:112-118.
94. McCracken M, O'Neal SJ. Dental erosion and aspirin headache powders: A clinical report. J Prosthodont 2000;9:95-98.
95. Grace EG, Sarlani E, Kaplan S. Tooth erosion caused by chewing aspirin. J Am Dent Assoc 2004;135:911-914.
96. Bahal P, Djemal S. Dental erosion from an excess of vitamin C. Case Rep Dent 2014;2014:485387.
97. Kenefick RW, Cheuvront SN. Hydration for recreational sport and physical activity. Nutr Rev 2012;70(suppl 2):S137-S142.
98. Sirimaharaj V, Brearley Messer L, Morgan MV. Acidic diet and dental erosion among athletes. Aust Dent J 2002;47:228-236.
99. Maughan RJ, Shirreffs SM. Dehydration and rehydration in competative sport. Scand J Med Sci Sports 2010;20(suppl 3):40-47.
100. Kane S KR. Tooth damage linked to public pool by Center for Disease Control. Fla Dent J 1983;54:12-13.
101. Geurtsen W. Rapid general dental erosion by gas-chlorinated swimming pool water. Review of the literature and case report. Am J Dent 2000;13:291-293.
102. Centerwall BS, Armstrong CW, Funkhouser LS, Elzay RP. Erosion of dental enamel among competitive swimmers at a gas-chlorinated swimming pool. Am J Epidemiol 1986;123:641-647.
103. Centers for Disease Control (CDC). Erosion of dental enamel among competitive swimmers—Virginia. MMWR Morb Mortal Wkly Rep 1983;32(28):361-362.
104. Buczkowska-Radlińska J, Łagocka R, Kaczmarek W, Górski M, Nowicka A. Prevalence of dental erosion in adolescent competitive swimmers exposed to gas-chlorinated swimming pool water. Clin Oral Investig 2013;17:579-583.
105. Noble WH, Donovan TE, Geissberger M. Sports drinks and dental erosion. J Calif Dent Assoc 2011;39:233-238.
106. Hannig M, Balz M. Protective properties of salivary pellicles from two different intraoral sites on enamel erosion. Caries Res 2001;35:142-148.
107. Ferguson MM, Dunbar RJ, Smith JA, Wall JG. Enamel erosion related to winemaking. Occup Med (Lond) 1996;46:159-162.
108. Mandel L. Dental erosion due to wine consumption. J Am Dent Assoc 2005;136:71-75.
109. Petersen PE, Gormsen C. Oral conditions among German battery factory workers. Community Dent Oral Epidemiol 1991;19:104-106.
110. Tuominen ML, Tuominen RJ, Fubusa F, Mgalula N. Tooth surface loss and exposure to organic and inorganic acid fumes in workplace air. Community Dent Oral Epidemiol 1991;19:217-220.
111. Ten Bruggen Cate HJ. Dental erosion in industry. Br J Ind Med 1968;25:249-266.
112. Tuominen M, Tuominen R. Dental erosion and associated factors among factory workers exposed to inorganic acid fumes. Proc Finn Dent Soc 1991;87:359-364.
113. Kim HD, Douglass CW. Associations between occupational health behaviors and occupational dental erosion. J Public Health Dent 2003;63:244-249.
114. Pioch T, Golfels D, Staehle HJ. An experimental study of the stability of irradiated teeth in the region of the dentinoenamel junction. Endod Dent Traumatol 1992;8:241-244.
115. Fränzel W, Gerlach R, Hein HJ, Schaller HG. Effect of tumor therapeutic irradiation on the mechanical properties of teeth tissue. Z Med Phys 2006;16:148-154.
116. Goncalves LM, Palma-Dibb RG, Paula-Silva FW, et al. Radiation therapy alters microhardness and microstructure of enamel and dentin of permanent human teeth. J Dent 2014;42:986-992.
117. Lieshout HF, Bots CP. The effect of radiotherapy on dental hard tissue—A systematic review. Clin Oral Investig 2014;18:17-24.
118. Soares CJ, Castro CG, Neiva NA, et al. Effect of gamma irradiation on ultimate tensile strength of enamel and dentin. J Dent Res 2010;89:159-164.
119. Soares CJ, Roscoe MG, Castro CG, et al. Effect of gamma irradiation and restorative material on the biomechanical behaviour of root filled premolars. Int Endod J 2011;44:1047-1054.
120. Cui FZ, Ge J. New observations of the hierarchical structure of human enamel, from nanoscale to microscale. J Tissue Eng Regen Med 2007;1:185-191.
121. Stefanski T, Postek-Stefanska L. Possible ways of reducing dental erosive potential of acidic beverages. Aust Dent J 2014;59:280-288.
122. Lussi A, Jäggi T, Schärer S. The influence of different factors on in vitro enamel erosion. Caries Res 1993;27:387-393.
123. Owens BM. The potential effects of pH and buffering capacity on dental erosion. Gen Dent 2007;55:527-531.
124. Birkhed D. Sugar content, acidity and effect on plaque pH of fruit juices, fruit drinks, carbonated beverages and sport drinks. Caries Res 1984;18:120-127.
125. Edwards M, Creanor SL, Foye RH, Gilmour WH. Buffering capacities of soft drinks: the potential influence on dental erosion. J Oral Rehabil 1999;26:923-927.
126. Ehlen LA, Marshall TA, Qian F, Wefel JS, Warren JJ. Acidic beverages increase the risk of in vitro tooth erosion. Nutr Res 2008;28:299-303.

127. Featherstone JD, Rodgers BE. Effect of acetic, lactic and other organic acids on the formation of artificial carious lesions. Caries Res 1981;15:377–385.
128. Lussi A, Megert B, Shellis RP, Wang X. Analysis of the erosive effect of different dietary substances and medications. Br J Nutr 2012;107:252–262.
129. Lussi A, Jaeggi T. Chemical factors. Monogr Oral Sci 2006;20:77–87.
130. Barbour ME, Parker DM, Allen GC, Jandt KD. Enamel dissolution in citric acid as a function of calcium and phosphate concentrations and degree of saturation with respect to hydroxyapatite. Eur J Oral Sci 2003;111:428–433.
131. Barbour ME, Parker DM, Allen GC, Jandt KD. Human enamel erosion in constant composition citric acid solutions as a function of degree of saturation with respect to hydroxyapatite. J Oral Rehabil 2005;32:16–21.
132. Ganss C, Lussi A. Diagnosis of erosive tooth wear. Monogr Oral Sci 2014;25:22–31.
133. Ganss C. Definition of erosion and links to tooth wear. Monogr Oral Sci 2006;20:9–16.
134. Hattab FN, Yassin OM. Etiology and diagnosis of tooth wear: A literature review and presentation of selected cases. Int J Prosthodont 2000;13:101–107
135. Sivasithamparam K, Harbrow D, Vinczer E, Young WG. Endodontic sequelae of dental erosion. Aust Dent J 2003;48:97–101.
136. Grippo JO, Simring M. Dental 'erosion' revisited. J Am Dent Assoc 1995;126:619–620,623–624,627–630.
137. Nascimento MM, Dilbone DA, Pereira PN, Duarte WR, Geraldeli S, Delgado AJ. Abfraction lesions: Etiology, diagnosis, and treatment options. Clin Cosmet Investig Dent 2016;8:79–87.
138. Barron RP, Carmichael RP, Marcon MA, Sandor GK. Dental erosion in gastroesophageal reflux disease. J Can Dent Assoc 2003;69:84–89.
139. Eckley CA, Costa HO. Comparative study of salivary pH and volume in adults with chronic laryngopharyngitis by gastroesophageal reflux disease before and after treatment. Braz J Otorhinolaryngol 2006;72:55–60.
140. Ranjitkar S, Kaidonis JA, Smales RJ. Gastroesophageal reflux disease and tooth erosion. Int J Dent 2012;2012:479850.
141. Valena V, Young WG. Dental erosion patterns from intrinsic acid regurgitation and vomiting. Aust Dent J 2002;47:106–115.
142. Adams DH. Sleisenger and Fordtran's Gastrointestinal and Liver Disease. Gut 2007;56:1175.
143. Vakil N, van Zanten SV, Kahrilas P, Dent J, Jones R. The Montreal definition and classification of gastroesophageal reflux disease: A global evidence-based consensus. Am J Gastroenterol 2006;101:1900–1920.
144. Marsicano JA, De Moura-Grec PG, Bonato RC, Sales-Peres Mde C, Sales-Peres A, Sales-Peres SH. Gastroesophageal reflux, dental erosion, and halitosis in epidemiological surveys: A systematic review. Eur J Gastroenterol Hepatol 2013;25:135–141.
145. Dent J, El-Serag HB, Wallander MA, Johansson S. Epidemiology of gastrooesophageal reflux disease: A systematic review. Gut 2005;54:710–717.
146. Richter JE. Gastroesophageal reflux disease. Best Pract Res Clin Gastroenterol 2007;21:609–631.
147. Machado NA, Fonseca RB, Branco CA, Barbosa GA, Fernandes Neto AJ, Soares CJ. Dental wear caused by association between bruxism and gastroesophageal reflux disease: A rehabilitation report. J Appl Oral Sci 2007;15:327–333.
148. Katz PO, Gerson LB, Vela MF. Guidelines for the diagnosis and management of gastroesophageal reflux disease. Am J Gastroenterol 2013;108:308–328.
149. Kaltenbach T, Crockett S, Gerson L. Are lifestyle measures effective in patients with gastroesophageal reflux disease? An evidence-based approach. Arch Intern Med 2006;166:965–971.
150. American Psychiatric Association. DSM-IV. Diagnostic and Statistical Manual of Mental Disorders, ed 4. Vancouver: American Psychiatric Association, 2000.
151. Herpertz-Dahlmann B. Adolescent eating disorders: Update on definitions, symptomatology, epidemiology, and comorbidity. Child Adolesc Psychiatr Clin N Am 2015;24:177–196.
152. Cândido Msm FM. Dental erosion caused by gastroesophageal reflux—A clinical case. Jornal Brasileiro de Dentística & Estética 2002;1:64–71.
153. Papadopoulos V, Mimidis K. The rumination syndrome in adults: A review of the pathophysiology, diagnosis and treatment. J Postgrad Med 2007;53:203–206.
154. Xhonga FA, Van Herle A. The influence of hyperthyroidism on dental erosions. Oral Surg Oral Med Oral Pathol 1973;36:349–357.
155. McLoughlin IJ, Hassanyeh F. Pica in a patient with anorexia nervosa. Br J Psychiatry 1990;156:568–570.
156. Fairburn CG, Stein A, Jones R. Eating habits and eating disorders during pregnancy. Psychosom Med 1992;54:665–672.
157. Katz S, Park KK, Palenik CJ. In-vitro root surface caries studies. J Oral Med 1987;42:40–48.
158. Nascimento FD, Minciotti CL, Geraldeli S, et al. Cysteine cathepsins in human carious dentin. J Dent Res 2011;90:506–511.
159. Tjäderhane L, Larjava H, Sorsa T, Uitto VJ, Larmas M, Salo T. The activation and function of host matrix metalloproteinases in dentin matrix breakdown in caries lesions. J Dent Res 1998;77:1622–1629.
160. Kato MT, Leite AL, Hannas AR, Buzalaf MA. Gels containing MMP inhibitors prevent dental erosion in situ. J Dent Res 2010;89:468–472.
161. Kato MT, Magalhães AC, Rios D, Hannas AR, Attin T, Buzalaf MA. Protective effect of green tea on dentin erosion and abrasion. J Appl Oral Sci 2009;17:560–564.
162. Magalhães AC, Wiegand A, Rios D, Hannas A, Attin T, Buzalaf MA. Chlorhexidine and green tea extract reduce dentin erosion and abrasion in situ. J Dent 2009;37:994–998.
163. Breschi L, Mazzoni A, Nato F, et al. Chlorhexidine stabilizes the adhesive interface: A 2-year in vitro study. Dent Mater 2010;26:320–325.
164. Carrilho MR, Geraldeli S, Tay F, et al. In vivo preservation of the hybrid layer by chlorhexidine. J Dent Res 2007;86:529–533.
165. Aguiar TR, Vidal CM, Phansalkar RS, et al. Dentin biomodification potential depends on polyphenol source. J Dent Res 2014;93:417–422.
166. Castellan CS, Pereira PN, Grande RH, Bedran-Russo AK. Mechanical characterization of proanthocyanidin-dentin matrix interaction. Dent Mater 2010;26:968–973.
167. Mirkarimi M, Toomarian L. Effect of green tea extract on the treatment of dentin erosion: An in vitro study. J Dent (Tehran) 2012;9:224–228.
168. Barbosa CS, Kato MT, Buzalaf MA. Effect of supplementation of soft drinks with green tea extract on their erosive potential against dentine. Aust Dent J 2011;56:317–321.
169. Magalhães AC, Wiegand A, Rios D, Buzalaf MA, Lussi A. Fluoride in dental erosion. Monogr Oral Sci 2011;22:158–170.
170. Comar LP, Gomes MF, Ito N, Salomão PA, Grizzo LT, Magalhães AC. Effect of NaF, SnF(2), and TiF(4) toothpastes on bovine enamel and dentin erosion-abrasion in vitro. Int J Dent 2012;2012:134350.
171. Basting RT, Leme AA, Bridi EC, et al. Nanomechanical properties, SEM, and EDS microanalysis of dentin treated with 2.5% titanium tetrafluoride, before and after an erosive challenge. J Biomed Mater Res B Appl Biomater 2015;103:783–789.
172. Bridi EC, Amaral FL, França FM, Turssi CP, Basting RT. Influence of dentin pretreatment with titanium tetrafluoride and self-etching adhesive systems on microtensile bond strength. Am J Dent 2013;26:121–126.
173. Mei ML, Ito L, Cao Y, Li QL, Chu CH, Lo EC. The inhibitory effects of silver diamine fluorides on cysteine cathepsins. J Dent 2014;42:329–335.
174. Mei ML, Li QL, Chu CH, Yiu CK, Lo EC. The inhibitory effects of silver diamine fluoride at different concentrations on matrix metalloproteinases. Dent Mater 2012;28:903–908.
175. Kim TH, Lee KJ, Yeo M, Kim DK, Cho SW. Pepsin detection in the sputum/saliva for the diagnosis of gastroesophageal reflux disease in patients with clinically suspected atypical gastroesophageal reflux disease symptoms. Digestion 2008;77:201–206.
176. Silbernagl S, Despopoulos A. Color Atlas of Physiology, ed 6. New York: Thieme, 2009.
177. Schlueter N, Ganss C, Pötschke S, Klimek J, Hannig C. Enzyme activities in the oral fluids of patients suffering from bulimia: A controlled clinical trial. Caries Res 2012;46:130–139.
178. Dung SZ, Li Y, Dunipace AJ, Stookey GK. Degradation of insoluble bovine collagen and human dentine collagen pretreated in vitro with lactic acid, pH 4.0 and 5.5. Arch Oral Biol 1994;39:901–905.
179. Schlueter N, Ganss C, Hardt M, Schegietz D, Klimek J. Effect of pepsin on erosive tissue loss and the efficacy of fluoridation measures in dentine in vitro. Acta Odontol Scand 2007;65:298–305.

Section III
Diagnosis and Treatment

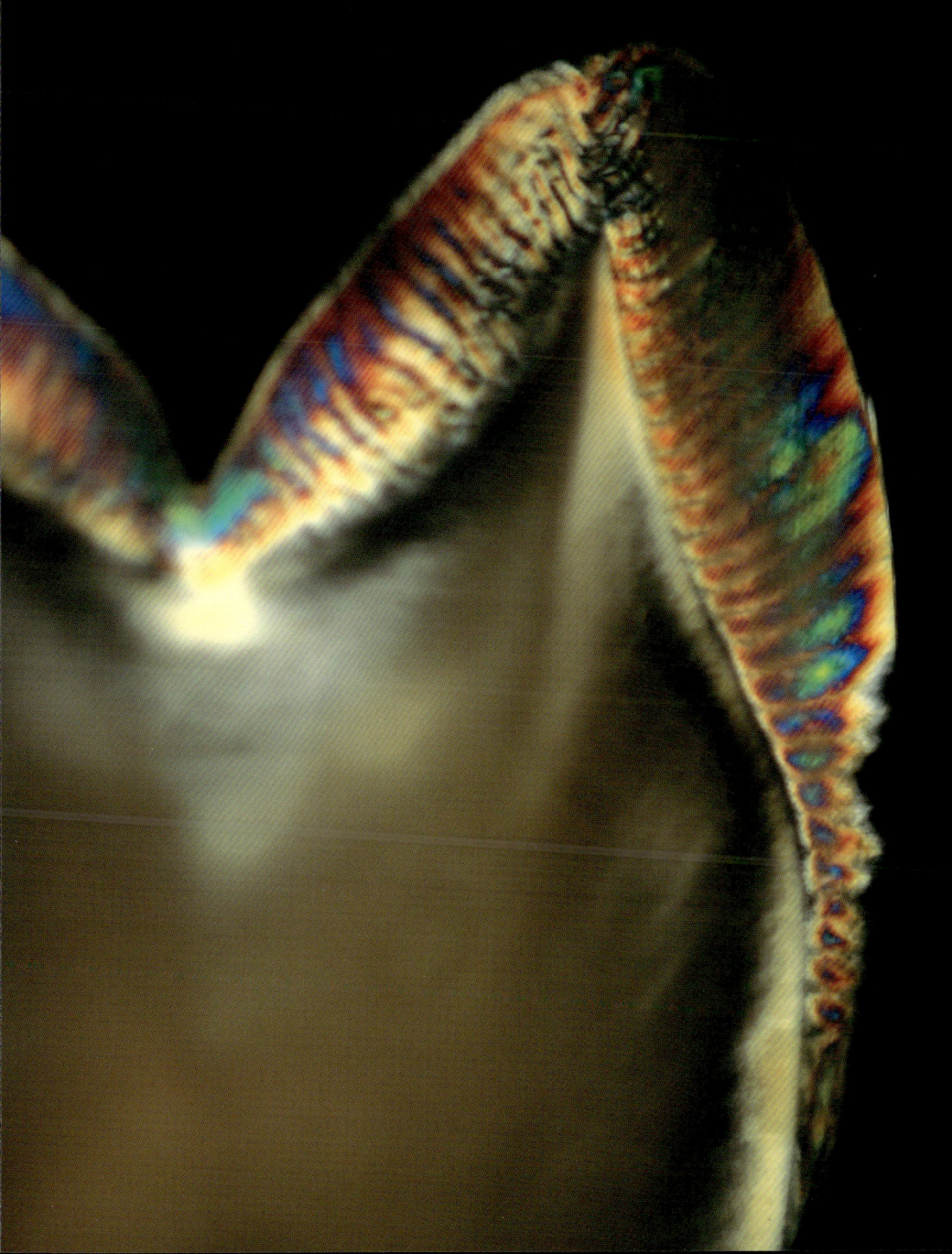

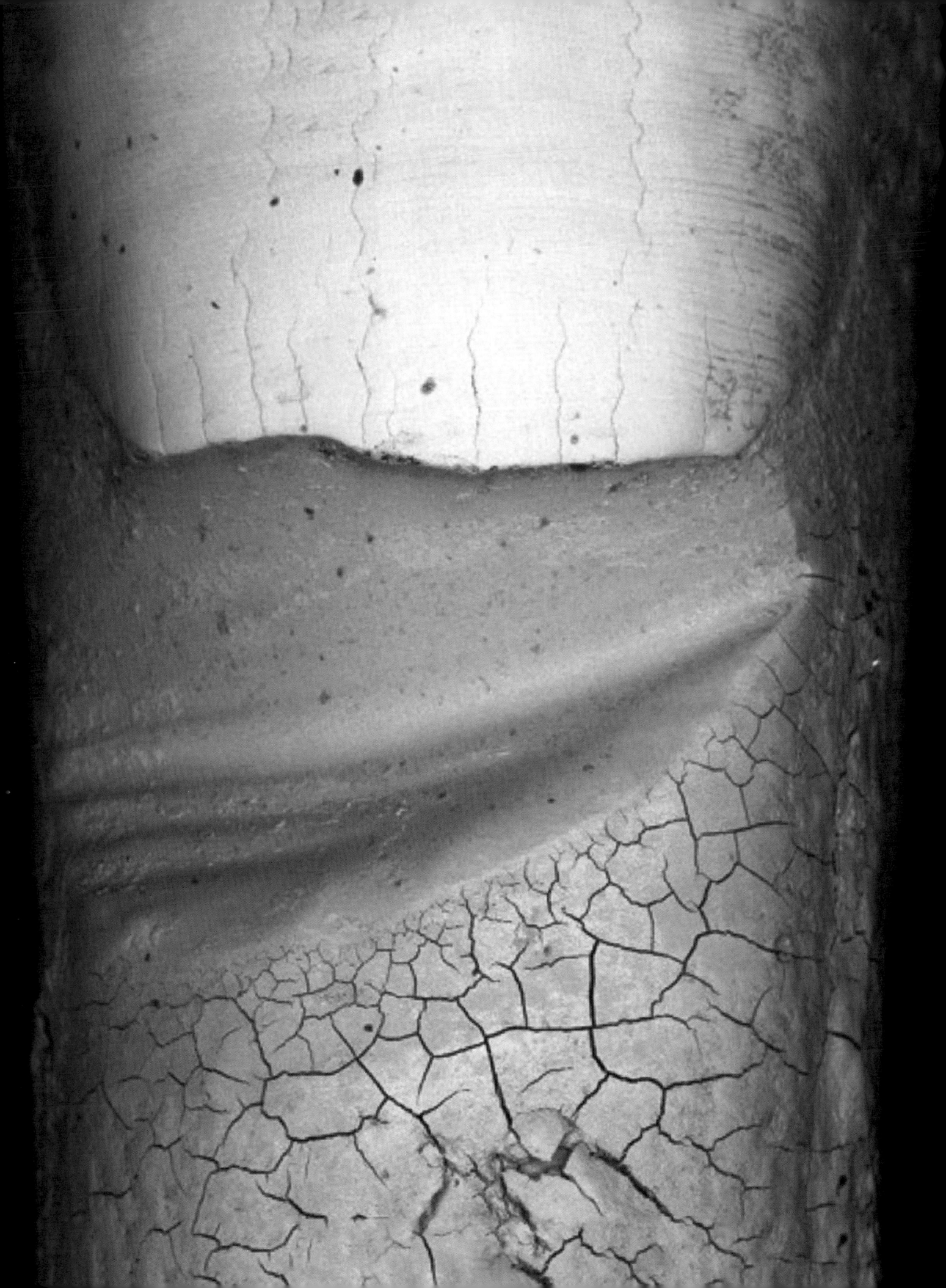

6

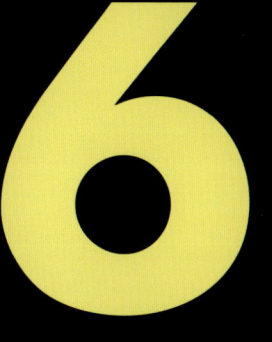

Morphologic Characteristics of NCCLs

The purpose of this chapter is to enable the clinician to identify and classify noncarious cervical lesions (NCCLs) based on their form. NCCLs have various morphologies, and it is important to elucidate the characteristics of each type of lesion to more precisely identify the etiologic mechanisms responsible. This chapter details clinical and histologic aspects involving macromorphology and micromorphology of NCCLs. Macromorphology includes the aspects that we can identify clinically in NCCLs, like form (geometry), dimensions, and anatomical location. Micromorphology includes histologic aspects of the tissues that are involved in the formation of these hard tissue lesions (Fig 6-1).

Macromorphology

Form/geometry

To determine the morphology of NCCLs, it is necessary to observe the geometry of the lost tooth structure in these lesions. First we must assign names to the walls constituting these lesions. The wall facing the occlusal surface is called the *coronal wall*. Walls facing the cervical region are called *gingival walls*, and the depth of the lesion is designated as the *pulp wall* or *apex* (Fig 6-2).

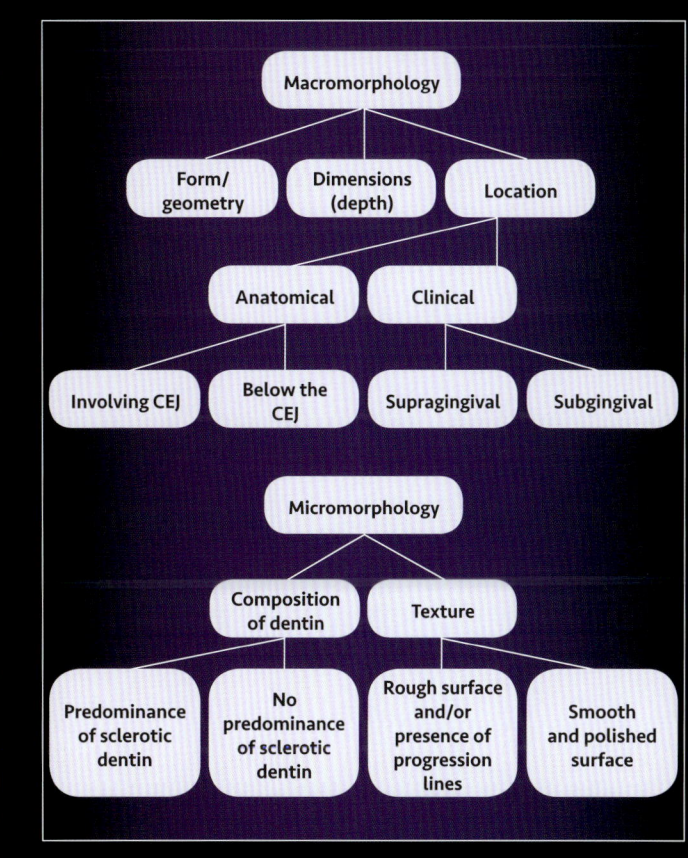

Fig 6-1 Classification scheme used for NCCLs. CEJ, cementoenamel junction.

6 Morphologic Characteristics of NCCLs

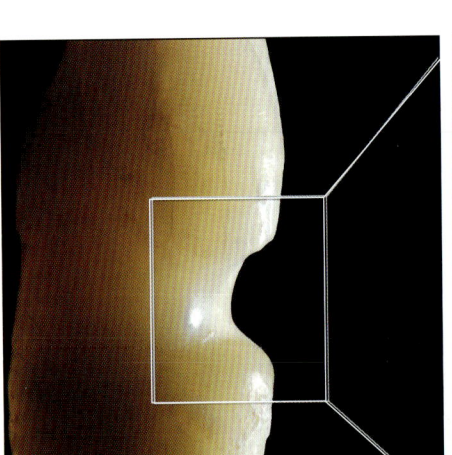

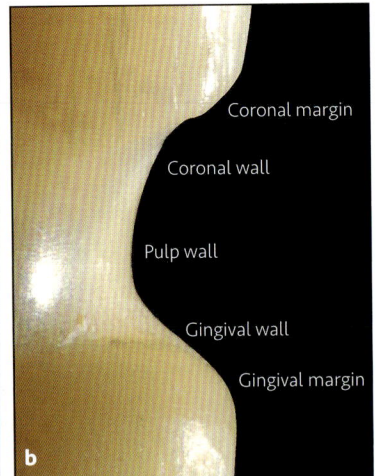

Fig 6-2 Nomenclature of the NCCL walls.

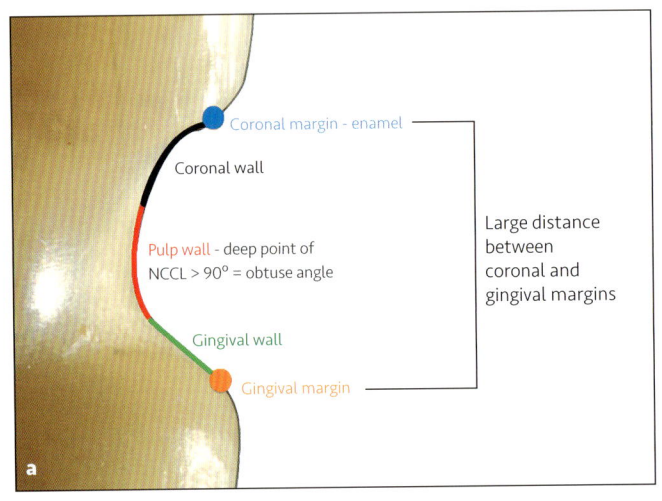

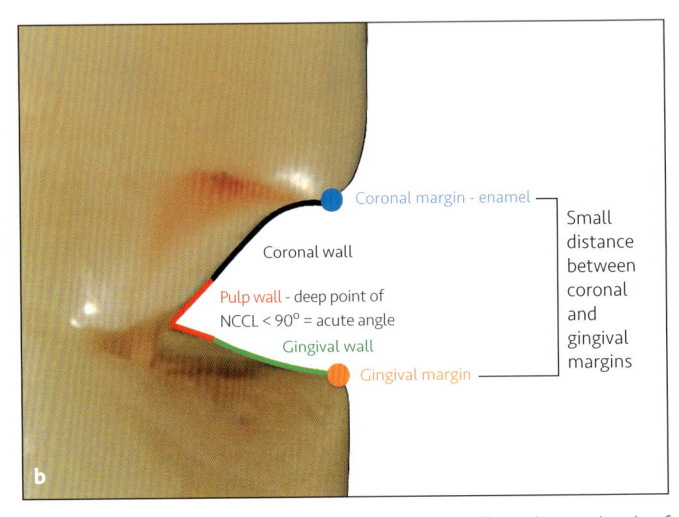

Fig 6-3 *(a)* Rounded NCCL. *(b)* Wedge-shaped NCCL. *Blue point*: upper limit of NCCL (coronal margin). *Black area*: coronal wall. *Red area*: depth of the NCCL (pulp wall). *Green curve*: base of the lesion (gingival wall). *Orange point*: lower limit of NCCL (gingival margin).

The morphologic features of NCCLs have been identified as two distinct patterns and can be categorized according to the type of angle found in the pulpal wall of the lesion.[1] One type has a more rounded form (Fig 6-3a), while the other has a sharp internal angle (Fig 6-3b). The morphology relates to the actions that take place in the area. When the stress is intense in the area of stress concentration for long period of time, then the lesion progresses pulpally, resulting in a deep angular lesion (see Fig 6-3b).

Based on these characteristics, there are two basic types of NCCL morphology: wedge-shaped and concave[1] (Figs 6-4a and 6-4b). Lesions can also be a combination of the two. This form takes into account the effects of biocorrosion, friction, and mechanical stress. This NCCL may have its base with rounded pulp wall but a flat gingival or coronal wall, thereby providing a composition of mixed type during its etiologic formation (Fig 6-4c). Epidemiologic studies have shown a slightly higher prevalence of wedge-shaped than concave NCCLs.[1-6]

Other classifications for NCCL morphology have been proposed, but they are all based on the angle characteristic of the pulp apex or wall of the lesion.[1,3,4,7-9] That is, the base of the lesion and the gingival wall will determine the morphologic classification.

Some teeth may even have two lesions with different forms. Because these lesions could have two or more pulp angles, some authors have classified them as being "irreg-

Macromorphology

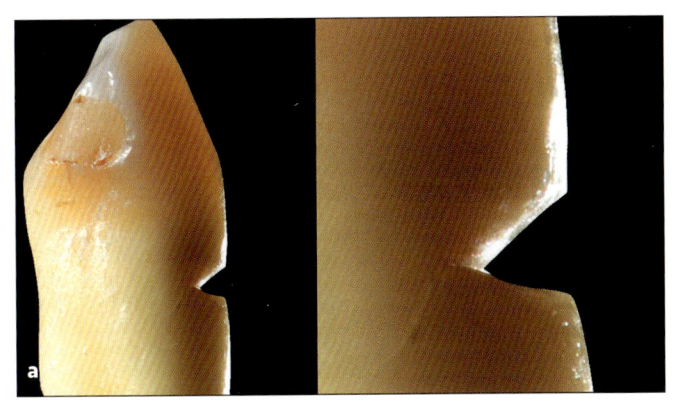

Fig 6-4 *(a)* Clinical wedge-shaped NCCL. *(b)* Concave NCCL. *(c)* NCCL with mixed morphology. (Courtesy of the NCCL Research Group, Uberlândia, Brazil.)

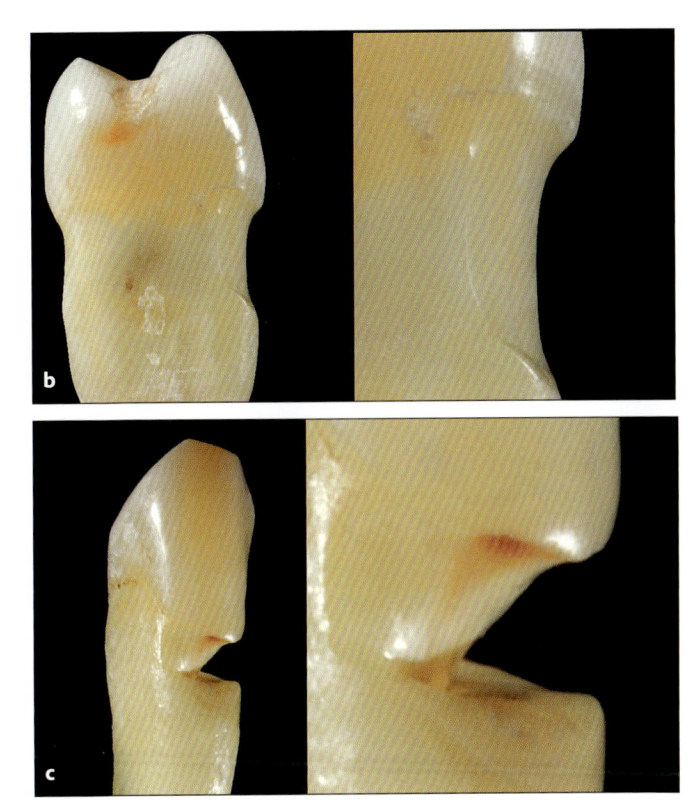

Fig 6-5 Example of irregular NCCL form.[7,9] *(a)* Lateral view. *(b)* Close-up frontal view. In this case, there are potential influences of stress concentration and biocorrosive injury. (Courtesy of the NCCL Research Group, Uberlândia, Brazil.)

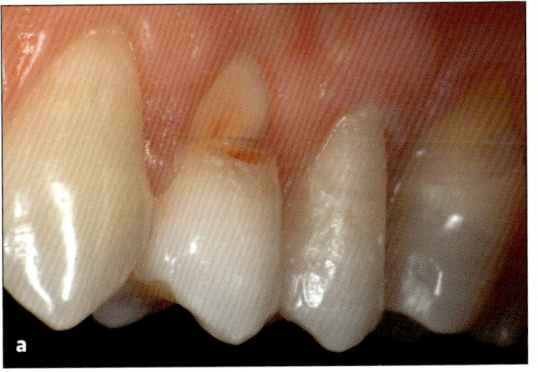

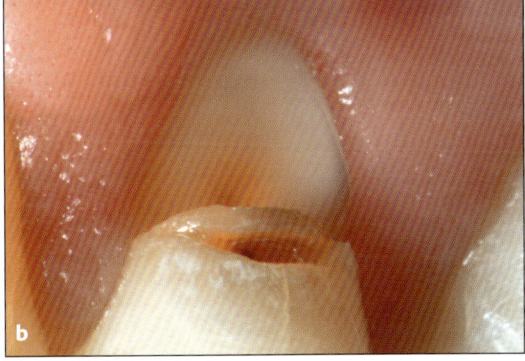

ular."[7] NCCLs with dual angles may differ in their base and occlusal wall angles, so it is appropriate to classify them as such (Fig 6-5).

Understanding the form of NCCLs may assist the clinician in diagnosing and treating these lesions. Researchers have found that the stress concentration in NCCLs is at the deepest recess of the lesion[10] (Fig 6-6). The presence of these deep NCCLs promotes further progression of hard tissue damage and may lead to fracture of a tooth from routine function, especially when combined with biocorrosive agents that degrade open dentin surfaces.

Grippo[4] avers that the irregularity of NCCLs occurs due to changes in periods of biocorrosive abfraction. For example, when bone and gingival attachment changes occur, the degradation will move in an apical direction at the fulcrum in areas of stress concentration. The longer the action occurs in an area of stress concentration, the deeper the lesion will progress. Conversely, if stresses are confined to the crown (as in a bruxer) and the bone is resistant, then the lesions will occur and move in a coronal direction. Simply stated, wedge-shaped NCCLs become areas of extremely high stress concentration levels that promote unfavorable biomechanical and biochemical behavior.

6 Morphologic Characteristics of NCCLs

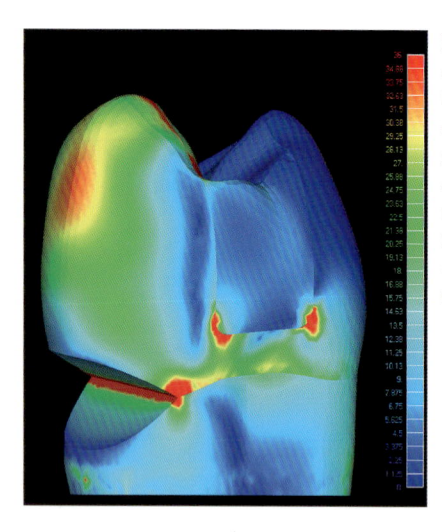

Fig 6-6 Results of finite element analysis shown by the von Mises criterion of stress concentration generated in the pulp angle of a deep NCCL. The mechanical stresses were made by occlusal load type and the presence of mesio-occlusodistal amalgam.

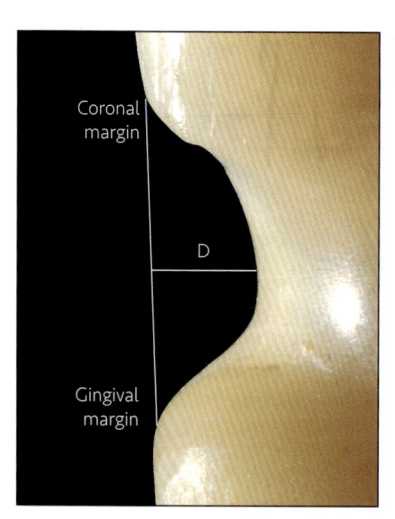

Fig 6-7 The depth (D) of an NCCL.

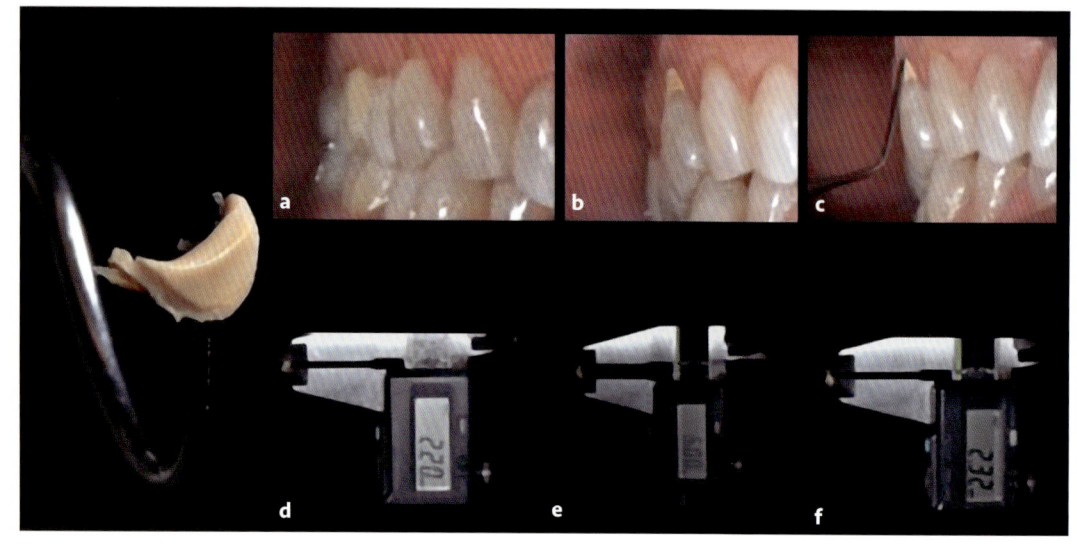

Fig 6-8 Protocol to measure the depth of an NCCL. *(a)* NCCL present in a maxillary premolar. *(b)* Insertion of impression material. *(c)* Removal of the excess impression material before its final curing. *(d)* Measurement of the cervical-occlusal dimension. *(e)* Measurement of the depth of the lesion. *(f)* Measurement of the mesiodistal length. (Protocol created by the NCCL Research Group, Uberlândia, Brazil.)

Dimension (depth)

The depth of an NCCL is a result of the extension of lost tooth structure measured perpendicular from a center line of the lesion to a straight line parallel to the long axis of the tooth drawn from the coronal margin to the gingival margin (Fig 6-7). The depth of the NCCL indicates the severity of the mechanisms involved in their genesis. Authors have used various quantitative and qualitative methods of classification or a scoring system designed to identify the increasing severity and progression of these lesions.[11]

The difficulty in quantifying complex cervical tooth substance loss rates is the lack of standardization in the measurement of NCCL severity. Depth measurements are often made clinically by placing a millimeter periodontal probe to the base of the lesion. The authors suggest instead that the dimensions and morphology of NCCLs can be measured with more accuracy by reproducing the depth of the lesion with impression material (Fig 6-8):

- Complete a prophylaxis in the NCCL region using pumice and water with a rubber cup.
- Isolate the region using gingival retraction cord and a cotton roll in the vestibule.
- Mix a silicone molding base and catalyst.
- Insert the silicone material, filling the cavity of the lesion, and remove the excess.
- Ensure final set prior to removing this segmental impression.
- Use a digital micrometer to measure the depth of the lesion.

Once the measurement is made, it is necessary to assign a score for classification. The literature identifies different

Macromorphology

Table 6-1 Smith and Knight[12] tooth wear index

Score	Surface	Criteria
0	B/L/O/I	No loss of enamel characteristics
	C	No loss of contour
1	B/L/O/I	Loss of enamel surface characteristics
	C	Minimal loss of contour
2	B/L/O	Loss of enamel exposing the dentin for less than one-third of the surface
	I	Loss of enamel just exposing the dentin
	C	Defect less than 1 mm deep
3	B/L/O	Loss of enamel exposing the dentin for more than one-third of the surface
	I	Loss of enamel and substantial loss of dentin
	C	Defect less than 2 mm deep
4	B/L/O	Complete loss of enamel, pulp exposure, and secondary dentin exposure
	I	Pulp exposure or exposure of secondary dentin
	C	Defect more than 2 mm deep, pulp exposure, and secondary dentin exposure

B, buccal; L, lingual; O, occlusal; I, incisal; C, cervical.

Table 6-2 Modified Smith and Knight tooth wear index used by the authors

Score	Depth of NCCL	Criterion
1	<1 mm	Shallow
2	1–2 mm	Moderate
3	>2 mm	Deep

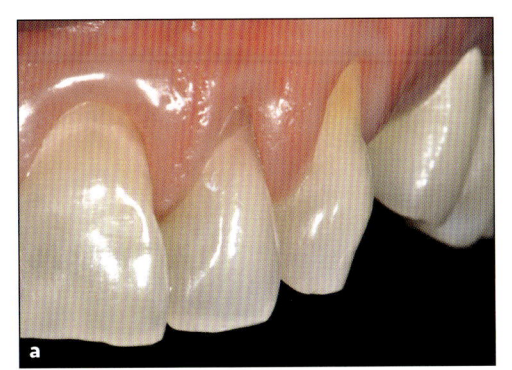

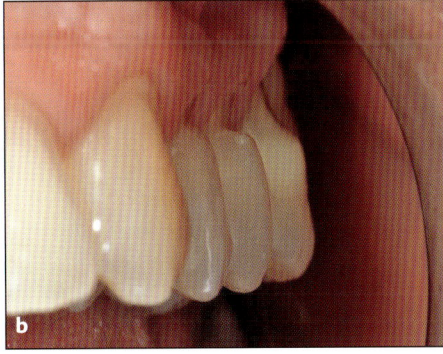

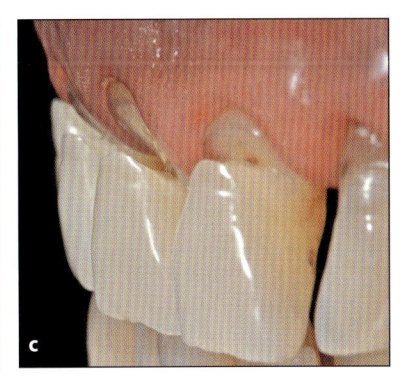

Fig 6-9 Classifications of NCCLs according to depth: *(a)* shallow, *(b)* moderate, and *(c)* deep. (Courtesy of the NCCL Research Group, Uberlândia, Brazil.)

levels for use in clinical and laboratory situations and specific values for these multifactorial NCCLs. However, a specific index can lead to confusion because of the difficulty in standardizing the terminology and translation to etiologic differences of opinion regarding tooth structure loss based on morphologic findings.

Smith and Knight[12] developed the first index to measure and monitor multifactorial tooth wear; the pioneering feature was the ability to distinguish acceptable and pathologic levels of wear. This index considers the size of the affected area (as a proportion of the sound surface and/or the depth of tissue loss) often expressed as a degree of dentin exposure. It includes a comprehensive system whereby all four visible surfaces (buccal, cervical, lingual, and occlusal-incisal) of teeth present are scored for wear, irrespective of how it occurred (Table 6-1). Because of the multifactorial nature of the formation and progression of NCCLs, most epidemiologic studies that measure the severity of tooth wear use this index.[13,14]

However, some problems have been identified with the Smith and Knight index, including the time applicable to the development of the lesions, the amount of data generated, and the comparisons with threshold levels for each age group; the thresholds proposed were high, erring toward understatement rather than exaggeration of pathologic wear. Thus, over time it became necessary to create adaptations to this index for standardization. The authors have used a modified Smith and Knight system to classify lesions as either shallow, moderate, or deep (Table 6-2 and Fig 6-9). With this system, a direct correlation can be made between the score and the clinical progression of the lesion during subsequent investigation.

6 Morphologic Characteristics of NCCLs

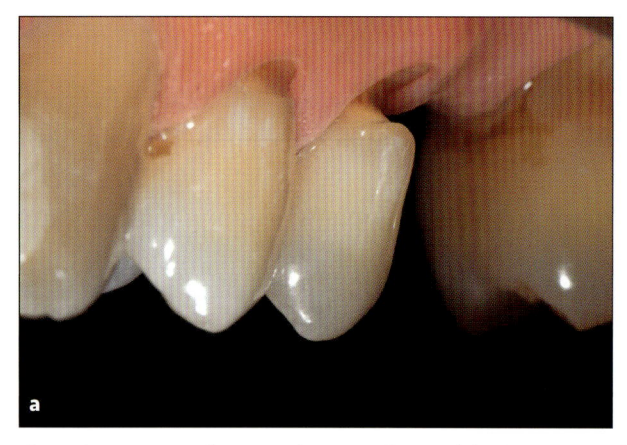

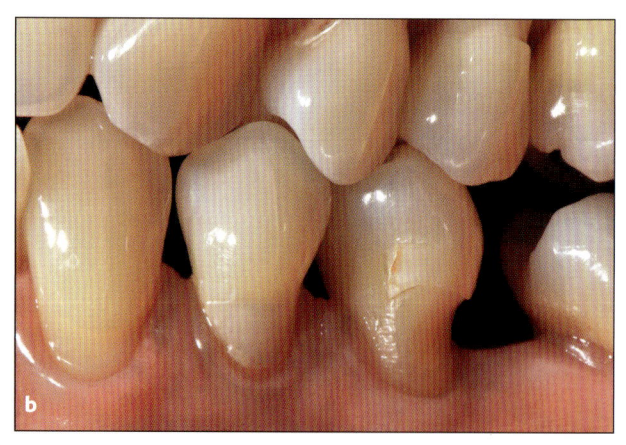

Fig 6-10 Locations of NCCLs relative to the CEJ. *(a)* Below the CEJ. *(b)* Involving the CEJ and crown.

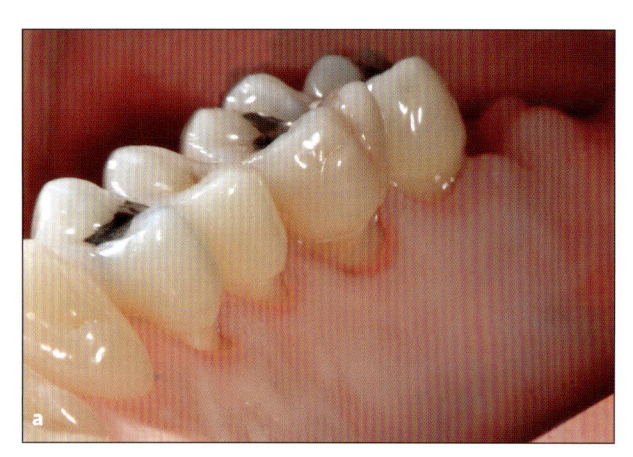

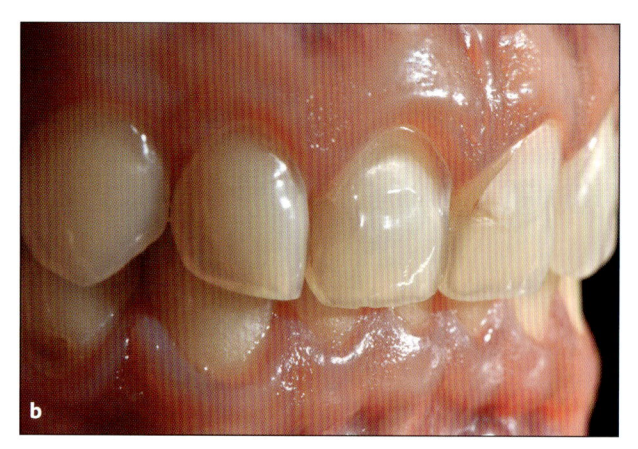

Fig 6-11 Locations of NCCLs relative to the gingival margin. *(a)* Subgingival. *(b)* Supragingival. (Courtesy of the NCCL Research Group, Uberlândia, Brazil.)

Location

Anatomical

The locations of NCCLs vary based on etiologic factors relative to bone loss and gingival recession. The presence of abfractive lesions indicates that stress concentration is acting at the site, creating wedge-shaped lesions.[4] Stress concentration initially produces microcracks in the brittle enamel, which can propagate through enamel and thereby start the formation of NCCLs. Combined mechanisms of stress and biocorrosion cause NCCLs in the cervical dentin that in many cases extend apically from the cementoenamel junction (CEJ) (Fig 6-10).

Clinical

NCCLs in teeth that are located under the free gingival margin apical to the CEJ may be classified as subgingival (Fig 6-11a). Those lesions occlusal to the gingival margin are designated as supragingival (Fig 6-11b). Subgingival margins of the NCCL, which are below the soft tissue margin, hamper their direct clinical access. Therefore, the location of the NCCL in relation to the gingival margin influences the type of isolation, choice of instrumentation, and clinical access for adhesive procedures.

Micromorphology

Composition

The micromorphology of the cervical region of teeth is especially vulnerable to physical and chemical injury.[15] In the scanning electron microscopic evaluation of cervical lesions performed by Levrini et al,[16] all main components of the tooth were damaged even when the CEJ was intact. When the enamel is subjected to stress, biocorrosion and to a minor degree toothbrush/dentifrice abrasion make it more fragile, resulting in microcracks,[10,16,17] and the odontoblasts generate sclerotic dentin that occludes the dentinal tubules.[18]

In the incipient phase, enamel is degraded without clinically detectable softening, but it bears microcracks and microporosity. Daley[18] reported that both the number of den-

Fig 6-12 Clinical view of sclerotic dentin in NCCLs. (Courtesy of the NCCL Research Group, Uberlândia, Brazil.)

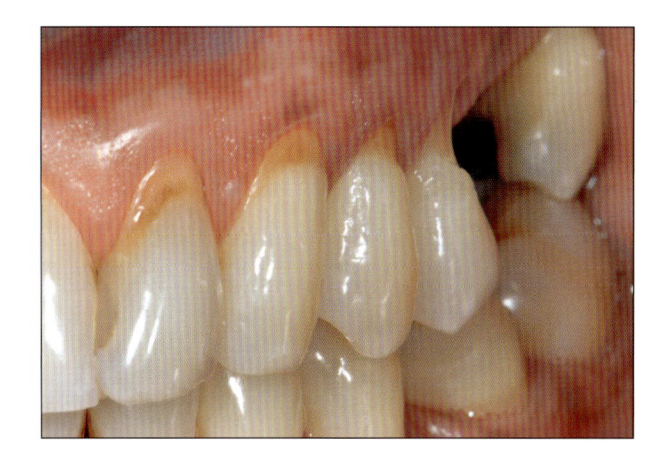

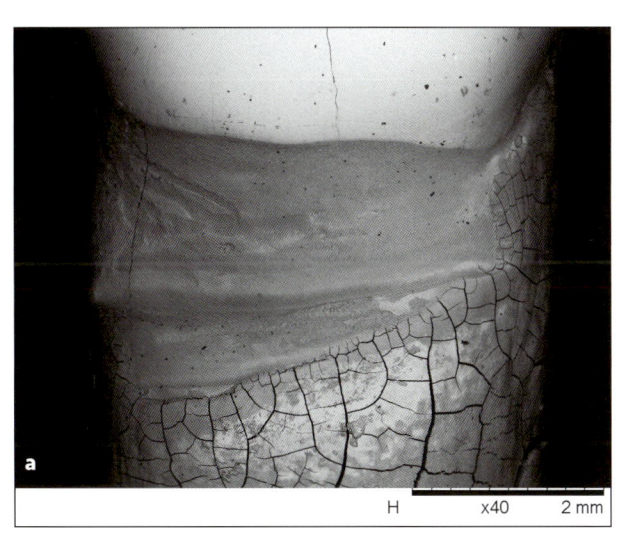

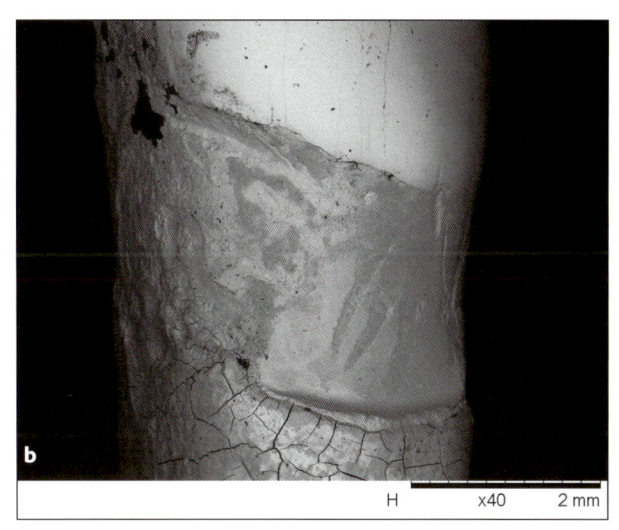

Fig 6-13 *(a)* Observe the angle in the NCCL, with irregular topography, scars, and surface roughness. *(b)* A shallow NCCL with smooth surfaces. (Courtesy of the NCCL Research Group, Uberlândia, Brazil.)

tinal tubules per square millimeter as well as the diameters of tubules were affected by intratubular dentin formation at different levels with respect to the NCCL. Within the gingival wall of the lesion, most tubules were obliterated. At the intermediate level between the lesion and the pulp, a smear layer frequently covered the surface of the dentin, and the characteristic tubules were not visible.[15]

We must also address the clinical characteristics of existing sclerotic dentin. These characteristics may be identified according to the color of the lesion within the dentin and its hardness before using a cutting instrument. Sclerotic dentin appears as yellow-brownish and has greater mineralization than secondary dentin (Fig 6-12).

Texture

Studies have reported that different surface textures can be found in NCCLs and appear as smooth or rough (scratched)[14,15,19] (Fig 6-13). The surface texture of NCCLs can be related to friction and/or biocorrosion mechanisms. Biocorrosive effects are characterized by smooth surfaces, with enamel showing a honeycomb structure and the dentin showing a waved or rippled surface.[19] Scratch marks on enamel and dentin are typical of abrasion due to agents such as toothbrush/dentifrice and hard foods, which can effect a high polish to the lesion and simultaneously generate scratches on the tooth substance.[14] Therefore, patients who use very abrasive toothpaste and toothbrushes with stiff bristles have lesions that look like scratches. In addition, acidic dietary patterns can be identified purely from the texture of the lesions. Deep parallel grooves known as *progression lines* (see Fig 3-10) signify high activity of mechanical etiologic factors in developing the NCCL.

Morphologic Characteristics of NCCLs

Box 6-1	New classification of NCCLs proposed by the authors

Form/geometry
- Concave
- Wedge-shaped
- Mixed

Severity
- Shallow (< 1 mm)
- Moderate (1–2 mm)
- Deep (> 2 mm)

Location
Relative to the CEJ (anatomical aspect)
- Involving the CEJ
- Apical to the CEJ

Relative to the gingival margin (clinical aspect)
- Supragingival
- Subgingival

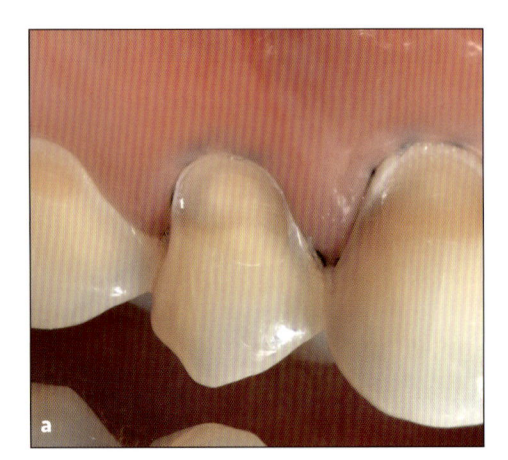

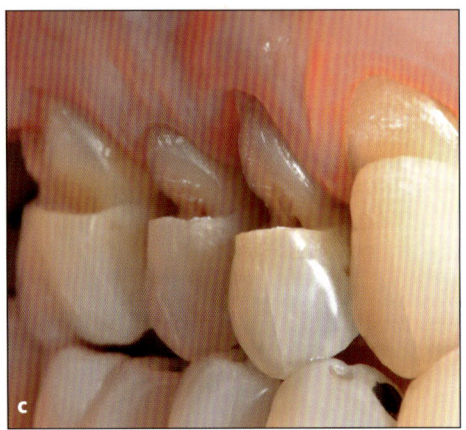

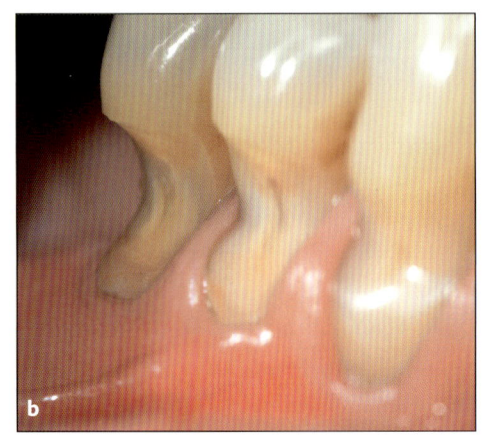

Fig 6-14 Examples of NCCL variations. *(a)* Concave, moderate NCCL that involves the CEJ and crown. Observe that the authors used retraction cord to access the gingival margin. *(b)* Concave, deep NCCL below the CEJ associated with significant gingival recession. *(c)* Mixed, deep NCCLs that involve the CEJ and crown. Observe the high concentration of sclerotic dentin and the pulp communication. Incredibly, this patient did not have cervical dentin hypersensitivity in these teeth.

Relationship Between Etiologic Factors and Morphology

If bone loss and gingival recession ensue, then the morphology of NCCLs changes in an apical location as the fulcrum relocates in that direction. In the presence of a biocorrodent, abfraction stresses occur in the direction of the fulcrum, creating long and shallow dish-shaped lesions.[20,21] On the other hand, the biocorrosive process associated with friction movements promotes flattening of the surface of NCCLs.

Box 6-1 provides a quick and effective classification for NCCLs based on form, severity, and location. However, it is important to remember that there are different combinations of geometry, severity, and location of NCCLs, as demonstrated in Fig 6-14. These variations lend credence to the proposed multifactorial nature of these lesions.

Note that other mammals have the same problem with NCCLs. The bovine tooth in Fig 6-15 was collected by researchers for study; observe the concave, deep lesion associated with a large wear facet on the incisal surface. This NCCL was likely created by stress concentration and facilitated by biocorrosion due to gastric acid. Cattle and other ruminants regurgitate partially digested food (cud) into their mouths for further chewing.

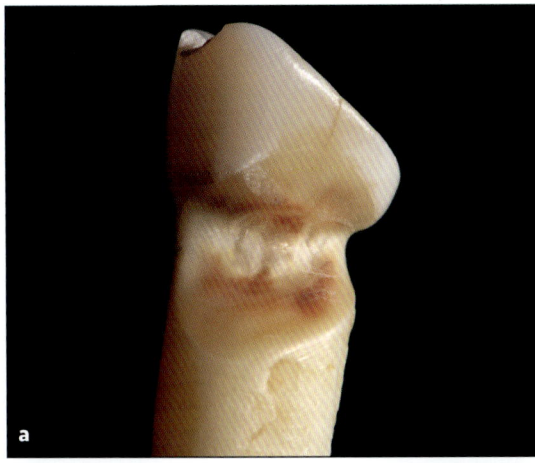

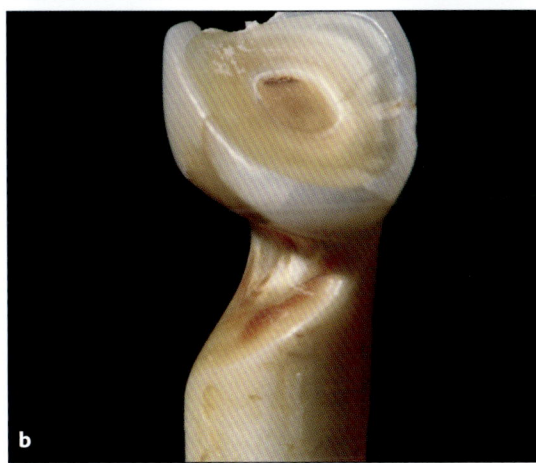

Fig 6-15 *(a and b)* NCCL in a bovine tooth.

Conclusion

Let's review what we have covered in this chapter:
- NCCLs have various morphologies.
- NCCLs can be rounded, wedge-shaped, or mixed.
- The depth of the NCCL indicates the severity and progression of the lesion.
- NCCLs can be located apical to or coronal to the CEJ.
- NCCLs can be located subgingivally or supragingivally.
- The surface texture of NCCLs can be smooth or rough. Smooth NCCLs are the result of biocorrosion, whereas rough surfaces are caused by abrasion and progression lines as a result of stress.
- The NCCL's morphology can help in diagnosis.

References

1. Hur B, Kim HC, Park JK, Versluis A. Characteristics of non-carious cervical lesions—An ex vivo study using micro computed tomography. J Oral Rehabil 2011;38:469–474.
2. Miller N, Penaud J, Ambrosini P, Bisson-Boutelliez C, Briançon S. Analysis of etiologic factors and periodontal conditions involved with 309 abfractions. J Clin Periodontol 2003;30:828–832.
3. Hong FL, Nu ZY, Xie XM. Clinical classification and therapeutic design of dental cervical abrasion. Gerodontics 1988;4:101–103.
4. Grippo JO. Abfractions: A new classification of hard tissue lesions of teeth. J Esthet Dent 1991;3:14–19.
5. Lussi A, Schaffner M. Progression of and risk factors for dental erosion and wedge-shaped defects over a 6-year period. Caries Res 2000;34:182–187.
6. Michael JA, Kaidonis JA, Townsend GC. Non-carious cervical lesions: A scanning electron microscopic study. Aust Dent J 2010;55:138–142.
7. Michael JA, Kaidonis JA, Townsend GC. Non-carious cervical lesions on permanent anterior teeth: A new morphological classification. Aust Dent J 2010;55:134–137.
8. Piotrowski BT, Gillette WB, Hancock EB. Examining the prevalence and characteristics of abfractionlike cervical lesions in a population of US veterans. J Am Dent Assoc 2001;132:1694–1701.
9. Soares PV, Santos-Filho PC, Soares CJ, et al. Non-carious cervical lesions: Influence of morphology and load type on biomechanical behaviour of maxillary incisors. Aust Dent J 2013;58:306–314.
10. Pereira FA, Zeola LF, de Almeida Millito G, Reis BR, Pereira RD, Soares PV. Restorative material and loading type influence on the biomechanical behavior of wedge shaped cervical lesions. Clin Oral Investig 2016;20:433–441.
11. López-Frías FJ, Castellanos-Cosano L, Martín-González J, Llamas-Carreras JM, Segura-Egea JJ. Clinical measurement of tooth wear: Tooth wear indices. J Clin Exp Dent 2012;4:e48–e53.
12. Smith BG, Knight JK. An index for measuring the wear of teeth. Br Dent J 1984;156:435–438.
13. Estafan A, Furnari PC, Goldstein G, Hittelman EL. In vivo correlation of noncarious cervical lesions and occlusal wear. J Prosthet Dent 2005;93:221–226.
14. Borcic J, Anic I, Urek MM, Ferreri S. The prevalence of non-carious cervical lesions in permanent dentition. J Oral Rehabil 2004;31:117–123.
15. Spranger H. Investigation into the genesis of angular lesions at the cervical region of teeth. Quintessence Int 1995;26:149–154.
16. Levrini L, Di Benedetto G, Raspanti M. Dental wear: A scanning electron microscope study. Biomed Res Int 2014;2014:340425.
17. Palamara D, Palamara JE, Tyas MJ, Pintado M, Messer HH. Effect of stress on acid dissolution of enamel. Dent Mater 2001;17:109–115.
18. Daley TJ, Harbrow DJ, Kahler B, Young WG. The cervical wedge-shaped lesion in teeth: A light and electron microscopic study. Aust Dent J 2009;54:212–219.
19. Nguyen C, Ranjitkar S, Kaidonis JA, Townsend GC. A qualitative assessment of non-carious cervical lesions in extracted human teeth. Aust Dent J 2008;53:46–51.
20. Sneed WD. Noncarious cervical lesions: Why on the facial? A theory. J Esthet Restor Dent 2011;23:197–200.
21. Soares PV, Souza LV, Veríssimo C, et al. Effect of root morphology on biomechanical behaviour of premolars associated with abfraction lesions and different loading types. J Oral Rehabil 2014;41:108–114.

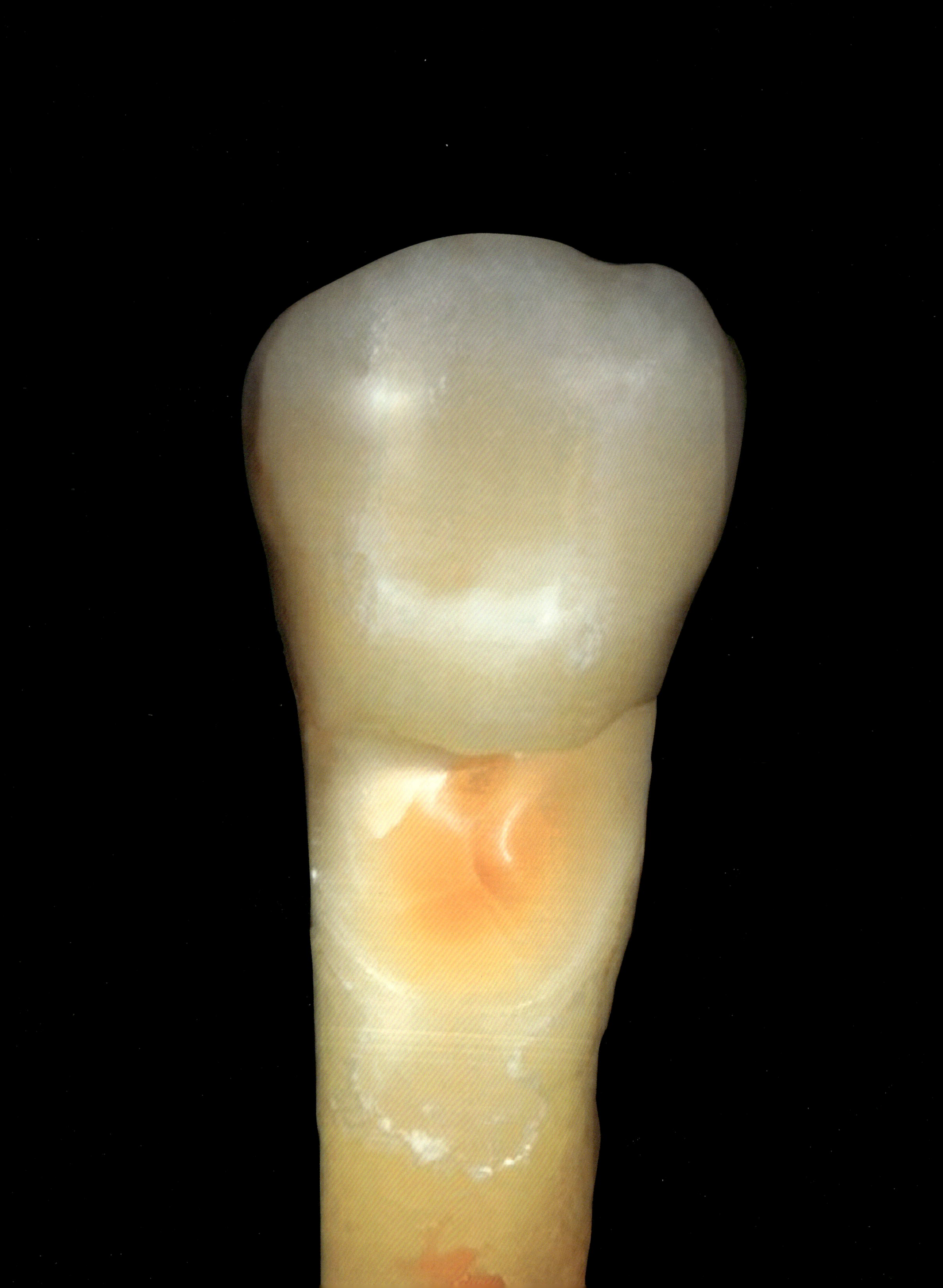

7

Clinical Analysis and Diagnosis of CDH and NCCLs

In the case of cervical dentin hypersensitivity (CDH) and noncarious cervical lesions (NCCLs), a thorough patient interview following a complete medical and dental history recorded by the patient serves as a starting point toward etiologic determination. Full-mouth radiographs and a complete oral examination yield information of value for establishing additional investigative tools or modalities to determine etiologies relating to CDH or NCCLs. Because these etiologies are often multifactorial,[1,2] the identification of current and past conditions is important for determining mechanism prominence during examination.[3] If the etiology is indeed multifactorial, then the dentist's clinical approach must also be multidisciplinary.

Patient History and Complaint

The first investigative step in the determination of CDH or NCCLs is to ask the patient in his or her own words to describe and record the chief complaint and symptoms, if any exist. The recording should include the duration, severity, and characteristics of the complaint. In this manner, the clinician will be better able to sort esthetic concerns of NCCLs from pain concerns of CDH. A minor source of oral pain or esthetic compromise generally appears to the individual as more severe over time. Likewise, the clinician may be able to rapidly assess the general psychologic status of the patient during this interview. Underlying systemic disease states are often identified by the dental health professional during this initial patient interaction.

It is essential that a written medical and dental history be carefully reviewed to determine if there is any indication of pathologies that can contribute to CDH or NCCL formation. Acidic dietary challenges, certain medications administered for systemic disease states, and environmental acid exposures contribute to exogenous biocorrosion, and endogenous biocorrosion from reflux diseases are not always diagnosed or reported by patients. Imbalances during masticatory system function, parafunctional activities, temporomandibular disorders (TMDs), muscular adaptation to the presence of occlusal prematurities (iatrogenic or otherwise), and evidence of occlusal disturbance can all produce transient or more permanent features of cervical stress concentration from excessive occlusal loading. The diagnosis is usually more accurate when the clinician completes a thorough interview and assesses the written medical or dental history.

Clinical Analysis and Diagnosis of CDH and NCCLs

Box 7-1 | Pathologies and questions to include on the medical history form

Have you had or do you currently have any of the following conditions?

- Alcoholism
- Allergy
- Anemia
- Asthma
- Bacterial endocarditis
- Cardiovascular disease
- Diabetes
- Epilepsy
- Fainting reflex
- Healing problems
- Hepatitis
- Herpes/thrush
- HIV
- Hypertension
- Kidney problems
- Psychologic disorder
- Rheumatic fever
- Smoking
- Syphilis
- Tuberculosis
- Tumor

Have you ever had surgery? If so, for what reason?
Have you ever been hospitalized? If so, for what reason?

Box 7-2 | Parafunction and TMD questions to include on the dental history form

Parafunction
- Do you usually grind your teeth?
- Do you press your tongue against your teeth?
- Do you usually clench your jaw?
- Do you often bite your lip, cheek, or tongue?
- Do you often bite objects such as pens, paper clips, etc?
- Do you usually bite your nails?

TMD
- Is it difficult for you to open your mouth?
- Is it difficult for you to move your jaw from one side to the other?
- Do you feel muscle fatigue when chewing?
- Do you often have headaches?
- Do you feel pain or tension in your neck?
- Do you feel pain in your skull and jaw joint?
- Does your jaw snap on opening and/or closing of your mouth?

Box 7-1 lists systemic pathologies and questions that should be included in the patient medical history. Box 7-2 lists other questions that should be included in the dental history.

Clinical Examination and Diagnosis

After concluding the patient interview and reviewing the medical/dental history, the clinician needs to discuss with the patient investigative tools that appear appropriate for his or her specific case. Full-mouth radiographic analysis and comprehensive oral examination are the basic tools for establishing an etiologic differential diagnosis for CDH and NCCLs, but additional resources such as magnetic resonance imaging, computed tomography, electromyography, or other diagnostic tools may be indicated to establish oral/muscular/temporomandibular joint health factors. Etiologic factors for CDH or NCCLs are commonly related to and/or produce complex head and neck as well as masticatory system pathologies. An understanding of how these factors can interact requires knowledge of anatomy, histology, biochemistry, periodontology, and occlusion.

Clinical examination

Extraoral examination

An extraoral examination should be performed first. The masticatory muscles should be palpated with 1 kg of force to determine if sensitive musculature exists in the presence of symptoms resulting from overwork or lactic acid buildup, which may indicate a sign of bruxism, other forms of parafunction, or muscular adaptation.

Intraoral examination

Intraoral examination includes an evaluation of the condition of any restorations (satisfactory or unsatisfactory) as

Fig 7-1 Note the extensive wear facet with curved surface in the maxillary right canine and the presence of a "dentin island"' in the first molar. Whereas the lesion at the cervical of the first premolar is a biocorrosive abfractive lesion, a dentin island is a cupping that appears on an occlusal surface.

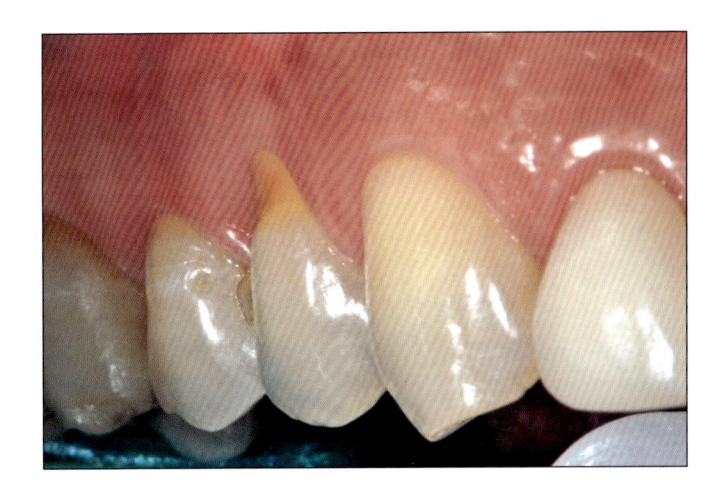

well as identification of any caries lesions. Of particular importance for diagnosis of NCCLs is the surface roughness of the enamel and dentin as well as the condition of the cementoenamel junction (CEJ) regions to determine if caries or the beginnings of NCCLs are present. Clinical recordings should include the descriptive location of any infractions present in enamel. These should be photographed and preserved as part of the record. They can also be used to enhance patient understanding and awareness of their oral condition prior to any treatment.

Periodontal examination

The presence of visible plaque or calculus can indicate the need for periodontal therapies prior to an occlusal determination. Gingival recessions should be noted on the basis of the Miller classification system.[4] All gingival recessions, which are considered the first stage of CDH and NCCLs, should be carefully investigated. They may be linked to mechanical trauma from occlusal interferences and the action of chemical biocorrosives, ill-fitting restorations in the cervical region with unsatisfactory margins, or lack of bony support.[5]

Occlusal examination

Mounted study casts in centric occlusion (CO) preserve the wear facets and can serve as an initial investigative tool by which to evaluate the occlusion. Manipulation of the mandible from a centric relation (CR) position may uncover prematurities in CO, lateral excursions, or protrusive interferences, all of which contribute to occlusal imbalance and thereby the development of CDH[6] and NCCLs.[4,7,8] The clinician also needs to determine if CO and maximal intercuspal position are coincident or not. If not, this may result in occlusal imbalance.

Conditions resulting in wear facets may suggest the presence of some type of active or inactive parafunctional habit, occlusal overload, or mandibular deviation due to occlusal interference. The presence of parafunctional habits (eg, bruxism) is considered a factor that may enhance the development of NCCLs.[9-11] Some wear facets present a "dentin island" that determines the most severe load factor (Fig 7-1).

Other examinations

Supplementary examinations for completing a diagnosis, such as a request for a computed tomography scan, can enhance analysis of anatomical features including buccal bone thickness, lingual bone height, or possible pulp involvement in cases with deep lesions. A laboratory analysis of salivary components can also be performed as a supplementary test to evaluate the pH, buffering capacity, and salivary flow rates.

Lesion analysis

Morphology

A multifactorial etiology of NCCLs results in different anatomical presentations, which are classified into three morphologies: wedge-shaped, concave, and mixed[12,13] (see chapter 6). The etiologic foundation of differences between these two forms has not been studied, but Coleman has postulated that wedge-shaped lesions result primarily from lateral occlu-

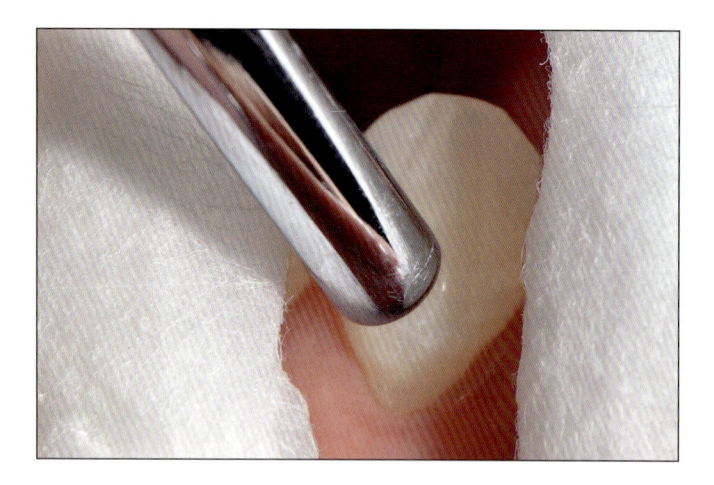

Fig 7-2 Air blast stimulus test with a three-way syringe according to Holland et al.[15] (Courtesy of the NCCL Research Group, Uberlândia, Brazil.)

sal force transmission upon tooth inclines, whereas concave NCCL defects occur from sagittal forces and resultant shear stress associated with flattened occlusal surfaces.[12]

Location

NCCLs may occur on any tooth in any nonocclusal surface region,[14] but studies suggest that depending on the predominant etiologic factor, they can be observed with greater prevalence in certain regions. Wedge-shaped NCCLs and CDH are primarily detected in buccal or labial regions.[12] Lesions in the canines, premolars, and first molars, which are subjected to prolonged contact with the toothbrush and with greater intensity during brushing, may suggest a strong correlation with friction. Similarly, NCCLs on posterior teeth are frequently related to occlusal excursive interferences, because lateral movements involving premolars or molars without contact on the canine can be harmful for the posterior teeth. The presence of lesions in the palatal region of anterior teeth indicates the likely etiology of biocorrosion,[14] while the presence of isolated lesions in the arch may be strongly linked to stress. Localized subgingival lesions are primarily associated with stress and biocorrosion.

Diagnostic protocols for CDH

By definition, CDH is characterized by short, sharp pain arising from exposed dentinal tubules in response to stimuli, typically thermal, that cannot be ascribed to any other form of dental defect or disease.[15-19] The investigation of objective CDH detection and quantification can be accomplished with the air indexing method combined with T-Scan (Tekscan) occlusal analysis.

Air indexing

Many stimuli will cause this pain, but not all are suited for quantifying CDH. Tactile, cold, and evaporative air stimuli are recommended because they are both physiologic and controllable. One example of a response-based method is the use of a timed air blast. The patient's response can be quantified by using a visual analog scale (VAS).[15] The interval between applications of the stimulus should be specified, because a prolonged blast of air causes pronounced desiccation, thereby reducing sensory response to dentinal fluid flow.[20,21] Patients with CDH will have a painful response to the stimuli at the site of the air blast. If pain is experienced at any site other than the site of the air blast, other potential etiologic factors may be at play.

Because patients have different pain thresholds and perceptions, in 1997 Holland proposed a method to standardize the air jet in order to facilitate quantification. First an air blast is directed to the buccal surface of teeth without CDH, so the patient will have a baseline for no pain (0 on VAS scale). Then the tooth with suspected CDH is isolated using cotton rolls, and the air-water syringe is used for 2 seconds from a distance of approximately 10 mm directed at the CEJ of the tooth.

Patients estimate their pain on a 10-point VAS (1–10): 0 = no pain; 1–3 = mild pain; 4–6 = moderate pain; and 7–10 = severe pain. Air blast stimuli were tested with a three-way syringe (Fig 7-2); the air was delivered from a standard dental unit air syringe at 40 psi (±5 psi).[22] The recognition of a patient threshold response is subsequently retested 1 minute later, such that only verified responses are recorded as an indication of further clinical etiologic determination.

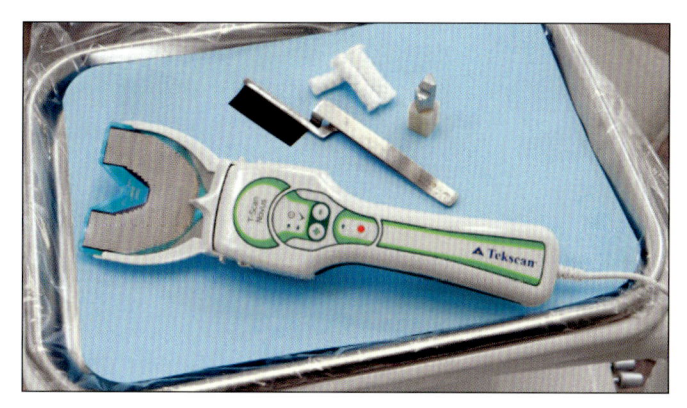

Fig 7-3 T-Scan apparatus.

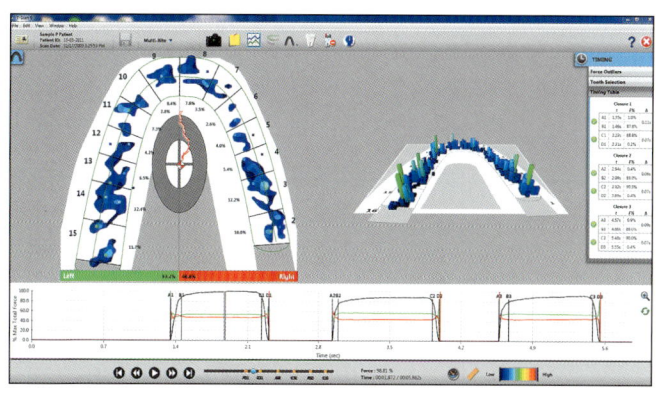

Fig 7-4 The T-Scan desktop display for occlusal analysis.

T-Scan occlusal analysis

T-Scan technology enables the clinician to measure the occlusion time, disocclusion time, and force distribution during full intercuspation (Fig 7-3). The T-Scan desktop display can be manipulated to capture occlusal force values for any time point during closure or excursive analysis (Fig 7-4). Values of force and timing have been extensively studied and used to establish optimal occlusion and disocclusion times for physiologic masticatory muscle contractile health.[23–43] Some studies concluded that less than 0.2 seconds is optimal for occlusion time (ie, the time elapsed from the first point of contact until static intercuspation is reached) and less than 0.5 seconds is optimal for disocclusion time (ie, the elapsed time required for all posterior teeth to disengage from each other during excursive movements). Values outside these norms may indicate excessive muscle load.

It was observed that periodontal and pulp neurosensory information received during function, hyperfunction, and/or parafunction regulate masticatory muscle contraction.[44–53] The presence of CDH denotes that pulp neurosensory input occurs during systemic regulation of masticatory muscle contractions, in the same way as does periodontal mechanoreceptor stimulation during intercuspation. Therefore, in the presence of chronic CDH, atypical T-Scan force recordings highlight masticatory muscle avoidance/adaptive contractions.[36,54–56] Furthermore, the combination of objective T-Scan analysis and the air indexing method to analyze occlusal contacts and CDH response expands the clinician's diagnostic and treatment capabilities compared with traditional, nondigital occlusal indicators.

Case Report

The patient presented with complaints about dentin sensitivity (Fig 7-5a). The first steps in making a diagnosis were to gather a complete medical and dental history, request a diet diary to be analyzed at the following consultation scheduled 1 week later, supervise the patient as he brushed his teeth, and perform prophylaxis and a clinical examination.

Reported history

- Athlete (soccer player)
- Highly anxious
- No systemic changes
- Maintains a balanced diet
- Consumes an excessive number of sports drinks
- Reports clenching during the day and night
- Brushes with excessive force

Clinical examination

- Pain during palpation of the right and left temporal muscle
- Obvious facial asymmetry
- Satisfactory Class I metal restorations on maxillary right second molar and mandibular left first molar
- Satisfactory Class III restoration on maxillary left canine
- Unsatisfactory metal-ceramic crown on mandibular right first molar (Fig 7-5b)
- NCCLs on maxillary right canine to first molar teeth, maxillary left lateral incisor to second premolar teeth, mandibular left canine to second molar teeth, and mandibular right canine to first molar teeth. Both wedge-shaped lesions (Figs 7-5c and 7-5d) and round-angled lesions (Fig 7-5e) were noted.

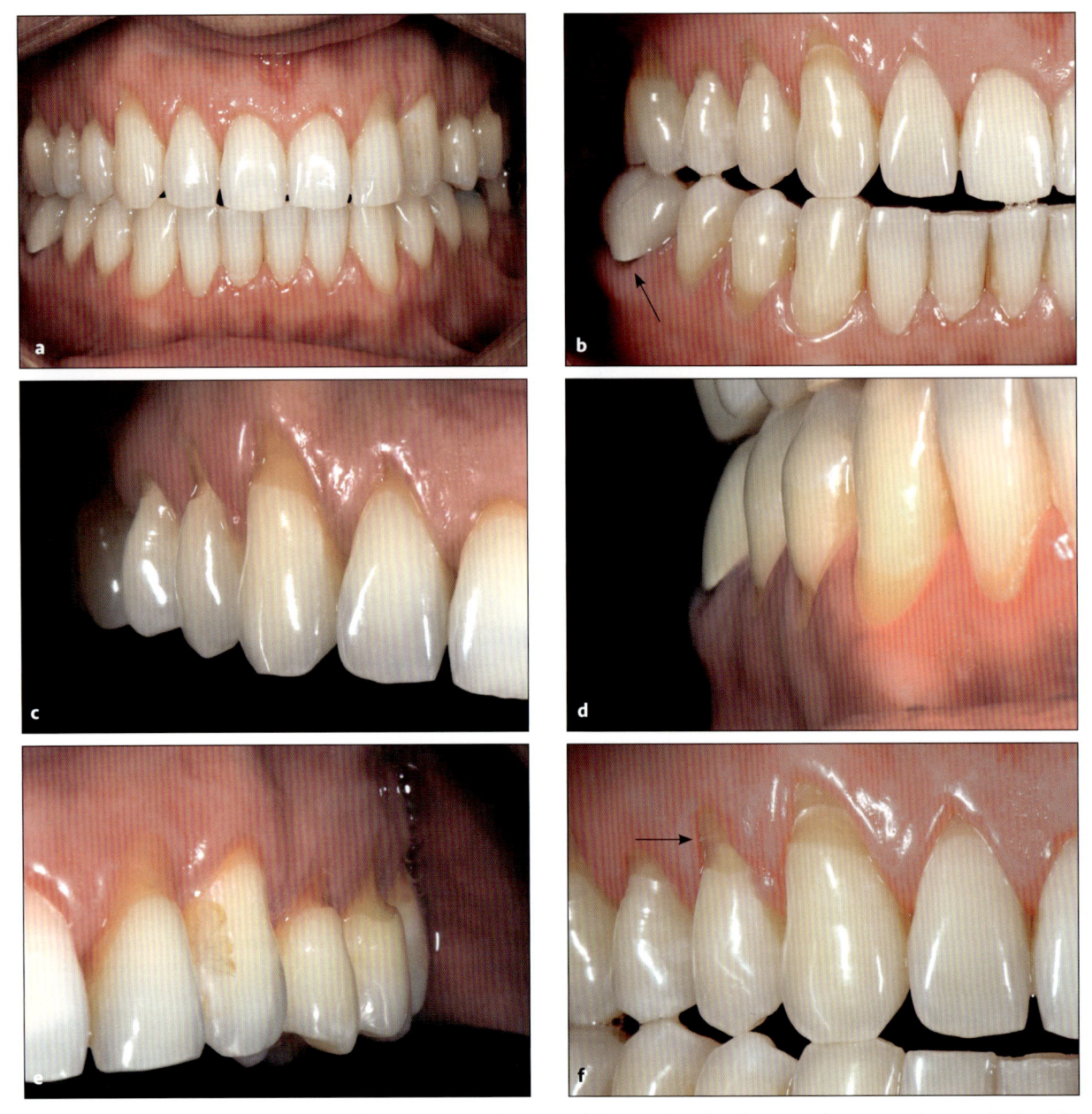

7 Clinical Analysis and Diagnosis of CDH and NCCLs

Fig 7-5 *(a)* Facial view at presentation. *(b)* Note the exposed margin of the porcelain-fused-to-metal crown on the mandibular right first molar. *(c)* Wedge-shaped lesions on the maxillary right canine to second premolar. *(d)* Wedge-shaped NCCLs on the mandibular right canine to first molar; there is little loss of dental structure, but the patient has severe CDH in these teeth. *(e)* Note the rounded angles of the NCCLs on the maxillary left lateral incisor to second premolar. *(f)* Right group function. Note the growth lines evident in the first premolar indicating active progression of the lesion associated with biocorrosive effects. →

- Dentin sensitivity that varies in intensity from tooth to tooth
- Class II, division 1 left subdivision malocclusion
- Premature contact in CR in the right first premolars
- Right group function (Fig 7-5f)
- Enamel cracks in the maxillary right canine and first premolar teeth (Fig 7-5g)
- Point wear facets on the maxillary right canine to first molar teeth (Fig 7-5h)
- Visible plaque

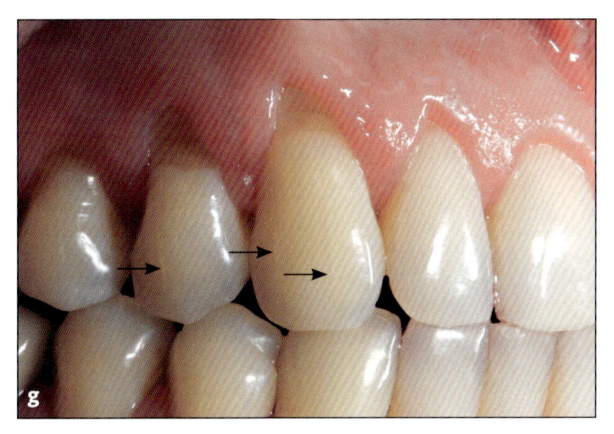

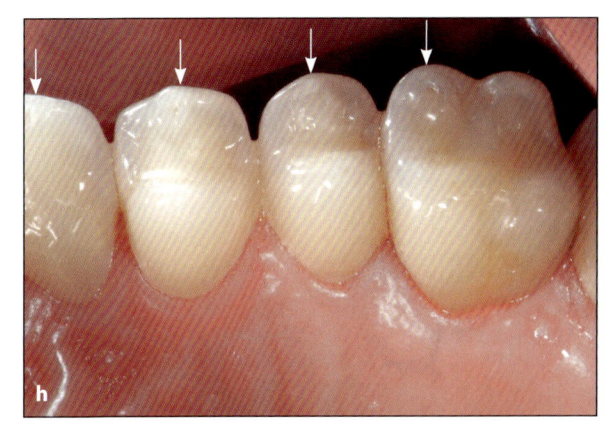

Fig 7-5 *(cont)* *(g)* Enamel cracks in the long axis of the maxillary right canine and first premolar *(arrows)*. *(h)* Wear facets on the maxillary right canine to first molar represented as a single point *(arrows)*. (Courtesy of the NCCL Research Group, Uberlândia, Brazil.)

Diagnosis

- Because the patient reports excessive consumption of sports drinks, verified by the presence of visible plaque during the clinical examination, biocorrosion is a major contributing factor. The presence of multiple lesions with rounded angles also suggests the influence of biocorrosion.
- The patient's self-reported history of clenching, the wear facets on the maxillary posterior teeth, and the enamel cracks in the maxillary right canine and first premolar indicate that biomechanical stress is a problem for this patient. The patient's response to muscle palpation confirms muscle overload, most likely generated by clenching, as well as occlusal instability that generates occlusal overload in several teeth. More severe occlusal overload is manifested as enamel cracks and wear facets.
- The patient is observed to brush with excessive force, resulting in frictional wear of the already weakened tooth structure.

All of these etiologic factors must be properly identified and eliminated in order to stem the progression of NCCLs and offer long-term treatment solutions.

Conclusion

Let's review what we have covered in this chapter:
- A thorough patient interview is essential for diagnosis.
- Full-mouth radiographic analysis and comprehensive oral examination are the basic tools for establishing an etiologic differential diagnosis for CDH and NCCLs.
- Additional imaging modalities or diagnostic tools may be indicated to establish other health factors.
- Clinical examination includes extraoral examination, intraoral examination, periodontal examination, and occlusal examination.
- The morphology and location of NCCLs should be considered as they relate to etiology.
- CDH can be diagnosed by a combination of air indexing and T-Scan occlusal analysis.

References

1. Reyes E, Hildebolt C, Langenwalter E, Miley D. Abfractions and attachment loss in teeth with premature contacts in centric relation: Clinical observations. J Periodontol 2009;80:1955-1962.
2. Takehara J, Takano T, Akhter R, Morita M. Correlations of noncarious cervical lesions and occlusal factors determined by using pressure-detecting sheet. J Dent 2008;36:774-779.
3. Grippo JO, Simring M, Coleman TA. Abfraction abrasion, biocorrosion, and the enigma of noncarious cervical lesions: A 20-year perspective. J Esthet Restor Dent 2012;24:10-25.
4. Miller N, Penaud J, Ambrosini P, Bisson-Boutelliez C, Briançon S. Analysis of etiologic factors and periodontal conditions involved with 309 abfractions. J Clin Periodontol 2003;30:828-832.
5. Lafzi A, Abolfazli N, Eskandari A. Assessment of the etiologic factors of gingival recession in a group of patients in Northwest Iran. J Dent Res Dent Clin Dent Prospects 2009;3:90-93.
6. Kornfeld B. Preliminary report of clinical observations of cervical erosions, a suggested analysis of the cause and the treatment for its relief. Dental Items of Interest 1932;54:905-909.
7. Madani AO, Ahmadian-Yazdi A. An investigation into the relationship between noncarious cervical lesions and premature contacts. Cranio 2005;23:10-15.
8. Brandini DA, Trevisan CL, Panzarini SR, Pedrini D. Clinical evaluation of the association between noncarious cervical lesions and occlusal forces. J Prosthet Dent 2012;108:298-303.
9. Ommerborn MA, Schneider C, Giraki M, et al. In vivo evaluation of noncarious cervical lesions in sleep bruxism subjects. J Prosthet Dent 2007;98:150-158.
10. Brandini DA, Pedrini D, Panzarini SR, Benete IM, Trevisan CL. Clinical evaluation of the association of noncarious cervical lesions, parafunctional habits, and TMD diagnosis. Quintessence Int 2012;43:255-262.
11. Telles D, Pegoraro LF, Pereira JC. Incidence of noncarious cervical lesions and their relation to the presence of wear facets. J Esthet Restor Dent 2006;18:178-183.
12. Hur B, Kim HC, Park JK, Versluis A. Characteristics of non-carious cervical lesions—An ex vivo study using micro computed tomography. J Oral Rehabil 2011;38:469-474.
13. Boricic J, Anic I, Urek MM, Ferreri S. The prevalence of non-carious cervical lesions in permanent dentition. J Oral Rehabil 2004;31:117-123.
14. Levitch LC, Bader JD, Heyman HO. Non-carious cervical lesions. J Dent 1994;22:195-207.
15. Holland GR, Narhi MN, Addy M, Gangarosa L, Orchardson R. Guidelines for the design and conduct of clinical trials on dentine hypersensitivity. J Clin Periodontol 1997;24:808-813.
16. Canadian Advisory Board on Dentin Hypersensitivity. Consensus-based recommendations for the diagnosis and management of dentin hypersensitivity. J Can Dent Assoc 2003;69:221-228.
17. Shiau HJ. Dentin hypersensitivity. J Evid Based Dent Pract 2012;12(suppl 3):220-228.
18. Lussi A, Hellwig E. Diagnosis and management of exposed cervical dentin. Foreword. Clin Oral Investig 2013;17(suppl 1):S1-S2.
19. Gernhardt CR. How valid and applicable are current diagnostic criteria and assessment methods for dentin hypersensitivity? An overview. Clin Oral Investig 2013;17(suppl 1):S31-S40.
20. Pashley DH. Mechanisms of dentin sensitivity. Dent Clin North Am 1990;34:449-473.
21. Matthews WG, Showman CD, Pashley DH. Air blast-induced evaporative water loss from human dentine, in vitro. Arch Oral Biol 1993;38:517-523.
22. Samuel SR, Khatri SG, Acharya S, Patil ST. Evaluation of instant desensitization after a single topical application over 30 days: A randomized trial. Aust Dent J 2015;60:336-342.
23. Kerstein RB, Radke J. Clinician accuracy when subjectively interpreting articulating paper markings. Cranio 2014;32:13-23.
24. Kerstein RB. Handbook of Research on Computerized Occlusal Analysis Technology Applications in Dental Medicine. Hershey, PA: IGI Global, 2015.
25. Qadeer S, Kerstein R, Kim RJ, Huh JB, Shin SW. Relationship between articulation paper mark size and percentage of force measured with computerized occlusal analysis. J Adv Prosthodont 2012;4:7-12.
26. Kerstein RB, Wright NR. Electromyographic and computer analyses of patients suffering from chronic myofascial pain-dysfunction syndrome: Before and after treatment with immediate complete anterior guidance development. J Prosthet Dent 1991;66:677-686.
27. Kerstein RB, Farrell S. Treatment of myofascial pain-dysfunction syndrome with occlusal equilibration. J Prosthet Dent 1990;63:695-700.
28. Kerstein RB. Disocclusion time-reduction therapy with immediate complete anterior guidance development to treat chronic myofascial pain-dysfunction syndrome. Quintessence Int 1992;23:735-747.
29. Kerstein RB. A comparison of traditional occlusal equilibration and immediate complete anterior guidance development. Cranio 1993;11:126-139.
30. Kerstein RB. Disclusion time measurement studies: A comparison of disclusion time between chronic myofascial pain dysfunction patients and nonpatients: A population analysis. J Prosthet Dent 1994;72:473-780.
31. Kerstein RB. Treatment of myofascial pain dysfunction syndrome with occlusal therapy to reduce lengthy disclusion time—A recall evaluation. Cranio 1995;13:105-115.
32. Kerstein RB, Chapman R, Klein M. A comparison of ICAGD (immediate complete anterior guidance development) to mock ICAGD for symptom reductions in chronic myofascial pain dysfunction patients. Cranio 1997;15:21-37.
33. Kerstein RB. Current applications of computerized occlusal analysis in dental medicine. Gen Dent 2001;49:521-530.
34. Kerstein RB, Wilkerson DW. Locating the centric relation prematurity with a computerized occlusal analysis system. Compend Contin Educ Dent 2001;22:525-528,530,532.
35. Kerstein RB. Sensitivity and repeatability of various occlusal indicators. J Prosthet Dent 2003;90:310.
36. Kerstein RB. Combining technologies: A computerized occlusal analysis system synchronized with a computerized electromyography system. Cranio 2004;22:96-109.
37. Kerstein RB, Lowe M, Harty M, Radke J. A force reproduction analysis of two recording sensors of a computerized occlusal analysis system. Cranio 2006;24:15-24.
38. Kerstein RB, Radke J. The effect of disclusion time reduction on maximal clench muscle activity levels. Cranio 2006;24:156-165.
39. Carey JP, Craig M, Kerstein RB, Radke J. Determining a relationship between applied occlusal load and articulating paper mark area. Open Dent J 2007;1:1-7.
40. Kerstein RB. Articulating paper mark misconceptions and computerized occlusal analysis technology. Dent Implantol Update 2008;19:41-46.
41. Watkin A, Kerstein RB. Improving darkened anterior peri-implant tissue color with zirconia custom implant abutments. Compend Contin Educ Dent 2008;29:238-240,242.
42. Kerstein RB. Reducing chronic masseter and temporalis muscular hyperactivity with computer-guided occlusal adjustments. Compend Contin Educ Dent 2010;31:530-534,536,538.
43. Kerstein RB, Radke J. Masseter and temporalis excursive hyperactivity decreased by measured anterior guidance development. Cranio 2012;30:243-254.
44. Sharav Y, Mcgrath PA, Dubner R. Masseter inhibitory periods and sensations evoked by electrical tooth pulp stimulation in patients with oral-facial pain and mandibular dysfunction. Arch Oral Biol 1982;27:305-310.
45. Riise C, Sheikholeslam A. The influence of experimental interfering occlusal contacts on the postural activity of the anterior temporal and masseter muscles in young adults. J Oral Rehabil 1982;9:419-425.
46. Xhonga FA. Bruxism and its effect on the teeth. J Oral Rehabil 1977;4:65-76.
47. Gremillion HA. The relationship between occlusion and TMD: An evidence-based discussion. J Evid Based Dent Pract 2006;6:43-47.
48. Laurell L, Lundgren D. Interfering occlusal contacts and distribution of chewing and biting forces in dentitions with fixed cantilever prostheses. J Prosthet Dent 1987;58:626-632.
49. Swenson HM. ABC's periodontics—"O" is for Occlusal adjustment. J Indiana Dent Assoc 1990;69:7-8.

50. Mohl ND, Zarb GA, Carlsson GE, Rugh JD. A Textbook of Occlusion. Chicago: Quintessence, 1991.
51. Burgett FG. Trauma from occlusion. Periodontal concerns. Dent Clin North Am 1995;39:301–311.
52. Ruiz JL. Achieving longevity in esthetic dentistry by the proper diagnosis and management of occlusal disease. Contemporary Esthetics 2007;11(6):24–30.
53. Suganuma T, Ono Y, Shinya A, Furuya R. The effect of bruxism on periodontal sensation in the molar region: A pilot study. J Prosthet Dent 2007;98:30–35.
54. Coleman TA, Grippo JO, Kinderknecht KE. Cervical dentin hypersensitivity. Part III: Resolution following occlusal equilibration. Quintessence Int 2003;34:427–434.
55. Ikeda T, Yasumura H, Yokoyama M, et al. A report of hypersensitive teeth induced by abnormal occlusal contacts. Nihon Hotetsu Shika Gakkai Zasshi 1987;31:36–42.
56. Harrel SK, Nunn ME, Hallmon WW. Is there an association between occlusion and periodontal destruction?: Yes—Occlusal forces can contribute to periodontal destruction. J Am Dent Assoc 2006;137:1380,1382,1384.

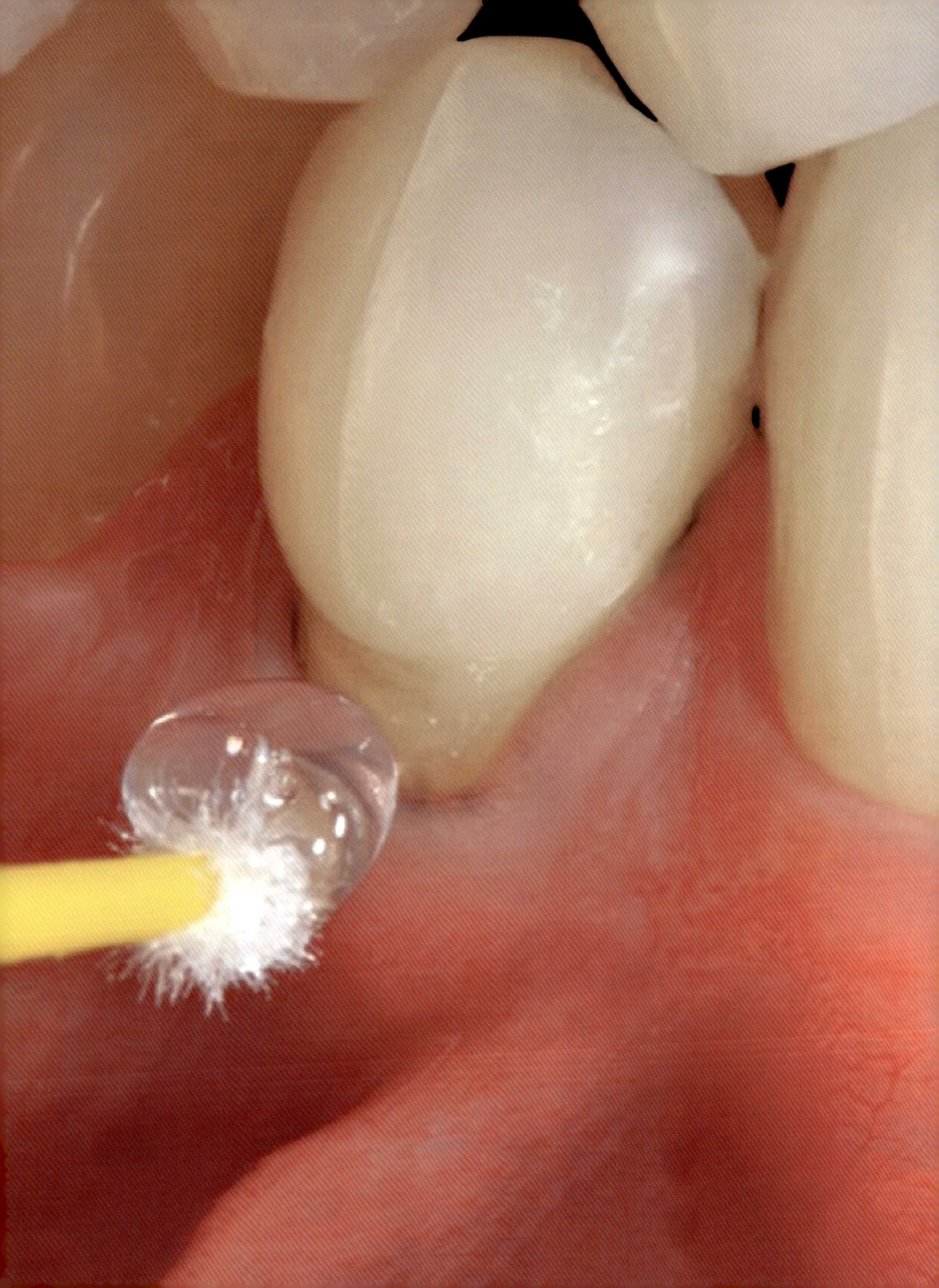

8

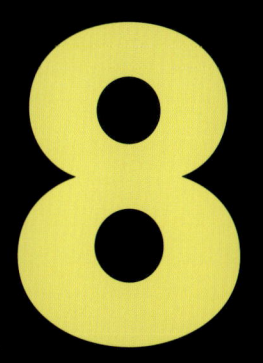

Nonrestorative Protocols: Occlusal, Chemical, and Laser Therapies

Etiologic determination is necessary prior to selecting treatment strategies for cervical dentin hypersensitivity (CDH) and noncarious cervical lesions (NCCLs). This allows treatment to focus on the cause of the problem rather than the symptoms. Furthermore, preventive investigation can reduce the environmental and systemic conditions that induce the oral nociception (pain) caused by biocorrosion, mechanical stress concentration, and/or friction mechanisms. Any preventive management strategy should consider the following:

- Control of parafunctional habits like bruxism and clenching
- Evaluation of occlusal prematurities, as they may relate to the initiation of CDH
- Avoidance of desensitizers prior to professional examination, which can mask CDH symptoms during its etiologic determination
- Treatment of periodontal factors
- Reduction of acidic diet and identification of gastroesophageal reflux disease, which promote control of exogenous or endogenous biocorrosion events, respectively
- Avoidance of toothbrushing with hard bristles and use of abrasive dentifrices and reduction in force used during brushing

Occlusal analysis, determination of active parafunction, diagnosis of endogenous or exogenous biocorrosion, treatment planning, and subsequent care prolong treatment time, so patients and clinicians may elect to use desensitizing agents to control the nociception of CDH primarily caused by dentin exposure.

Occlusal Therapy

Studies have documented that excessive occlusal force leads to stress generation in the cervical area and consequent breakage

8 Nonrestorative Protocols: Occlusal, Chemical, and Laser Therapies

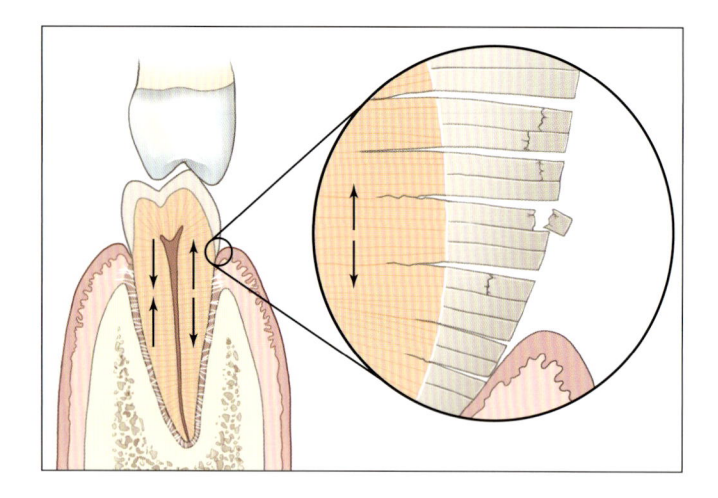

Fig 8-1 Schematic drawing demonstrating the onset of the abfractive process due to excessive occlusal loading. These cyclic occlusal forces produce stress and strain from tension and compression, which lead to enamel crystalline failure.

of enamel prisms[1,2] (Fig 8-1). This enamel breakdown facilitates the development of CDH and NCCLs as stress leads to tooth degradation (see chapter 3). However, occlusal therapy can mitigate this process by reducing the forces imposed on the teeth.

Occlusal imbalance

Occlusal imbalance may be caused by a number of factors. Natural factors include defects in craniofacial development, defects in tooth structure and/or tooth eruption, and tooth drifting, tilting, or supereruption resulting from the lack of an opposing counterpart. Restorative dental procedures or orthodontic treatment may also lead to unbalanced occlusal force patterns, producing deflective contacts and/or changes in the force vectors on the occlusal table.[3] Because stress is a function of force over area ($S = F/A$),[4] minor forces with small intercuspal contact areas have the potential to create severe stresses to the enamel and cervical regions of teeth, and chronic microtrauma has been associated with CDH and the formation of NCCLs from abfraction.[5–8]

Muscular adaptation

Investigations by Ikeda et al[9,10] and Riise and Sheikholeslam[11] showed that the masticatory musculature adapts to different situations. In the first week, increased contractility of muscles on the ipsilateral side followed by increased tonus of the contralateral musculature occurred in consequence of artificial prematurities. Electromyographic (EMG) values returned to normal once these prematurities were removed. Less severe occlusal disorders can result in major masticatory signs and/or symptoms of occlusal pathology.

Indications for occlusal therapy

Occlusal therapy is indicated for the following clinical situations:

- To treat microtraumatic occlusion (causing tooth pain, CDH, periodontal bone loss, abfractive lesions, and other forms of occlusal disease [OD])
- To treat muscular temporomandibular joint disorders (diagnosed by the presence of pain or parafunctional habits)
- As a refinement to clinical procedures (orthodontic, surgical, restorative)

Recording media for occlusal therapy

Time, expense, recording viability, training, and learning curve needs may all be factors related to the type of occlusal analysis performed in a given practice. Because of the relationship between occlusion/intercuspation and vertical bone loss, CDH, NCCLs, wear facets, temporomandibular joint and muscular pain, tooth or restorative fractures, and other manifestations of OD, Christensen has repeatedly called for improved professional education in occlusal knowledge during professional training.[12,13] This section therefore outlines several recording media and techniques that can be used in occlusal therapy. After all, the accuracy of the recording medium and protocol used in large part determines the effectiveness of occlusal therapy. Clinicians are not expected to use all of these protocols on a daily basis, but they should be able to select different materials or techniques when confronted by clinical failures and recognize signs and symptoms of CDH and NCCL progression related to occlusal pathologies and treat them.

Occlusal Therapy

Fig 8-2 Various books of articulating paper.

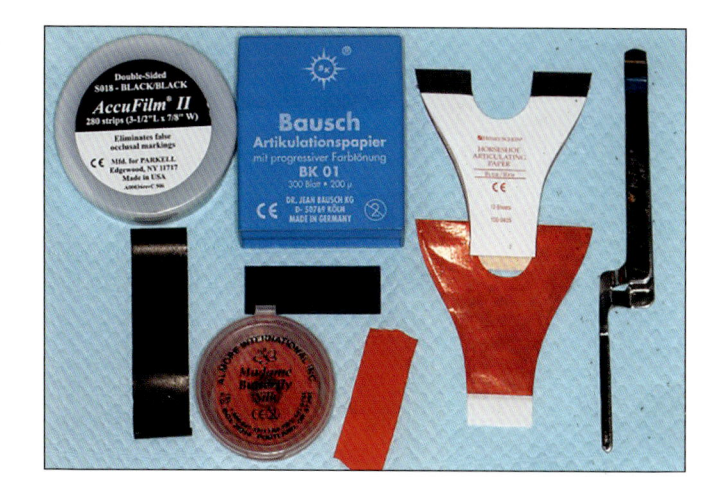

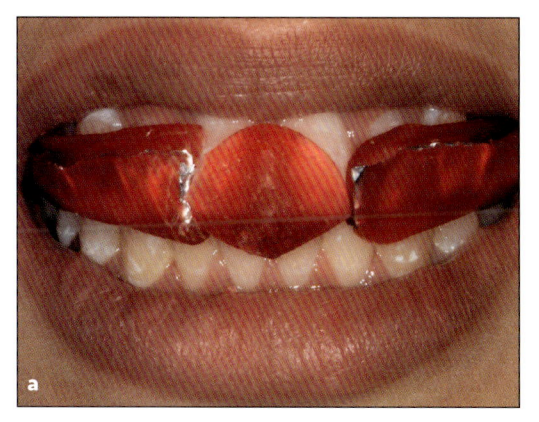

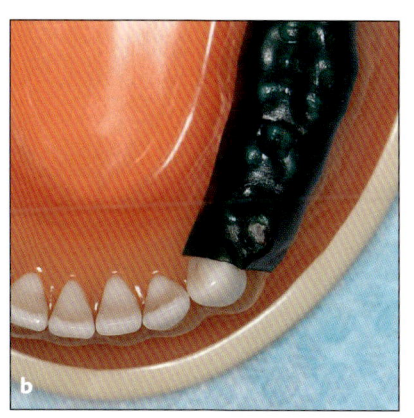

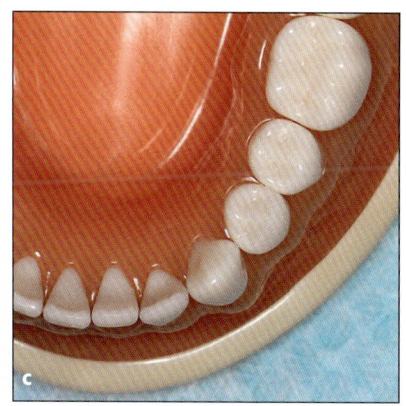

Fig 8-3 *(a)* Occlusal wax associated with Lucia JIG. *(b and c)* Wax indicators.

Occlusal indicating papers

Articulating papers (Fig 8-2) are available in thin or thick versions and are used to register occlusal dimensions. Low cost, easy access, disposability, and the possibility of visual analysis are some of the technical advantages. A potential for moisture contamination and deflection by the tongue or cheek are some disadvantages. The dental auxiliary can support the operator in reducing muscular or moisture difficulties.

In 2012, Qadeer et al[14] showed few associations between articulating papers and recordings with T-Scan (Tekscan) digital occlusal analysis (see later section and chapter 7). This same investigation of occlusal recordings found no relationship between force values and the thickness of articulating papers.

Occlusal wax indicators

Occlusal wax indicators (Fig 8-3) help the clinician and patient visualize the intercuspation. Like articulating papers, they offer an inexpensive investigative tool for intercuspal recording. Bending wax over dried teeth helps to fixate the wax prior to mandibular closing movements. Although wax markings do not record force or timing values, registrations may detect initial points of intercuspation that require further investigation. Waxes are a useful medium for enhancing patient visualization of existing contacts when occlusal diagnostic work-ups are in progress. However, the clinician needs to use a method to mark the occlusal surfaces that correspond to regions of anticipated occlusal modification prior to removing the wax. Assistance from auxiliary staff is helpful to avoid wax record distortion.

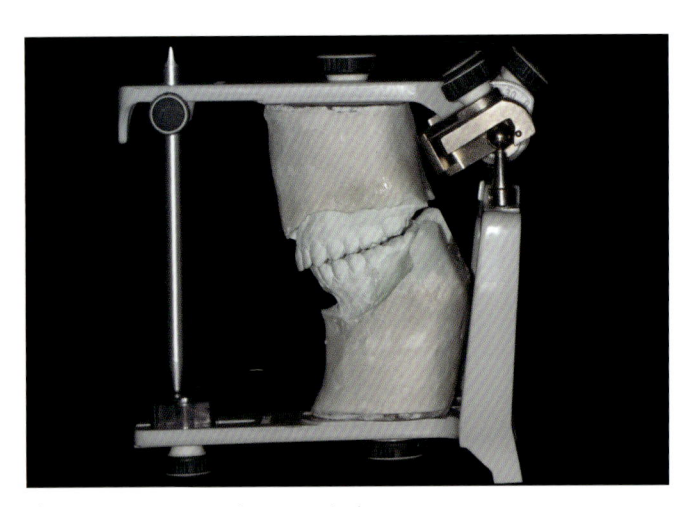

8 Nonrestorative Protocols: Occlusal, Chemical, and Laser Therapies

Fig 8-4 Casts mounted on an articulator.

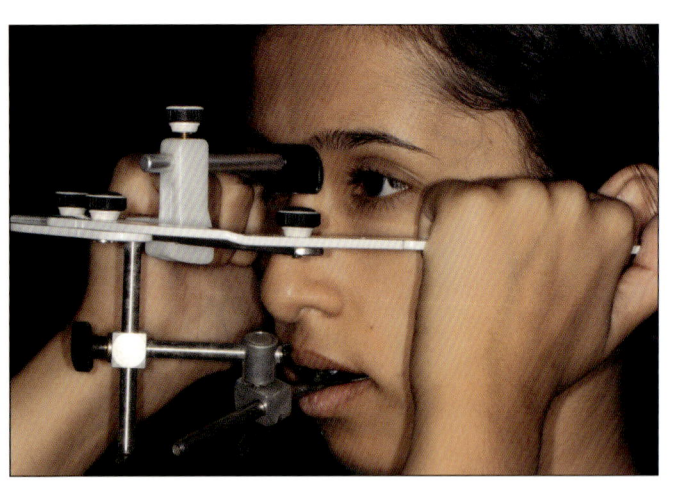

Fig 8-5 Facebow recording of the maxillary arch relative to the Frankfort plane to facilitate the orientation of the maxillary study cast on the articulator.

One disadvantage of occlusal wax recording is that once used, the further recording of occlusal contacts with articulating papers can be restricted. On the other hand, the use of articulating paper prior to wax occlusal registration does not restrict this intercuspation modality. Holders for articulating paper and wax are useful for their placement on occlusal surfaces prior to clinical occlusal registration activities.

Articulating foils

Articulating foils are another low-cost medium for intercuspal occlusal recordings. As with occlusal wax recordings, they most often require a marking medium during oral use and enable the patient and clinician to visualize intercuspal recordings. Foils do not register timing or force values, but unlike waxes they do not restrict the subsequent use of articulating paper. However, they carry no distinct advantage over articulating papers or waxes during occlusal analysis.

Use of articulators

Benchtop evaluation of mounted study casts is an expensive alternative for occlusal evaluation and treatment planning (Fig 8-4). The articulator allows the clinician to visualize and manipulate the intercuspal relationships of the dentition, which is a necessary step for any occlusal therapy. The casts can also be used to track occlusal wear as well as the progressive effects of chronic microtrauma or biocorrosion for NCCLs. These casts may help to detect progressive internal temporomandibular joint (TMJ) pathologies when dental diastemas appear over time, especially when they are related to distalization of molars.[15,16] Mounted study casts are a necessity for comprehensive orthodontic or prosthetic treatment planning[17] as well as for fabrication of occlusal guards. They can also serve as tools for patient-clinician communication.

Auxiliary personnel generally take the preliminary impressions; manufacturer instructions must be followed precisely to ensure the accuracy of study casts. Before the maxillary cast is mounted on the articulator, an accurate facebow recording of the maxillary arch must be performed to establish the relationship of this arch to the horizontal (Frankfort) plane[18] (Fig 8-5). Precise registration of interarch occlusal relationships must then be recorded prior to mounting the mandibular study cast on the articulator (Fig 8-6). Lateral mandibular records must be precisely recorded and transferred to the respective articulator for accuracy. Clinicians must choose between semi- and fully adjustable articulators depending on specific treatment needs. The advantages and disadvantages of the various types of articulators are beyond the scope of this text and available elsewhere.

T-Scan digital analysis

T-Scan digital technology is an expensive investment for the clinician with a steep learning curve, but it offers objective timing and force values specific to each patient's masticatory system and occlusal patterns (see chapter 7 for details). The combination of timing and force values with muscular

Fig 8-6 Mounting of maxillary and mandibular casts on the articulator.

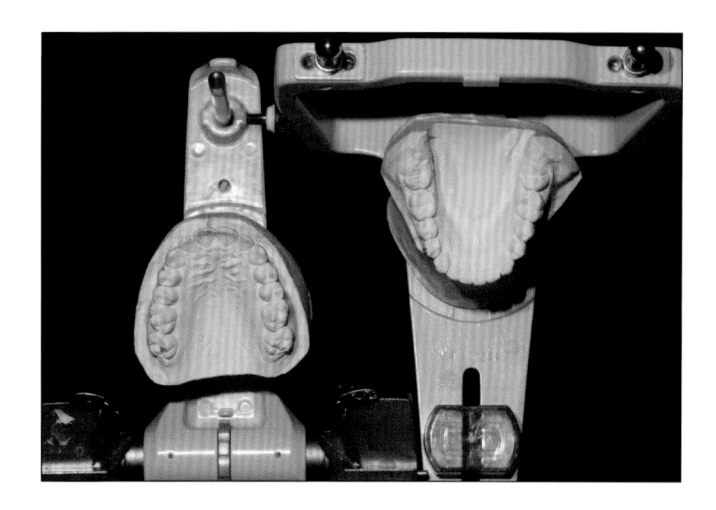

contractility signals provides the clinician with useful information for determining occlusal therapy needs.

Choices for occlusal therapy

Occlusal therapy can be additive or subtractive. That is, tooth height is either added or removed to adjust the occlusion. Once a recording medium has been selected and intercuspal recordings have been evaluated by the clinician, he or she needs to determine if these markings need adjustment to maintain or improve masticatory system balance.

Additive therapy

Canine or anterior guidance[19] along with rapid disarticulation of posterior teeth during lateral mandibular movement[20-24] have been advocated as effective occlusal schemes. Techniques for achieving canine guidance include the following:

- Apply an acid-etched composite resin on the lingual surfaces of maxillary canines or the incisal regions of maxillary or mandibular canines.
- Use computer-aided design/computer-assisted manufacturing (CAD/CAM) in-office technology.
- Fabricate porcelain or zirconia overlays for canines in the laboratory.

Interruption of TMJ health or production of increased masticatory muscle tension is a signal to reduce iatrogenic lateral excursion interference by additive therapy treatment. Additive materials must be inspected on a routine basis to ensure that their integrity is not compromised, which can inhibit physiologic mandibular excursive movements.

Subtractive therapy

Subtractive and selective adjustment is routine in restorative treatment. It is the duty of the clinician to detect and correct prematurities associated with the treatment of caries, esthetic reconstruction, or dental hard tissue loss. The diagnosis of CDH, NCCLs, and other forms of OD require a careful occlusal analysis because minor dimension alterations can result in these major pathologic consequences.[6,8,25,26]

Subtractive occlusal therapy involves chairside modification of vertical height or lateral excursion refinements with low- or high-speed tools. It is most often performed with minimal occlusal adjustment (< 0.1 mm). Premature recordings beyond this dimension may exist during iatrogenic placement of restorative materials. Clinicians often find articulated study casts to be of benefit during occlusal analysis prior to chairside subtractive modification.

Selective occlusal adjustment

Occlusal adjustment refers to subtractive therapy to specific intercuspations of teeth or regions of contacts not involving the entire dentition. Clinicians with good working knowledge of OD may be able to provide localized occlusal adjustments to resolve specific pathologies such as CDH from cervical stress concentration. Selective occlusal modification is indicated

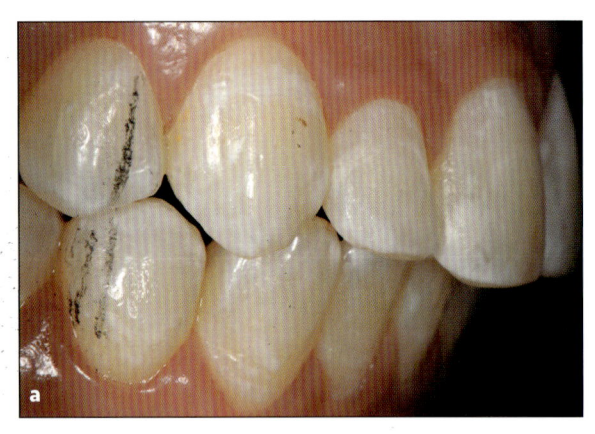

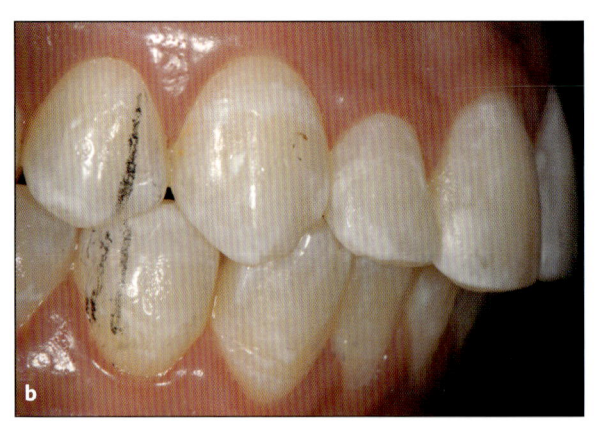

8 Nonrestorative Protocols: Occlusal, Chemical, and Laser Therapies

Fig 8-7 Note the discrepancy between CR *(a)* and MIP *(b)* resulting from a deflective contact. (Courtesy of the NCCL Research Group, Uberlândia, Brazil.)

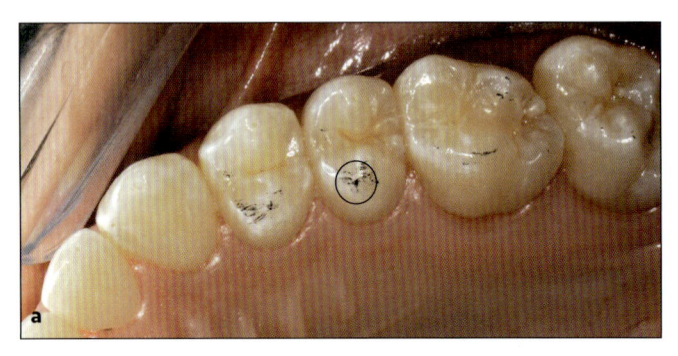

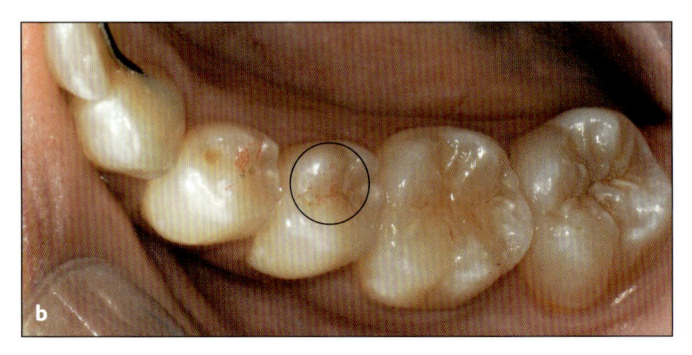

Fig 8-8 *(a and b)* The deflective contact indicated with articulating paper *(circled)*. (Courtesy of the NCCL Research Group, Uberlândia, Brazil.)

for cases in which there are no demands for changes in bony support or tooth positioning or the recovery of lost tooth structure. In this context, the following principles are applied for executing this technique safely:

- Eliminate contacts deflecting the mandible from centric relation (CR) to maximal intercuspal position (MIP) (Fig 8-7).
- Reorient the force vectors to the long axis of posterior teeth.
- Avoid changes in the height of functional cusps, thus avoiding changes in the vertical dimension.
- Refine the lateral contacts of posterior teeth, which restrict anterior disocclusions during lateral excursive or protrusive movements of the mandible.
- Obtain stability in centric occlusion (CO) and avoid further changes in the functional cusps.

Selective occlusal adjustment should always be minimal in nature to enhance masticatory system health rather than detract from it. It is strongly suggested that the complete procedure be mapped and recorded first on an articulator to ensure that the intraoral procedure follows a preestablished sequence.[27,28] Selective occlusal adjustment involves three steps: *(1)* occlusal adjustment in CO, *(2)* occlusal adjustment for lateral excursion prematurities, and *(3)* occlusal adjustment in protrusion.

1. Occlusal adjustment in centric occlusion

Before undertaking this step, the centric relation must be recorded on an articulator. The primary goal of this procedure is to determine in the mouth which teeth have initial points of contact that deflect the mandible away from a CO position. These points of contact are termed *centric prematurities* and are most often associated with deflection on inclines in the sagittal plane. They are commonly detected by the use of articulating papers, foils, or occlusal indicator waxes (Fig 8-8). If this contact is reproduced on the articulator, it means that the mounting is correct. If not, the mounting position should be revised so that any mapping done on the articulator can be reproduced in the mouth. Disparities between articulator recording and oral verification of prematurity data present a challenge for the clinician during the identification of CO deflections. Ultimately, the goal is to make CO coincident with MIP while *(1)* achieving the greatest number of interocclusal contacts independent of the TMJs, *(2)* preserving the vertical dimension of occlusion, *(3)* minimizing or correcting active OD forms, and *(4)*

Occlusal Therapy

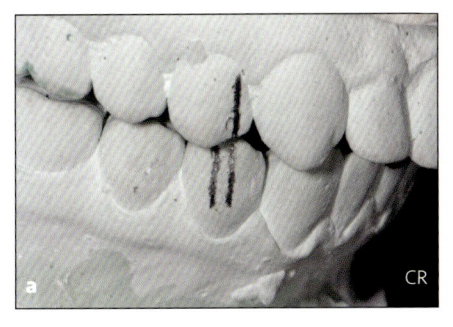

Fig 8-9 Occlusal mapping performed on the articulator. *(a and b)* Verification of CR and MIP on the mounted casts. *(c)* Locating the interfering contact and marking it with articulating paper. *(d and e)* Contact marked on each arch. (Courtesy of the NCCL Research Group, Uberlândia, Brazil.)

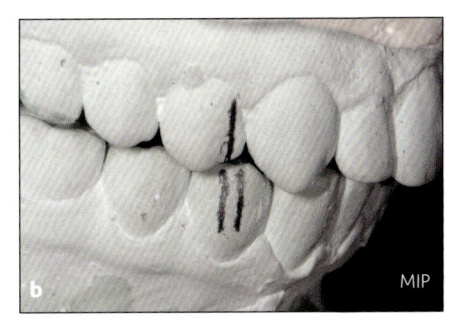

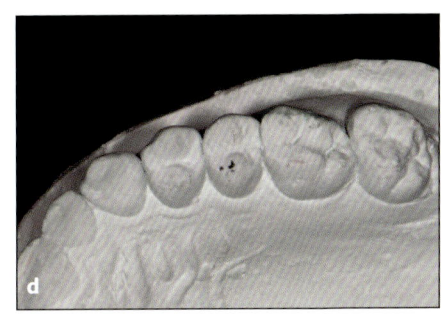

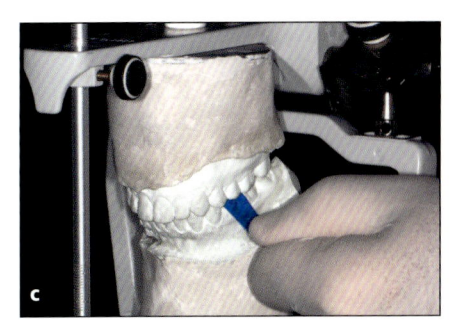

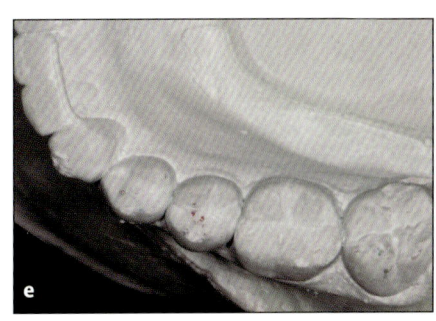

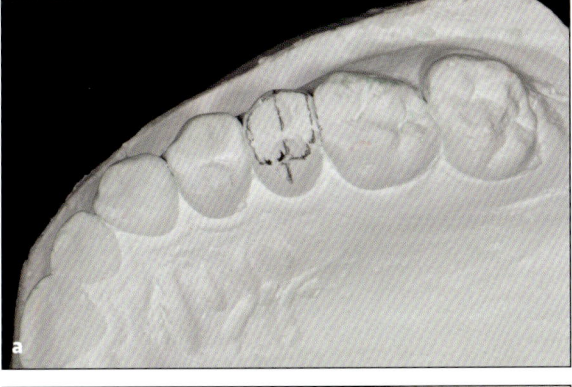

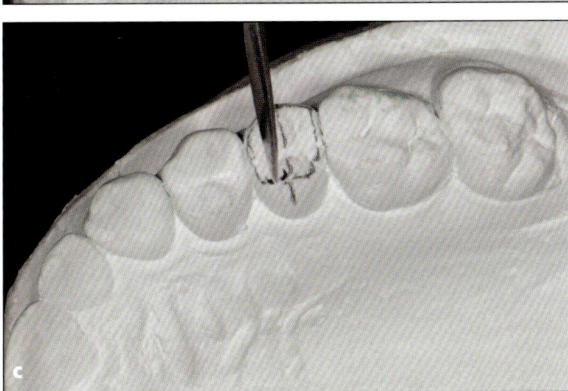

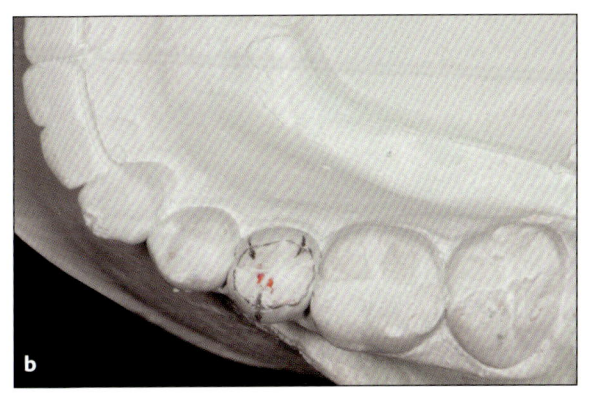

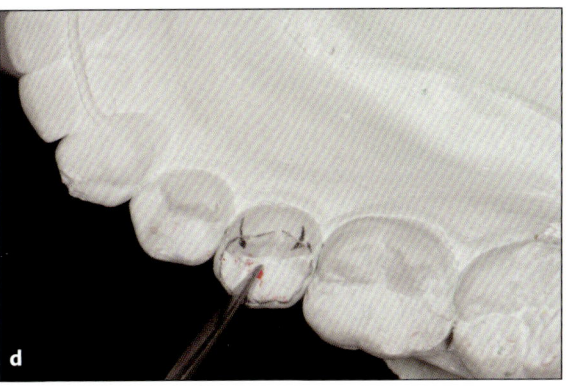

Fig 8-10 *(a and b)* Identification of the structure to be relieved on the occlusal anatomy. *(c and d)* Grinding of both teeth. (Courtesy of the NCCL Research Group, Uberlândia, Brazil.)

enhancing function. Both comfort and functional hinge closure positions should be ensured to reduce the incidence of pain and improve occlusal intercuspal balance.

On the articulator, every contact should first be registered with the articulating paper and then adjusted on the stone cast (Fig 8-9). These contacts must be recorded by the tooth number(s), cusp(s), and specific incline(s) involved in the prematurity. For example, there can be a premature contact between the mesial nonworking incline of the mesiolingual cusp of tooth no. 30 (mandibular right first molar) and the distal working incline of the lingual cusp of no. 4 (maxillary right second premolar). This record identifies where the stone should be shaved to relieve the contact on the articulator (Fig 8-10). The clinician must avoid excessive grinding of tooth stone that could translate to exposed dentin in the mouth.

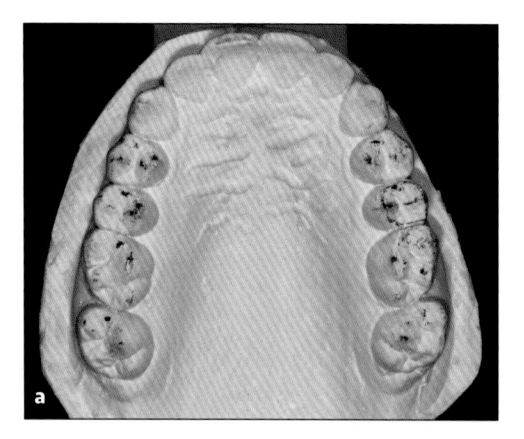

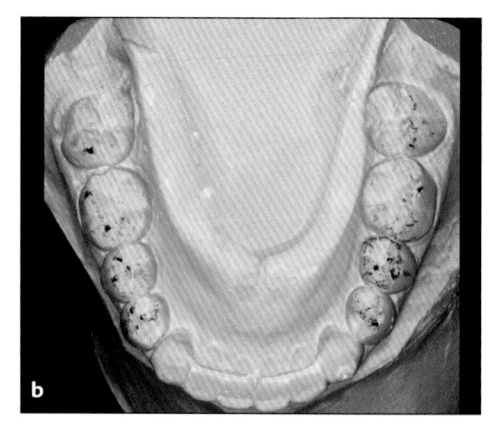

Fig 8-11 *(a and b)* Occlusal adjustment finished in the mounted study casts. Note the contact in all posterior teeth to confirm feasibility in the clinical situation. (Courtesy of the NCCL Research Group, Uberlândia, Brazil.)

Selective grinding is performed based on the type of premature contact:

- *Contact deflecting the mandible away from the midline:* This occurs between two working cusps (both on working inclines). Because both cusps have the same functional importance, the contact closest to the cusp tip should be ground, if necessary, until it reaches the top of the cusp. If this action does not relieve the deflection, the coronoplasty procedure should be performed on the opposite tooth.
- *Contact deflecting the mandible toward the midline:* This occurs between a functional cusp (on the nonfunctional incline) and a nonfunctional cusp (on the functional incline). In this case, the nonfunctional incline should be ground first until the contact achieves the tip of the functional cusp; if the premature contact is still present, the functional incline of the opposite tooth should be ground.
- *Contact deflecting the mandible toward an anterior position:* This occurs between the mesial incline or the transverse ridge of the maxillary tooth (functional cusp) and the distal incline or the transverse ridge of the mandibular tooth (functional cusp). This type of contact can lead to trauma on the anterior teeth, so both teeth must be ground.
- *Premature contact with no deflection of the mandible:* This contact occurs between the tip of a functional cusp and the fossa/marginal ridge of the opposing tooth. It may also happen between the functional cusp and a plateau on the functional incline of the opposing tooth, generated after adjusting other deflective contacts. If the functional cusp is interfering with the working movement, this cusp must be ground; if not, the fossa or plateau must be widened to accommodate the opposing functional cusp.

After grinding this first contact, any further contacts should be mapped and selective grinding performed. All found contacts should be mapped and adjusted until maximal intercuspation is achieved (Fig 8-11). If, for any reason, any tooth remains without contact, it may be necessary to add tooth structure to achieve this particular contact. Furthermore, the anterior guidance must be respected and functional before any procedure is performed on the patient, as this guidance is essential for occlusal balance and TMJ health[29] (Fig 8-12).

2. Occlusal adjustment for lateral excursion prematurities

Once CO is coincident with MIP, the occlusion must be evaluated for eccentric movements.

For adjustment on the working side, the first determination to be made is whether a patient's disocclusion pattern is by canine guidance (Fig 8-13) or group function:

- *Canine guidance:* Only the working canines should be in contact, with no other teeth contacting. If posterior contacts exist, then subtractive therapy of nonworking cusp inclines may be necessary to achieve a canine-rise lateral excursion. If the canine is displaced, twisted, or has some sort of structural loss (eg, bruxism, fractures), it may be necessary to rebuild its functionality before any further adjustment procedure is performed.
- *Group function:* During lateral excursions, canine-rise or canine-protected lateral mandibular contacts exist on posterior teeth as well as the occlusal or incisal surfaces of the canines. These contacts may exist unilaterally or bilaterally depending on respective surface loss. In general, if the group function is not on the canines, the risk of OD pathology increases from chronic micro-

Occlusal Therapy

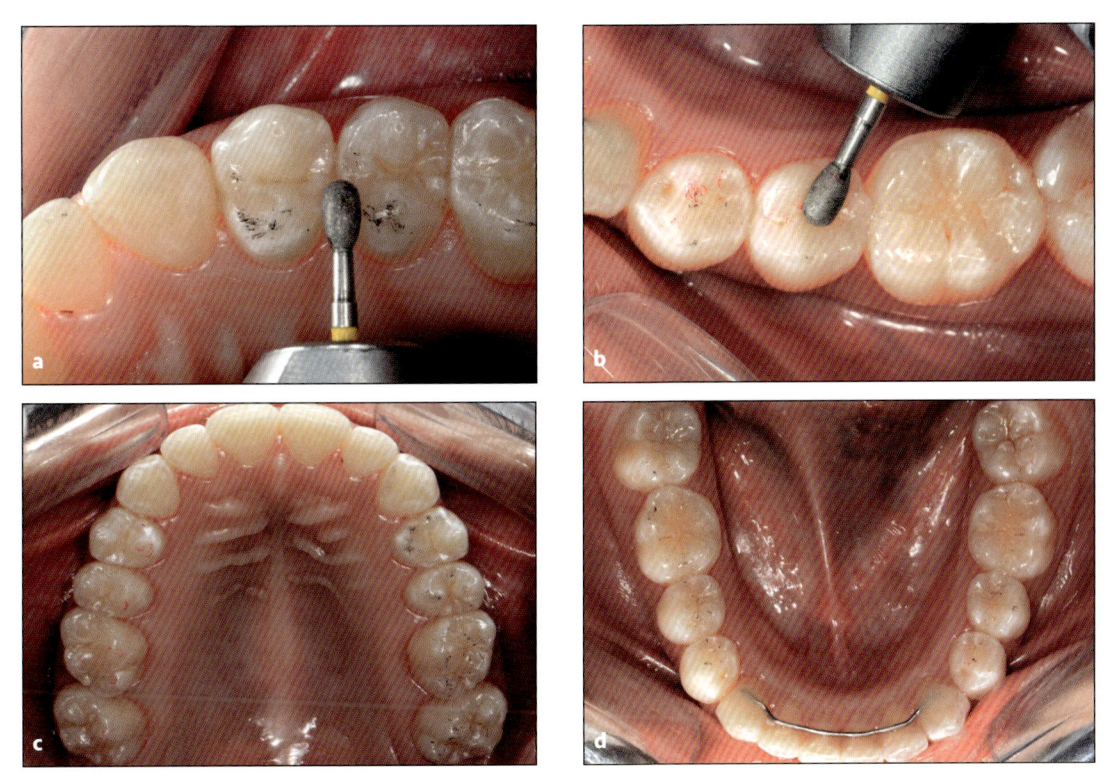

Fig 8-12 *(a and b)* Clinical occlusal adjustment after confirmation in the mounted study casts. As planned on the casts, both teeth were adjusted. *(c and d)* Occlusal adjustment finished in the patient's mouth. Note the contact in all posterior teeth as observed in the mounted study casts. (Courtesy of the NCCL Research Group, Uberlândia, Brazil.)

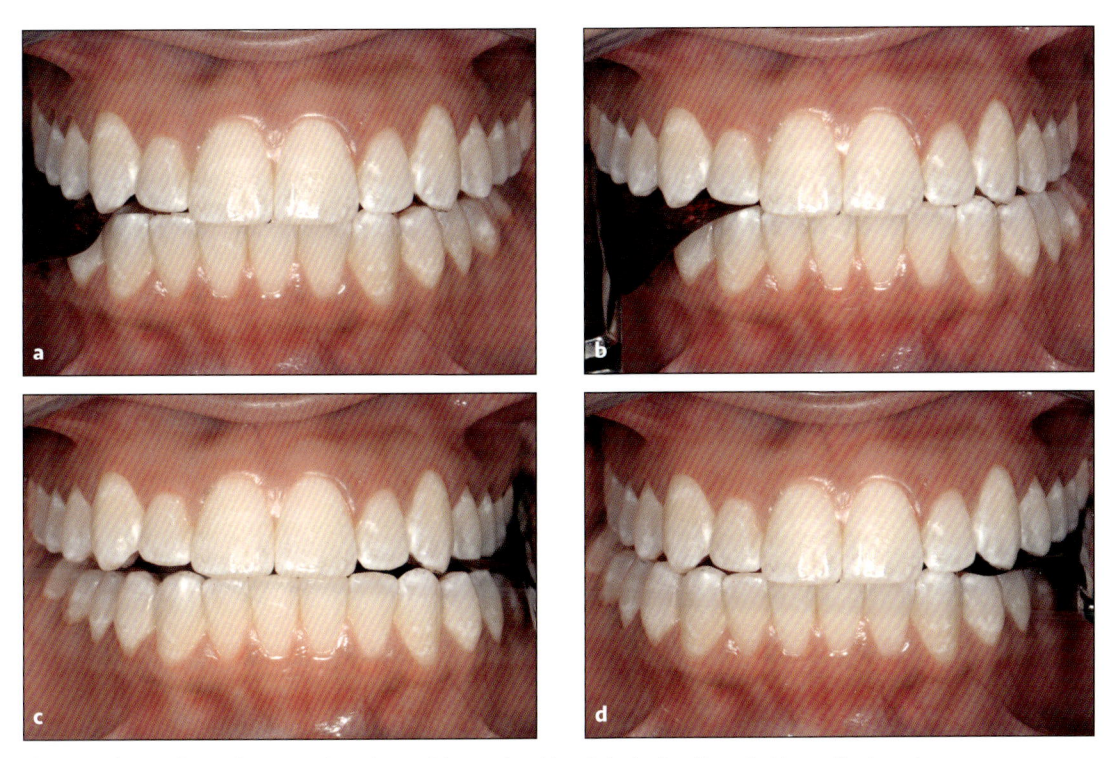

Fig 8-13 *(a to d)* Verification of canine guidance. In this clinical situation, further adjustment was unnecessary. (Courtesy of the NCCL Research Group, Uberlândia, Brazil.)

103

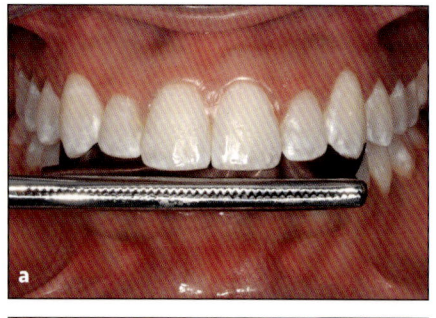

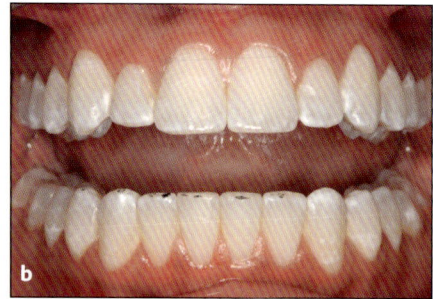

Fig 8-14 *(a to c)* Verification of protrusion with a small interference at the beginning of the movement. *(d)* Performing the necessary adjustment. (Courtesy of the NCCL Research Group, Uberlândia, Brazil.)

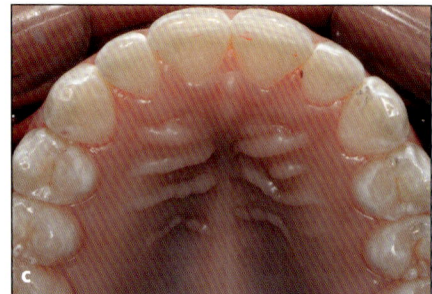

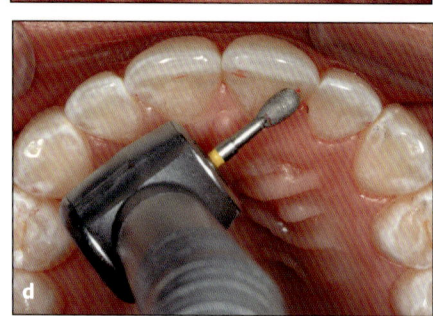

trauma. Any signs or symptoms of OD must be carefully inspected, and any lateral contact adjustment must not interrupt CO.

For adjustment on the balancing side, every posterior tooth that interferes or restricts working-side lateral TMJ translation must be adjusted. Chronic restriction to a contralateral canine-rise excursion can result in meniscus stress, tooth fractures (as well as other forms of OD), or muscular imbalances. Corrective adjustments to ipsilateral occlusal surfaces often give rise to contralateral canine guidance and decreased muscular tonus, so occlusal adjustment to working cusps should be avoided.

3. Occlusal adjustment in protrusion

During protrusive movements from CO, there should be no contacts on posterior teeth because they deflect physiologic TMJ anterior movements. Shearing forces on teeth can result in restoration dislodgement or enamel/dentin fractures if not corrected by occlusal adjustment (Fig 8-14). The clinician must be aware that sudden protrusive interferences arising during these anterior mandibular movements connote internal TMJ derangement.

Conclusion

Clinicians are often confounded by the different approaches to occlusal therapy. A recording of occlusal contacts needs to fall within normal limits of accommodation by the masticatory system to prevent OD. Both CDH and NCCL formation are OD issues resulting from occlusal microtrauma and biocorrosion. Clinicians should become familiar with all occlusal treatment options in order to provide the most favorable functional and esthetic result for each patient.

Chemical Therapy

Chemical desensitizers and occluding agents can be used to prevent further dentin sensitivity and block the mechanism of action of CDH prior to restorative or surgical treatment. These chemical agents can be classified into in-office products and at-home products based on their characteristics and indications. In-office agents are delivered in a professional treatment environment, whereas at-home agents can be applied by the patient. (See Table 1 in the Appendix for scientific data on their effectiveness.) Box 8-1 introduces the three types of desensitizing agents based on their mechanism of action: neural agents, tubule-blocking agents, and mixed agents. Unless otherwise indicated, the following sections discuss in-office agents.

Neural agents: Potassium

A single neural desensitizing agent, potassium (K^+) acts in the process of depolarization and prevents repolarization of the nerve fibers. Neural activity is divided into three stages: resting, depolarization, and repolarization. Nerve transmission occurs when the membrane-induced potential of polarization is reached. When that happens, the membrane instantly becomes permeable to sodium (Na^+) ions, thereby allowing a large number of positively charged Na^+ ions to diffuse into the interior of the axon. The resting polarized

Chemical Therapy

> **Box 8-1 Mechanisms of action of in-office chemical agents**
>
> **Neural agents**
> Potassium-based agents act on nerve impulse transmission. The extracellular concentration of ions depolarize neural elements and prevent repolarization, thereby decreasing reactivity of CDH.[30,31]
>
> **Tubule-blocking agents**
> Tubule-blocking agents act by sealing the dentinal tubules through protein precipitation, remineralizing the structure, plugging tubules, and reducing the dentin fluid flow (dentin permeability).[32–42] These actions deliver *(1)* materials such as particulates that occlude the tubules or *(2)* agents that will interact with the oral environment to promote the formation of mineral in the dentinal tubules.
>
> **Mixed**
> These agents have the capabilities of neural agents as well as tubule-blocking agents in a single manufactured product.

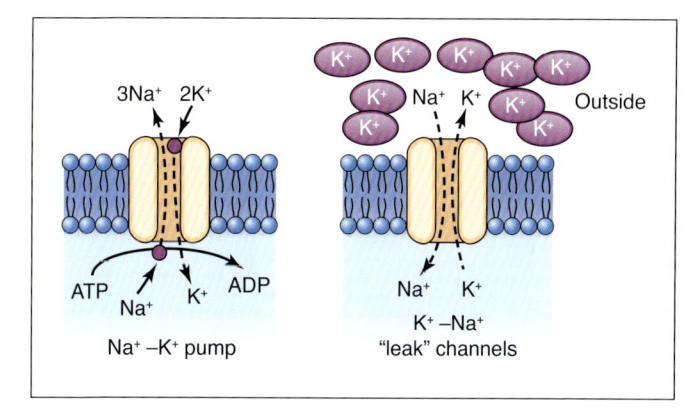

Fig 8-15 Potassium mechanism on membrane of nerve ending.

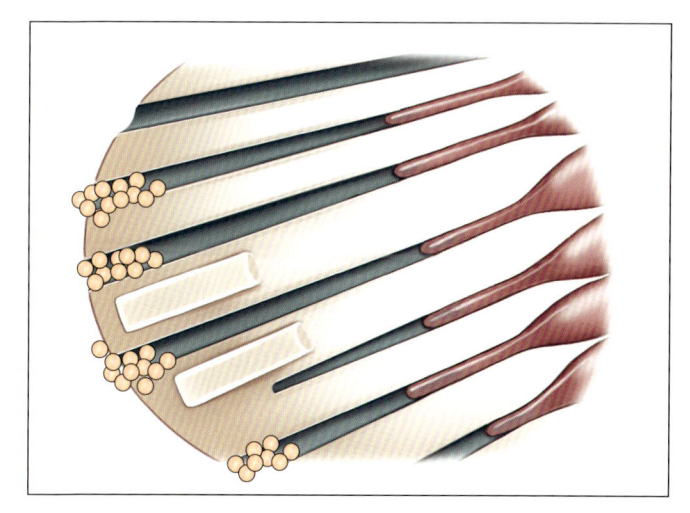

Fig 8-16 Oxalate precipitates on the tubule walls.

state of the axon is immediately neutralized by these Na⁺ ions, and as the potential rises rapidly in the positive direction, depolarization results. After this stage, the neural fibers return to the resting stage, the sodium channels begin to close, and the potassium channels open more than normal. Rapid diffusion of potassium ions to the exterior reestablishes the normal negative resting membrane potential.[43]

The application of extra-axionic potassium at the depolarization stage raises the concentration gradient of potassium outside the fiber, thereby making repolarization more difficult. This means that nerve impulses are not generated as easily, which relieves CDH (Fig 8-15).

Potassium is frequently associated with oxalates and nitrates.[31,44–46] During the 1980s, in vitro studies demonstrated that potassium nitrate was not efficient in terms of a reduction in dentin fluid flow and was instead characterized exclusively by neural action.[32,33] More recent studies have shown that whereas a 5% potassium nitrate solution resulted in no CDH reduction,[47] 10% potassium nitrate gel resulted in a 35% reduction in CDH within 48 to 96 hours,[48] and 35% potassium nitrate gel resulted in a 91% reduction in CDH immediately.[49] Potassium iodide can also be considered a potential desensitizing agent for CDH.[50]

At-home potassium

Potassium nitrate toothpaste and mouthwash are available over the counter. In a clinical study comparing dentifrices with and without potassium nitrate, the former showed statistically significant decreases in CDH.[51]

Tubule-occluding agents

There are many types of tubule-occluding agents. The following discussion outlines the characteristics, composition, and properties of the agents most commonly used by professionals.

Oxalates

Oxalates were introduced as agents to treat CDH in the late 1970s. Several in vitro studies reported significant decreases in hydraulic conductance across dentinal tubules treated with oxalates, suggesting that oxalates limit fluid flow in exposed dentin due to their ability to form precipitates on the walls of the tubules[30,52] (Fig 8-16). In vivo studies supported this proposed action of oxalates to occlude dentinal tubules and thereby reduce pain.[30,32,52–54] Oxalates have the ability to block more than 98% of the dentinal tubule permeability.[55,56] The formation of calcium oxalate crystals occurs 30 seconds after the application of oxalate-based solutions.[53,57]

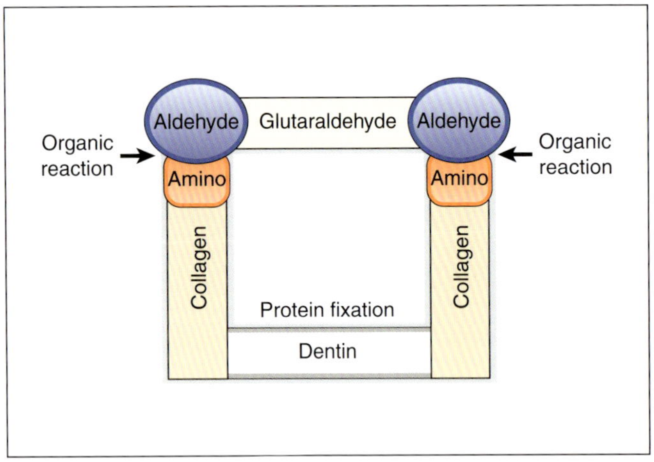

Fig 8-17 The two aldehyde groups of glutaraldehyde interlace with the amino groups of dentin collagen, forming a barrier that blocks the dentinal tubule.

Studies have shown wide variability regarding the effectiveness of oxalates. One clinical study evaluating the degree of CDH after periodontal root planing and scaling concluded that applying 3% potassium oxalate promoted statistically significantly greater relief compared with a placebo in postoperative reduction of CDH.[56] In regard to dentin permeability, potassium oxalate was found to be as effective as sodium fluoride varnish and more effective than titanium tetra-fluoride using experimental models.[58] In a comparison of five desensitizing agents (potassium oxalate, glutaraldehyde/hydroxyethyl methacrylate [HEMA], dimethacrylate and trimethacrylate resin, 2.59% sodium fluoride, and low-intensity laser therapy), potassium oxalate was found to be as effective as the other agents in a 24-week follow-up period and particularly effective for immediate relief. While another study showed potassium binoxalate gel to be effective in managing CDH, a 9-month postoperative evaluation showed the neodymium-doped yttrium aluminum garnet (Nd:YAG) to be more effective in CDH reduction. Whereas both methods of treatment resulted in recurrence of CDH, the gel may be considered a better treatment modality in the short term for its limited armamentarium, ease of application, and fewer precautions.[57]

A systematic review with meta-analysis of clinical studies up to July 2009 evaluating the oxalates concluded that this dentinal tubule–occluding agent should be considered in the treatment of CDH.[54]

Strontium

Strontium salts have been shown to occlude open dentinal tubules, thereby altering the permeability of sodium and potassium.[30,59,60] The application of strontium chloride by chemical reactivity has demonstrated their ability to precipitate protein in the dentinal tubules.[39,61–63] In addition, following the substitution of calcium ions with strontium, the dentinal tubules are blocked by recrystallization of the strontium within the tubules.[64]

Strontium compounds have been an active ingredient in toothpastes since 1960 and are widely used today.[65,66] Furthermore, Bekes et al[67] concluded that tooth demineralization was reduced by the use of strontium chloride following toothbrushing due to its resistance to plaque buildup. In a clinical study, strontium resulted in a reduction in discomfort and pain in 95 patients (72%) after treatment and at the 24-week follow-up. Statistical analysis showed a significant positive effect of this agent compared with the placebo group. Therefore, strontium chloride is an effective alternative to existing agents for desensitizing hypersensitive dentin.[64]

At-home strontium. Strontium is found in several over-the-counter toothpastes as a desensitizing agent. Studies have shown that 8% strontium acetate toothpaste presented greater CDH reduction than 8% arginine toothpaste under strong dietary acidic challenge[68] and that toothpastes with strontium decreased dentin permeability but did not completely occlude the dentinal tubules.[69]

Glutaraldehyde

This commercial product is present in aqueous formulation of glutaraldehyde 5% associated with 35% HEMA.[70–76] Being water soluble, HEMA promotes deep penetration of glutaraldehyde into the tubules, leading to the formation of a peripheral intrinsic barrier consisting of multiple thin septa within the dentinal tubule lumen.[72] The proposed mechanism of glutaraldehyde involves a reaction with serum albumin from dentinal tubular fluid, leading to precipitate formation, coagulation,[76] and subsequent narrowing or blocking of the orifice.[30] The 35% HEMA is a hydrophilic monomer capable of infiltrating acid-etched and moist dental hard tissue.[75]

Fig 8-18 Fluoride reaction blocking open dentinal tubules.

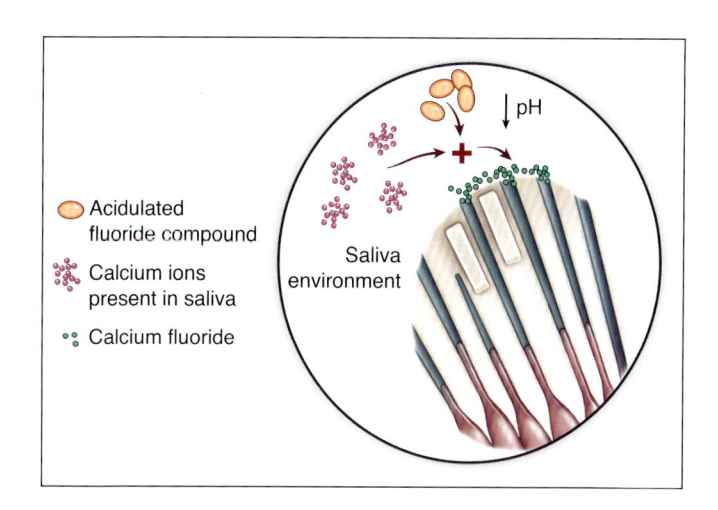

Studies with glutaraldehyde/HEMA have shown mixed results. An in vitro study demonstrated that glutaraldehyde has lower resistance than other compounds such as arginine for topical use.[76] Another in vitro permeability investigation showed that glutaraldehyde/HEMA was highly efficacious both when applied as an aqueous solution and in a gel formulation. It was proposed that the clinical advantage of the gel formulation is a well-controlled application, limiting the contact of the desensitizing agent to the target area and preventing inadvertent exposure to neighboring gingival tissue, wherein prolonged contact may result in a localized inflammatory response[74] (Fig 8-17).

Several in vivo studies have demonstrated that glutaraldehyde agents have a highly significant immediate relief effect.[73,77] A clinical study that evaluated four different desensitizing agents showed that all desensitizing treatments, including glutaraldehyde, provided relief in patients with CDH during a 6-month follow-up. Further, the glutaraldehyde immediately relieved the patient's pain.[70] Another study that compared glutaraldehyde/HEMA desensitizer with an oxalate and a placebo found that the glutaraldehyde was more effective than the placebo, whereas the placebo showed better results than the oxalate throughout a 6-month evaluation period.[78]

Varnishes

Varnishes are resin-based vehicles for fluoride, chlorhexidine,[79] or other preparations and are highly adhesive to the tooth structure. The application of varnish creates a mechanical barrier after drying and effectively seals the dentinal tubules with no known adverse side effects. Varnishes allow a slow and continuous release of whatever agent they carry. While varnishes are easy to apply and low in cost, they require reapplication periodically and often detract temporarily from preexisting tooth color.[80]

When compared with an oxalate gel in a clinical study, two different fluoride varnishes presented better results in reducing CDH 30 days after application.[81] Another study showed that a chlorhexidine-containing varnish and a glutaraldehyde-containing varnish are able to reduce CDH for a period of at least 3 months.[79]

A recent study introduced a novel material for CDH treatment: a varnish containing 10% potassium chloride and 10% fluoridated hydroxyapatite (FHA). This varnish is deemed effective based on its release of potassium ions for neural desensitization and dentinal tubule occlusion by FHA. The in vitro data of the varnish properties and biologic responses suggest this material's potential for use in CDH management.[82]

Fluorides

Fluoride products have demonstrated positive effects in blocking dentinal tubules and offering clinical CDH relief.[30] Sodium fluoride (NaF) is one of the most commonly used agents in the treatment of CDH.[58] Fluorides precipitate calcium fluoride crystals inside dentinal tubules, thereby decreasing the dentinal permeability because these crystals are almost insoluble in the oral environment from exogenous biocorrosion.[30,31,83]

Acidulated NaF is used in the clinical setting at a 2% concentration. Saliva or mechanical abrasion can remove the precipitate formed by NaF, so acid has been added to the formula to facilitate formation of precipitates inside the dentinal tubules (Fig 8-18). When these precipitates of apatite fluoride form, they can resist the effects of low-pH saliva, toothbrushing, and dietary substance challenges.[31] Stannous fluoride has the same effect as NaF.

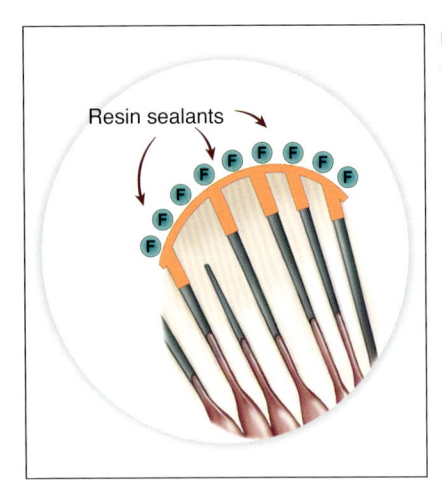

Fig 8-19 Mechanism of action of resin sealants.

Fluorides and fluorosilicates are also used in combination with iontophoresis,[31] a technique in which fluoride is transferred under electrical pressure deep into the dentinal tubules.[72] A comparison between 2% NaF local application, 2% NaF iontophoresis, and glutaraldehyde/HEMA desensitizers showed that 2% NaF iontophoresis and glutaraldehyde/HEMA were equally effective. Topical 2% NaF without iontophoresis did not provide an immediate effect, but results showed modest relief of CDH after 2 weeks.[72] Whereas both applications of NaF were effective up to 4 weeks, 2% NaF iontophoresis was comparatively more efficient at 12 weeks, indicating a longer-lasting effect.

At-home fluoride. Fluoride has been a component of toothpastes and mouthwashes for decades because of its ability to prevent caries.[84] More recently, stannous fluoride and NaF have been advertised as desensitizing agents in toothpastes. A clinical study showed that stannous fluoride–containing dentifrices provide significantly greater protection from dietary challenge than conventional fluoride-containing dentifrices.[85] Preparations with greater concentration of fluoride are also available but require a prescription and professional monitoring.[86]

Sealants

The use of sealants to prevent dental demineralization is not new. Since the 1970s, silanes, coupling agents, and unfilled or composite resins have been used to reduce demineralization and to seal etched enamel.[87] Resin sealants are often combined with glass-ionomer cements because of their bonding capability with tooth structure and potential to reduce bacterial growth. Glass ionomers release fluoride and maintain its effluence for an extended period of time. Glass-ionomer formulations are therefore indicated as cementing agents, adhesives for bonding orthodontic brackets, sealing of pits and fissures, as a base for pulp protection, direct core fabrication, and treatment of CDH. The adhesion mechanism primarily involves chelation of the carboxylic groups of polyacrylic acid to the calcium of enamel and apatite of dentin.[88] In the treatment of CDH, the glass ionomer adheres to exposed dentin, thereby occluding any open dentinal tubules (Fig 8-19).

An in vitro study evaluating the effects of different desensitizing agents on the prevention of root caries found that fluoride-containing resin-based desensitizers protected exposed root surfaces from demineralization.[89] Another study comparing the remineralization effect of different desensitizers showed that glass-ionomer cement–based dental materials can promote more remineralization of the artificial enamel lesions than can NaF-based dental materials. Resin-modified glass-ionomer cement–based materials have the potential for more controlled and sustained release of remineralizing agents.[90]

Selected calcium compounds

Casein phosphopeptide–amorphous calcium phosphate (CPP–ACP). CPP-ACP was primarily developed for the control of dental caries because it easily attaches to the tooth surface as well as bacterial colonizations. CPP–ACP deposits a high concentration of ACP in close proximity to the tooth surface.[42,91] In addition to its ability to remineralize hard tissue, it can occlude open dentinal tubules.[92] It is therefore indicated for reduction of the effects of biocorrosion in patients with gastroesophageal reflux disease (GERD) and relief of CDH.

While an in vitro study concluded that CPP–ACP yields only a short-term therapeutic effect for treating CDH and should be considered only for remineralization,[93] clinical studies showed that CPP-ACP resulted in rapid reduction of CDH at 6 months with high patient satisfaction.[94,95]

Bioglass. Bioglasses are commonly found in toothpastes as well as in-office prophylaxis pastes.[30] They have been studied as a treatment for CDH since the 1990s. Bioglasses composed of calcium, phosphorus, sodium, silicon, and oxygen react in the presence of water to release $Ca^{2+}(PO_4)_3$, thereby forming a thin layer of calcium phosphate crystals to occlude open dentinal tubules (Fig 8-20). The fine particulates formed have a median size of < 20 μm.

In a study comparing the efficiency of 15% calcium sodium phosphosilicate (CSPS) with or without 2.7% NaF and a placebo prophylaxis paste, the single application of both fluoridated and nonfluoridated prophylaxis pastes containing 15% CSPS provided a significant reduction of CDH for at least 4 weeks.[98]

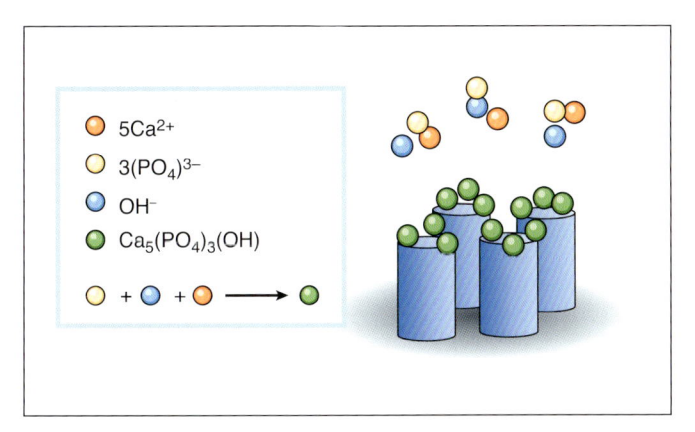

Fig 8-20 Sodium phosphosilicate is found in many toothpastes. This preparation is formed from 25% calcium, 25% sodium, and 6% to 8% phosphate; silica makes up the remainder.[96] The bonding process initiates with the bioglass reaction when calcium and phosphate react with calcium hydroxide (OH^-). Sodium ions exchange with hydrogen ions from saliva, causing a pH increase. Calcium and phosphate subsequently migrate from the glass, forming a calcium phosphate–rich surface layer on top of a silica-rich layer from the loss of calcium sodium phosphate ions.[97]

Fig 8-21 Mechanism of arginine: Saliva transports calcium and phosphate ions in close proximity of dentinal tubules to induce occlusion as a substitute for salivary glycoproteins (ie, pellicle).

At-home bioglass. Toothpastes with CSPS are available over the counter and have been found to occlude dentinal tubules better than glutaraldehyde/HEMA.[99,100] Another study showed that bioglass in toothpaste significantly reduced dentin permeability after 7 days and provided excellent resistance to acid challenge.[101] Compared with potassium nitrate–based toothpaste, CSPS-based toothpaste showed better results for CDH relief over 8 weeks.[102]

Arginine. Commonly used in toothpastes, arginine has little use in office. As a tubule-occluding desensitizing agent, arginine bicarbonate combines with calcium carbonate to form deposits that plug open dentinal tubules and physically block fluid flow, thereby relieving CDH[103] (Fig 8-21).

A clinical study found arginine to be more effective in desensitizing teeth after root scaling than NaF.[104] Other studies have reported that arginine-based dentifrices result in statistically significant reductions in CDH compared with potassium-based[105-108] or NaF-based[109] dentifrices.

Mixed agents

Mixed agents combine the capabilities of neural and tubule-blocking agents in a single product.

Potassium oxalate

Potassium oxalate combines two common desensitizer agents, the neural agent of potassium and the tubule-blocking oxalate. When these agents are combined, the oxalate acts initially as a carrier, enabling the potassium to contact the odontoblast endings. Oxalates are formed by neutralization of oxalic acid with a corresponding base or by exchanging the cation. Thus, potassium oxalate results from combining oxalic acid and potassium hydroxide (Fig 8-22).

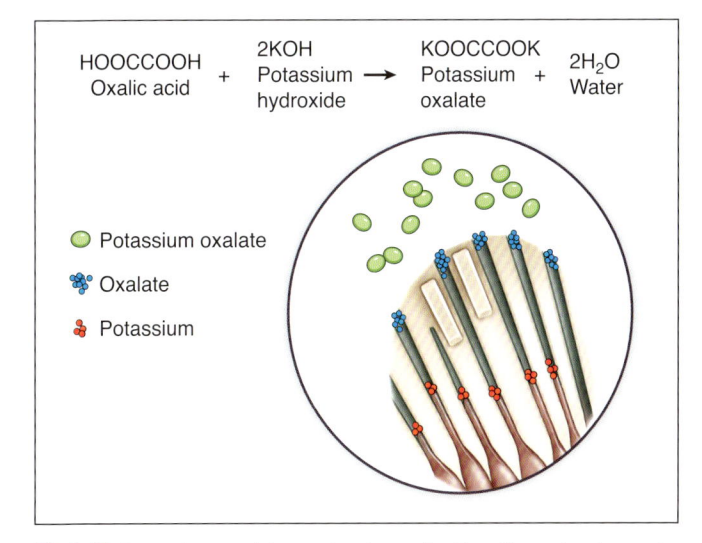

Fig 8-22 Potassium oxalate mechanisms of action: The potassium acts as a neural agent while the oxalate occludes the dentinal tubules.

At-home potassium oxalate. As an at-home treatment, 1.4% potassium oxalate mouthrinse resulted in reduction of CDH within 5 days.[110] An in vitro study similarly reported this agent to occlude dentinal tubules more effectively than other desensitizing products without oxalate.[111]

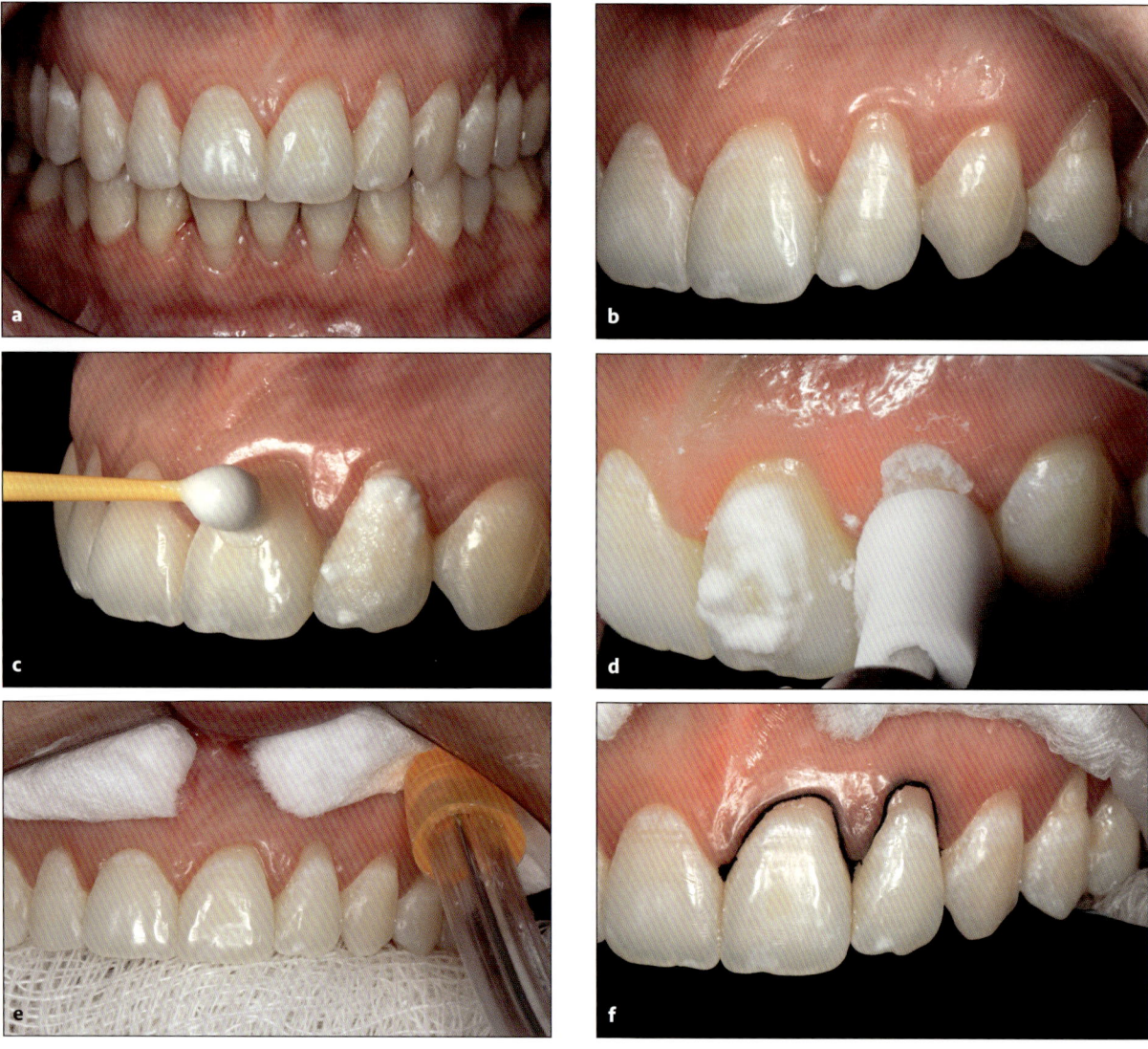

8 | Nonrestorative Protocols: Occlusal, Chemical, and Laser Therapies

Fig 8-23 *(a)* Initial clinical view of a 30-year-old woman with a high level of CDH primarily in teeth on her left side. Occlusal interferences were detected on that side, which she reported was her dominant side for mastication. Her diet report indicated that she had an acidic diet. *(b)* Occlusal adjustments were made, and the acidic diet was controlled by the patient. There was no loss of dental structure that justified the use of a composite, and the periodontology staff had no reason to surgically cover the area. Therefore, the clinician advised the use of 5% potassium oxalate gel over two to four clinical sessions. The number of sessions depends on the size of the exposed dentin and the degree of CDH. *(c)* Before the application of the desensitizer, it is very important to perform surface prophylaxis and apply a paste of 2% chlorhexidine and pumice powder. Commercial prophylaxis pastes containing glycerin or Vaseline should be avoided because they can interfere with the action of the desensitizer. *(d)* It is important to avoid friction from a rubber cup and pumice powder by using intermittent gentle movements. *(e)* Partial isolation and control of humidity. *(f)* Insertion of cotton cord size #000. →

Potassium nitrate and NaF

The combination of potassium nitrate and NaF acts as a neural desensitizing medicament to odontoblast processes as well as a tubule-blocking agent.[112]

Conclusion

Although protocols and agents can alleviate nociception of CDH, the clinician must establish an etiologic diagnosis prior to recommending these chemical therapies. In-office or at-home desensitizing agents are appropriate for the management of CDH when an etiologic diagnosis cannot be found or when the responsible oral conditions cannot be resolved (Fig 8-23). Table 8-1 lists desensitizing agents recommended by the authors.

Figure 8-24 illustrates the authors' multiple-session treatment protocol for use of mixed desensitizing agents. This protocol employs high concentrations of neural agents associated with dentinal tubule–occluding agents applied over multiple sessions to manage CDH. Figure 8-25 shows a clinical case following a combined protocol with five clinical sessions using neural and tubule-occluding agents.

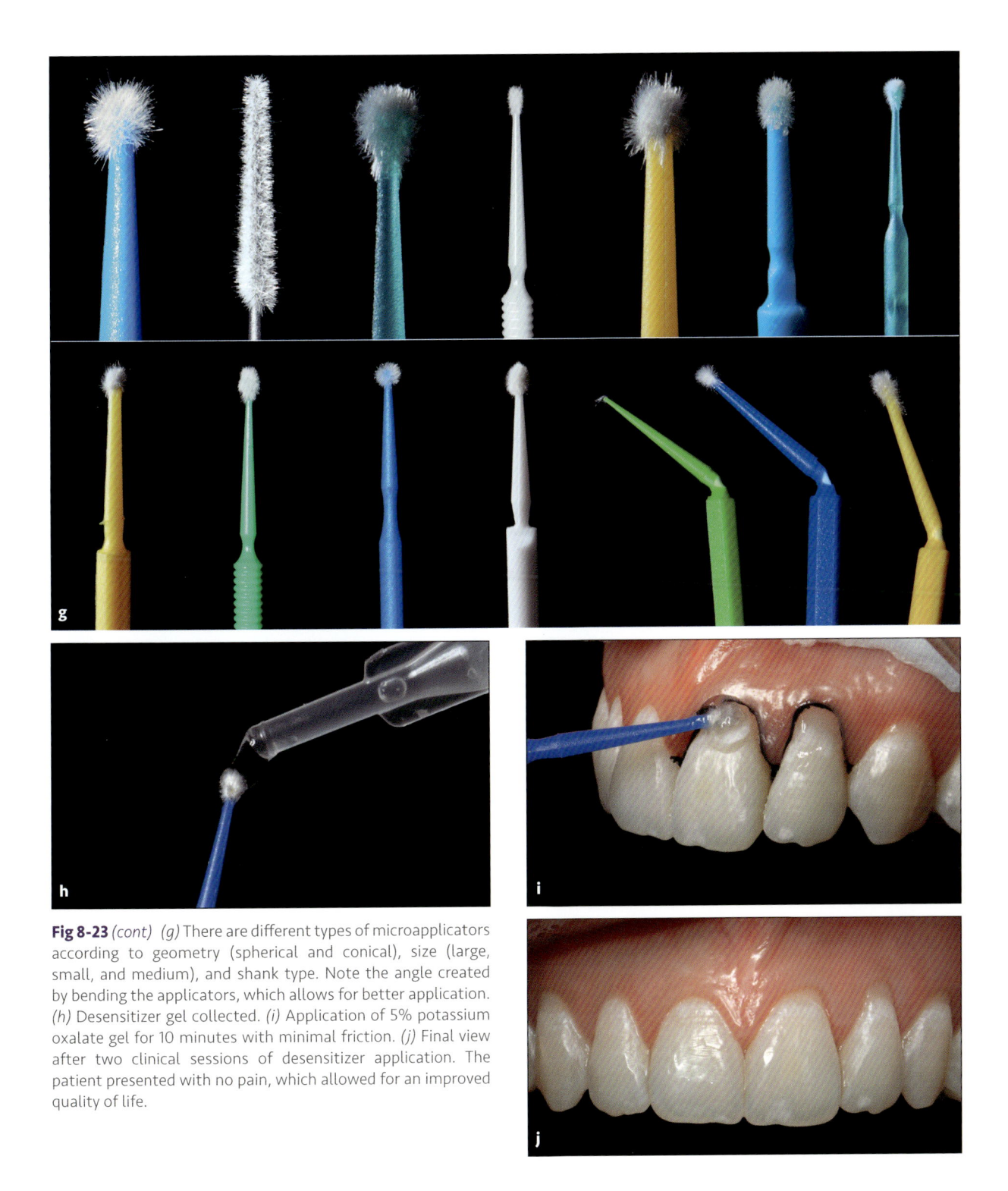

Chemical Therapy

Fig 8-23 *(cont)* *(g)* There are different types of microapplicators according to geometry (spherical and conical), size (large, small, and medium), and shank type. Note the angle created by bending the applicators, which allows for better application. *(h)* Desensitizer gel collected. *(i)* Application of 5% potassium oxalate gel for 10 minutes with minimal friction. *(j)* Final view after two clinical sessions of desensitizer application. The patient presented with no pain, which allowed for an improved quality of life.

8 Nonrestorative Protocols: Occlusal, Chemical, and Laser Therapies

Table 8-1 Chemical desensitizers recommended by the authors

Material	Classification	Manufacturer
Neural agents		
Ultra EZ	Potassium nitrate	Ultradent
Soothe	Potassium nitrate	SDI
Isodan	Potassium nitrate	Septodont
Tubule-occluding agents		
Isodan	Sodium fluoride/HEMA	Septodont
Clinpro XT Varnish	Sealant/fluoride release	3M ESPE
Riva Star	Silver, iodide, fluoride	SDI
Gluma Desensitizer	Glutaraldehyde/HEMA	Heraeus Kulzer
BisBlock	Oxalic acid	Bisco
Shield Force	SR monomer	Tokuyama
Teethmate Desensitizer	Hydroxyapatite	Kuraray
Bifluorid	Fluoride varnish	Voco
Clinpro White Varnish	Fluoride varnish	3M ESPE
Enamelast	Fluoride varnish	Ultradent
Cervitec Plus	Chlorhexidine and thymol	Ivoclar Vivadent
Seal & Protect	Sealant/fluoride release	Dentsply
Admira Protect	Sealant/ormocer	Voco
Calm-it	Sealant	Dentsply

First session	Neural agent
Second session	Neural agent
Third session	Tubule-occluding agent (eg, glutaraldehyde or oxalate/calcium derivative)
Fourth session	Tubule-occluding agent (eg, glutaraldehyde or oxalate/calcium derivative)
Fifth session	Sealing agent (eg, fluoride varnish or self-adhesive sealer)

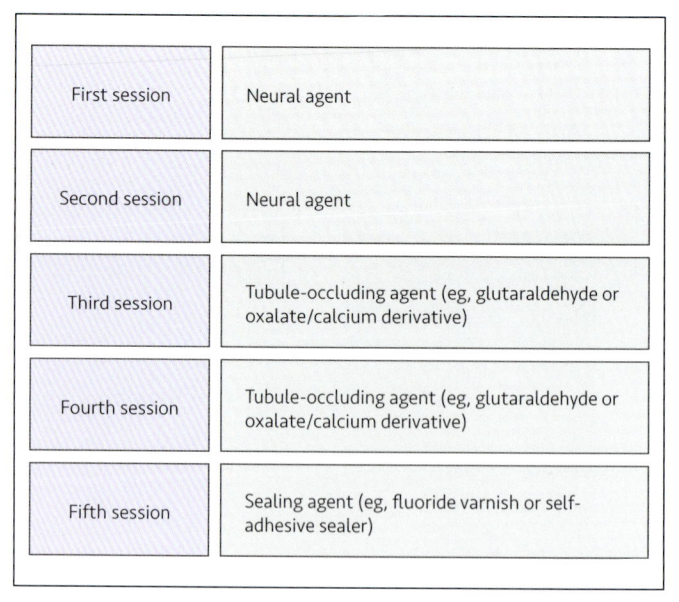

Fig 8-24 The NCCL Research Group's chemical protocol to treat CDH in five sessions using desensitizing agents. This protocol employs high concentrations of neural agents followed by dentinal tubule–occluding agents applied over multiple sessions to manage CDH. The authors recommend 48 to 72 hours as the minimum interval between the sessions. Laser therapy can also be incorporated into this protocol. In sessions 3 and 4, different materials are suggested based on etiologic factor: glutaraldehyde if biocorrosion is the predominant factor, and oxalate/calcium derivative if stress or friction is the predominant factor.

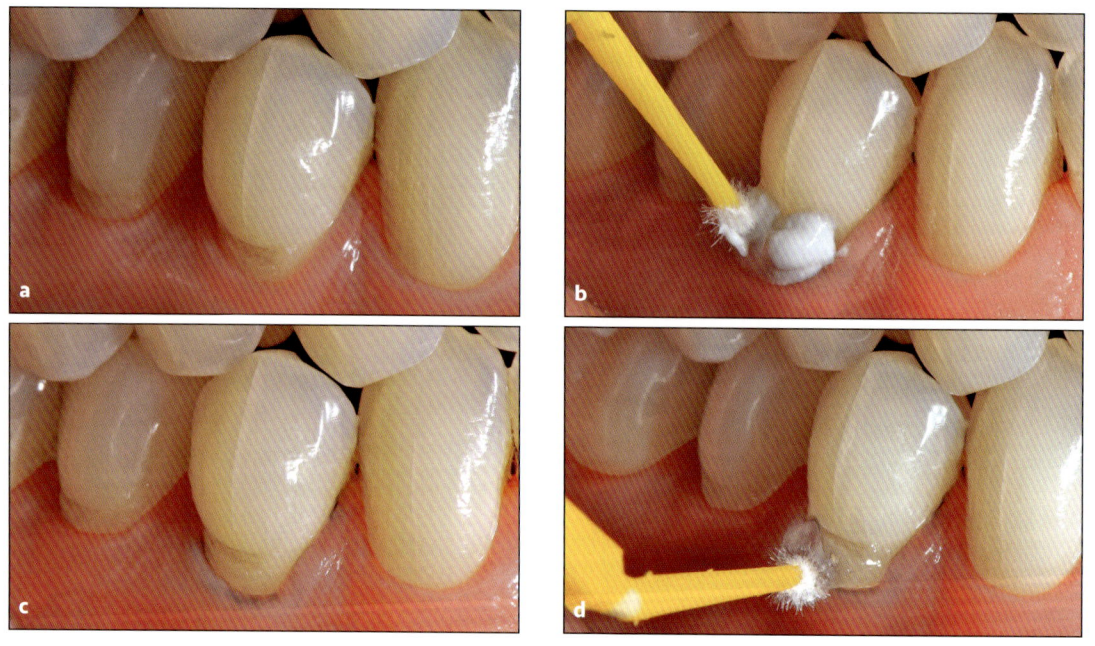

Fig 8-25 In this clinical case, the patient presented with high levels of CDH in the mandibular premolars. The main etiologic factors were detected and controlled. The treatment protocol included a combination of desensitizing agents: potassium agents and tubule-blocking agents. *(a)* Initial clinical view of a mandibular premolar with exposed dentin, lack of space to build a composite resin restoration, and a high level of CDH. *(b)* Prophylaxis as well as application of 2% chlorhexidine and pumice powder. *(c)* Insertion of cotton cord size #000. *(d)* Sessions 1 and 2: Application of 5% potassium nitrate gel. The gel should be applied gently with the microapplicator, and any excess should be removed.

Fig 8-25 *(cont) (e)* Sessions 3 and 4: Dentinal tubule–blocking agents are utilized. Options are 5% glutaraldehyde, 5% potassium oxalate, nanoparticles of phosphates, 5% fluoride varnish, or specific self-adhesive sealants. In this case, 5% potassium oxolate was used. *(f to h)* At the fifth clinical session, a self-adhesive sealant was applied, and any excess was removed with the microapplicator. After waiting 5 minutes for the chemical reaction, the sealant was light cured for 40 seconds. *(i)* Final view.

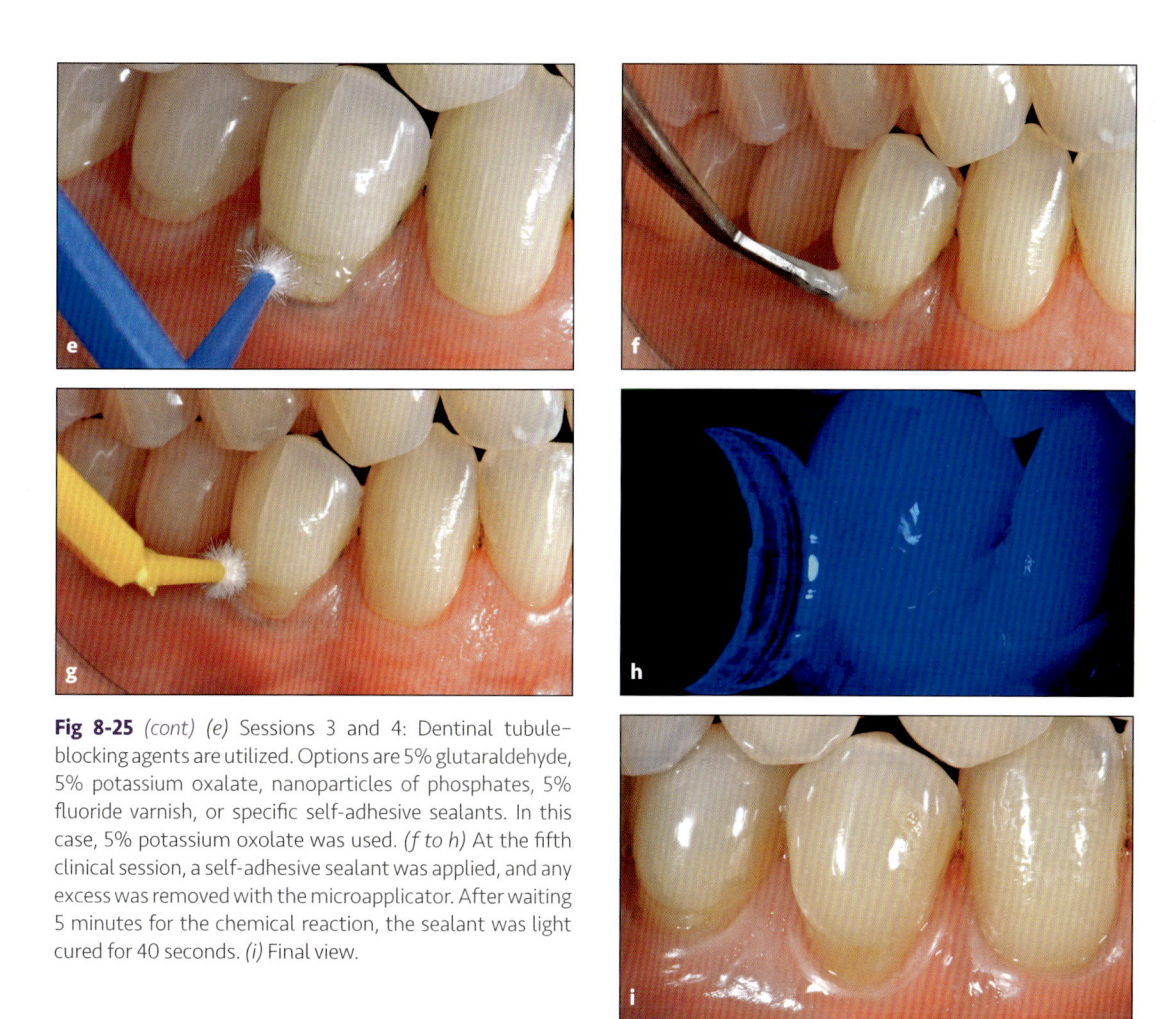

Laser Therapy

Lasers were introduced as an innovative, conservative, and effective alternative for the treatment of CDH. Dentin desensitization with lasers depends on the wavelength, parameters, and protocols used (ie, power, repetition rate, energy density, irradiation time, and frequency).[113,114]

Literature review

Studies have shown mixed results with laser therapy to treat CDH. Lin et al showed that laser therapy leads to better treatment results than occlusal therapy.[115] Another study confirmed these findings.[116] A systematic review indicated that laser therapy showed a clinical advantage over topical treatments without adverse effects.[117] However, another review reported that irradiation with high- and low-power lasers in the treatment of CDH has a minimal clinical advantage over topical treatments.

The one consistent conclusion from systematic reviews is this: Well-designed randomized clinical trials over time with controlled studies are needed to assess the effectiveness of laser therapy in the treatment of CDH.[118] That is, the treatment of CDH with lasers seems to reduce pain,[119] but evidence for the effectiveness of this modality is still weak due to the large variation in the methods used.[113,120]

Both low-power lasers and high-power lasers have advantages and disadvantages that can be overcome when using protocols and irradiation parameters appropriately, but the duration of desensitizing effects from laser therapy is still unclear. Multiple studies have shown that pain reduction levels after irradiation with low-power diode and Nd:YAG lasers are maintained for at least 6 months after treatment.[121–123] However, clinical results after 2 to 3 years would be interesting.

Despite the paucity of high-level research into laser treatment for CDH, clinically there is a positive effect in terms

Table 8-2 Lasers for the treatment of CDH and their respective wavelengths and mechanisms

Laser	Wavelength	Mechanism(s)
Low-power		
HeNe	632.8 nm	Decrease of intradental excitability, tertiary dentin formation
GaAlAs diode	Infrared: 780, 830, and 900 nm	Decrease of intradental excitability, tertiary dentin formation
InGaAsP	Red: 660 nm	Decrease of intradental excitability, tertiary dentin formation
High-power		
CO_2	10,600 nm	Occlusion of dentinal tubules
Nd:YAG	1,064 nm	Occlusion of dentinal tubules, decrease of intradental excitability
Er:YAG	2,940 nm	Occlusion of dentinal tubules, evaporation of dentinal fluid
Er,Cr:YSGG	2,780 nm	Occlusion of dentinal tubules, evaporation of dentinal fluid

HeNe, helium-neon; GaAlAs, gallium aluminum arsenide; InGaAsP, indium gallium arsenide phosphide; CO_2, carbon dioxide; Er:YAG, erbium-doped yttrium aluminum garnet; Er,Cr:YSGG, erbium, chromium–doped yttrium, scandium, gallium, and garnet.

of decreasing pain, as observed in the Special Laboratory of Lasers in Dentistry at the University of São Paulo School of Dentistry, where more than 1,000 patients have been successfully treated since 1995. Table 8-2 outlines the various types of low-power and high-power lasers as well as their respective wavelengths and mechanisms for dentin desensitization in clinical practice.

Low-power lasers

Low-power lasers were initially used in dentistry to accelerate the process of healing, reduce pain, and biomodulate the inflammatory response.[124,125] Compared with high-power lasers, low-power lasers cost less and are simpler to use. In general, low-power lasers involve the release of energy from absorbed photons through photochemical, photophysical, or photobiological effects on cells and tissues without generating heat.[114]

The first low-power dental laser described was a helium-neon (HeNe) unit emitting a wavelength of 632.8 nm and low power (5 to 30 mW). Because the wavelength produced by the HeNe laser was highly absorbed by soft tissue, it provided limited penetration.[113] Therefore, modern low-power lasers are composed of a crystal semiconductor diode that allows higher power and wavelengths that can penetrate into soft tissue without damaging it. The diode lasers are usually variants of GaAlAs (gallium aluminum arsenide) that emit in the near infrared spectrum (780, 830, and 900 nm), with a power output ranging from 20 to 100 mW, or InGaAsP (indium gallium arsenide phosphide) that emit in the red visible spectrum (600 to 680 nm), with a power output ranging from 1 to 50 mW. Figure 8-26 presents some commercially available low-power lasers.

Low-power lasers have many effects at the cellular level: stimulation of mitochondrial activity, DNA or RNA synthesis, intracellular as well as extracellular pH change, acceleration of metabolism, protein production, and encouragement of enzyme activity.[125-128] The mechanism by which low-power lasers reduce pain symptoms (desensitization) is based on stimulation of nerve cells. More specifically, the laser interferes with the polarity of the Na^+/K^+ pump by increasing the amplitude of the action potential, thereby blocking transmission of painful stimuli.[114,129-131] Other effects such as anti-inflammatory, vascular, muscle relaxant, and healing responses have also been attributed to low-power laser irradiation. In addition, capillary vasodilation and vascular neoformation occurs, leading to an increased blood flow to the irradiated area.[114,132]

There is also evidence in the literature that low-power lasers help to reduce the inflammatory process and form reactive dentin, thereby reducing the pulp tissue repair time and consequently promoting patient comfort.[133,134] The formation of reactive dentin could be an advantage because of its resistance to bacterial insult and covering of the pulp tissues.

In 1993, Groth[135] supported the use of low-power lasers in the treatment of CDH. The protocol, consisting of a 15-mW laser applied for 10 seconds each at four different points (mesial, distal, central, and cervical) over three sessions with a 72-hour interval, found statistically significant improved results in the resolution of CDH and is still used today (Fig 8-27). Similar protocols were carried out by other authors with satisfactory results.[121,123,136-140]

Another study analyzing the effectiveness of two lasers with different wavelengths (660 and 830 nm) for desensitization found that the diode red laser at 660 nm was more effective than the infrared laser at 830 nm. It was observed that a higher level of desensitization occurred 15 and 30 minutes after irradiation.[141] In a comparison of different treatments for CDH, low-power laser irradiation showed a gradual reduction of pain, reaching similar levels as those presented by other desensitizing agents (ie, gels) after three sessions of irradiation.[121] Similarly, in an in vivo study comparing a low-power laser with a sodium fluoride varnish, the laser showed superior long-term results in reducing the levels of pain in the treatment of CDH.[142] Lopes et al[123] showed that low-power lasers

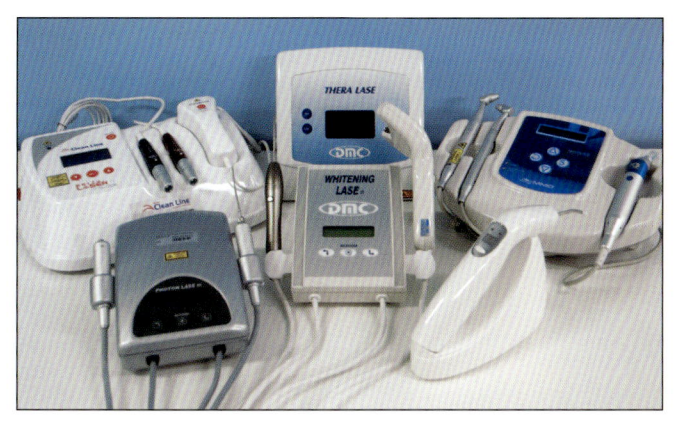

Fig 8-26 Low-power diode lasers.

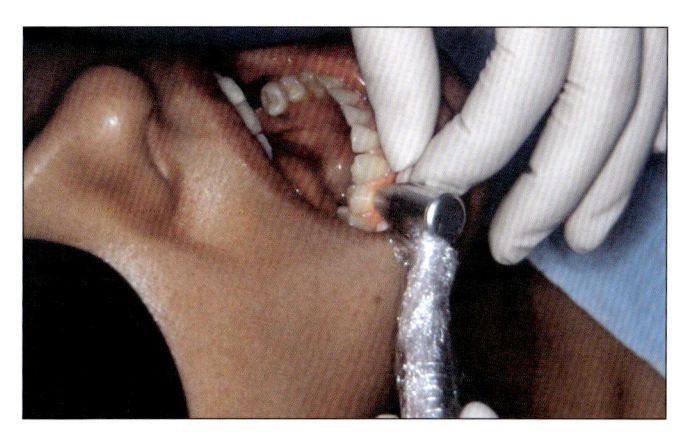

Fig 8-27 Low-power laser irradiation with a 780-nm laser positioned in the cervical area.

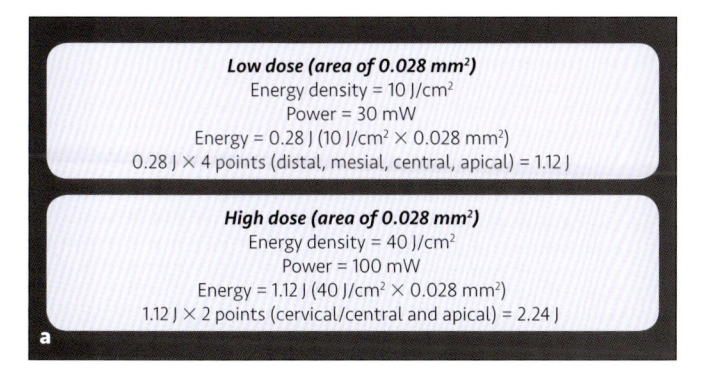

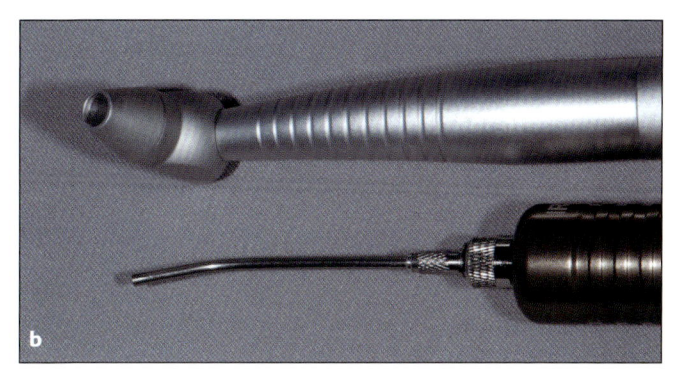

Low dose (area of 0.028 mm²)
Energy density = 10 J/cm²
Power = 30 mW
Energy = 0.28 J (10 J/cm² × 0.028 mm²)
0.28 J × 4 points (distal, mesial, central, apical) = 1.12 J

High dose (area of 0.028 mm²)
Energy density = 40 J/cm²
Power = 100 mW
Energy = 1.12 J (40 J/cm² × 0.028 mm²)
1.12 J × 2 points (cervical/central and apical) = 2.24 J

Fig 8-28 Differences in clinical parameters of low-power laser usage. *(a)* Dosimetry differences (low and high doses). *(b)* Handpiece size of two different lasers. Knowing the correct spot size and diameter of the beam is extremely important to determine the correct dose.

used in conjunction with desensitizing gel resulted in immediate pain reduction, whereas the use of a low-power laser alone was efficient in reducing pain for up to 6 months.

This combination of protocols (laser with desensitizing agent) is particularly effective[122,143,144] and has been adopted by the authors. The use of at-home desensitizing agents (eg, toothpastes) in combination with a professionally applied irradiation treatment is recommended as a first line of treatment because it is noninvasive and has fewer associated costs.[145,146] However, as mentioned previously, the etiology of the CDH must be determined before desensitizing agents are prescribed or used, as desensitizers do not treat the underlying cause of CDH but rather reduce the pain symptoms associated with CDH.

There is a great variability among the protocols used with low-power lasers because of differences in parameters such as dosage (Fig 8-28a), methodology, beam size (Fig 8-28b), and source diameter, and this variation hinders the establishment of an ideal irradiation treatment protocol for CDH resolution. That being said, it can be concluded from the literature that lower irradiation doses are indicated for lower levels of CDH pain and that higher doses should be reserved for patients with higher pain levels. The response of the patient in each session should be taken into consideration in order to adequately individualize the applied dosage.

High-power lasers

High-power lasers have been used to obliterate dentinal tubules through melting and resolidification of the dentin surface (Fig 8-29). This phenomenon has been described as a mechanism involved in reducing pain and dentin permeability, supporting the hydrodynamic theory.[147–161] Some authors speculate that the occlusion of dentinal tubules may also result from coagulation of proteins, producing immediate relief as a result of denaturation of proteins present in dentinal fluids.[162–164] Figure 8-30 presents some commercially available high-power lasers.

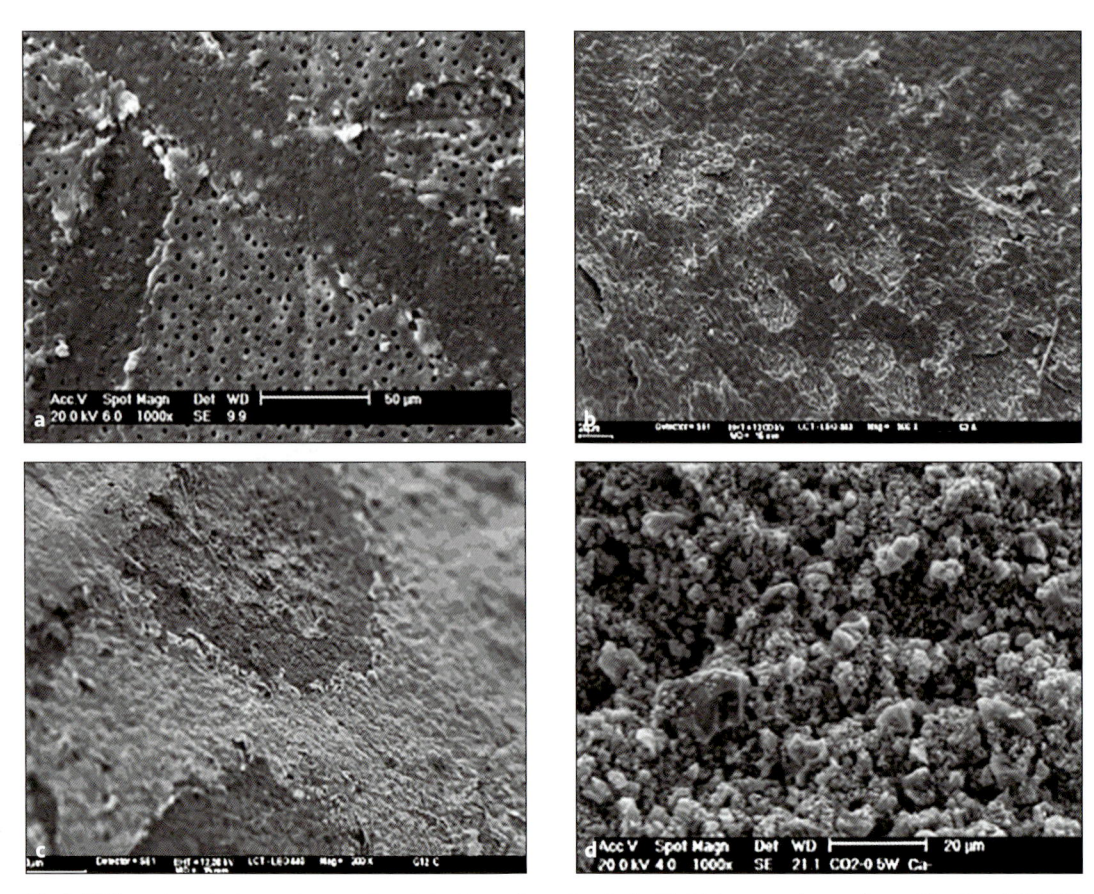

8 Nonrestorative Protocols: Occlusal, Chemical, and Laser Therapies

Fig 8-29 Scanning electron micrographs of dentin surfaces treated with high-power lasers (magnification ×1,000). *(a)* CO_2 laser associated with calcium hydroxide paste. *(b)* Erbium-doped yttrium aluminum garnet laser. *(c)* Erbium, chromium–doped yttrium, scandium, gallium, and garnet laser. *(d)* Nd:YAG laser.

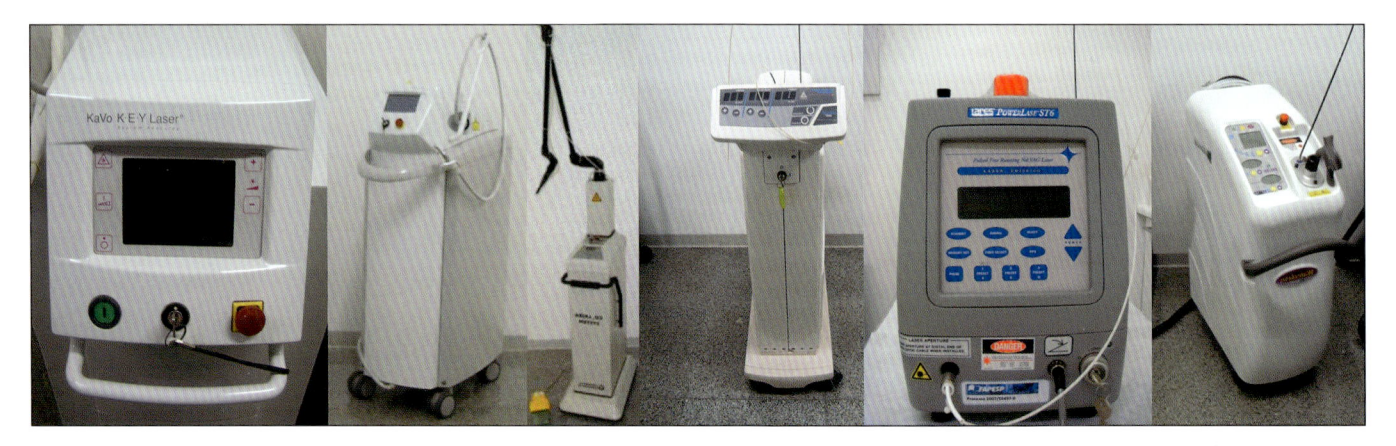

Fig 8-30 High-power lasers.

Noteworthy is that the use of the Nd:YAG laser melts the hydroxyapatite structure of dentin, which upon cooling resolidifies to form hydroxyapatite crystals larger than those of the initial structure.[151,154,161] Research into the recrystallized structure of the dentin surface shows a "glazed," nonporous obliteration of dentinal tubules (Fig 8-31). In addition, some authors have proposed that the Nd:YAG laser causes a blockage of the neural transmission mechanism by interfering with the Na^+/K^+ pump, reducing the cell membrane permeability of nerve fibers and/or changing the endings of sensory axons temporarily.[114,148,155]

All acidic beverages contribute to the exposure of and increase in the diameter of dentinal tubules, but irradiation with an Nd:YAG laser produces obstruction and reduction in the number of patent dentinal tubules, thus modifying the original structure and making it resistant to acidic challenge.[161] Unlike other in-office desensitizing agents, the Nd:YAG laser is able to immediately seal the dentinal tubules.[165]

Fig 8-31 Scanning electron micrograph of a dentin disc treated with an Nd:YAG laser (100 mJ, 10 Hz, 1W, ~40 J/cm^2; magnification ×2,000).

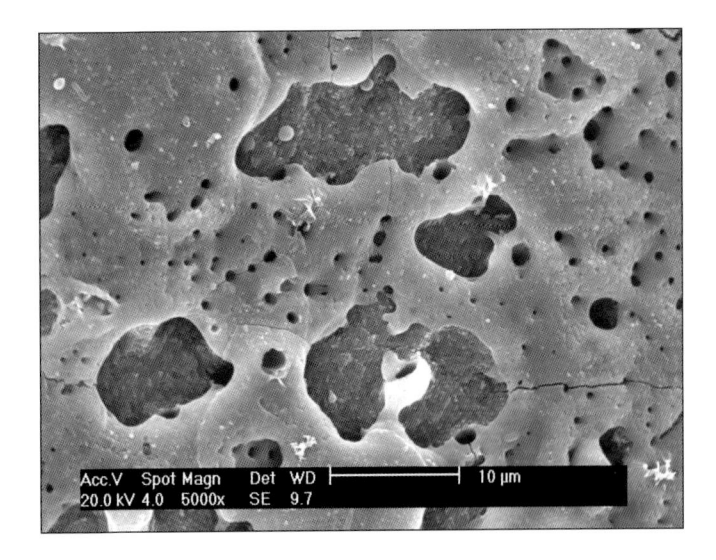

Like the Nd:YAG laser, other high-power lasers (eg, CO_2 laser) produce significant changes in dentin and are indicated for the treatment of CDH. These changes include the occlusion and narrowing of dentinal tubules as well as a reduction in dentin permeability, resulting in positive clinical CDH reduction.[164,166–168] When combined with calcium hydroxide paste, the CO_2 laser has shown promising results in terms of reducing dentin permeability and sealing dentinal tubules (see Fig 8-29a), and this protocol is safe for the treatment of CDH.[169] A clinical study reported that 94.5% of patients irradiated with a CO_2 laser remained without symptoms for a period of 12 months after the initial irradiation when combined with stannous fluoride gel. The authors concluded that the CO_2 laser is recommended and ideal for dentin desensitization.[167,168]

Despite their high water and hydroxyapatite absorption and thus their indication for the ablation of dentin hard tooth tissue, the erbium lasers (erbium-doped yttrium aluminum garnet [Er:YAG] and erbium chromium–doped yttrium, scandium, gallium, and garnet [Er,Cr:YSGG]) are also indicated for the treatment of CDH. In 2002, Schwarz et al stated that irradiation with the Er:YAG laser reduced the movement of dentinal fluid through evaporation of its superficial layers. The authors concluded that the Er:YAG laser was effective for dentin desensitization.[170] Other studies have corroborated this finding.[162] A preliminary clinical study with the Er:YAG laser reported that it was effective in reducing pain from CDH,[171] whereas another clinical study found that while low energy densities were effective in the treatment of CDH, a partial limitation in the effect of treatment with Er:YAG lasers exists due to the recurrence of pain.[172]

Both the Nd:YAG and Er:YAG lasers have been shown to be useful in reducing dentin permeability and consequently reducing CDH.[160] A clinical comparison of the effects of the Nd:YAG and Er:YAG lasers reported that the Nd:YAG laser is more effective in reducing CDH pain but that both can be used as a treatment for this common oral condition.[173] Another study confirmed these findings.[143] Recently, Belal and Yassin[174] have shown that the Er:YAG laser, at the predetermined power settings of 40 mJ/pulse and 10 Hz, can significantly reduce CDH symptoms. The current protocol adopted by the authors is 60 mJ, 2 Hz at four applications of 20 seconds each 6 mm from the dentin surface (Fig 8-32).

Few studies have reported on the efficacy of the Er,Cr:YSGG laser. Although it has been shown that this high-power laser can cause irreversible damage to dentin and/or pulp tissues,[175] a clinical study found that the Er,Cr:YSGG laser protocol (0.25 W, 20 Hz, 0% water and 10% air) was effective in the treatment of CDH. This same research group compared the effects of the Er,Cr:YSGG laser with a low-power laser and found that both were effective in promoting dentin desensitization immediately after irradiation.[176] Another study compared the effects of an Er,Cr:YSGG laser with a desensitizing dentifrice containing nanocarbonate apatite and found that both treatments were effective in reducing CDH; the laser had a superior initial desensitizing effect, while the dentifrice maintained its effects for a relatively longer period of time.[177] Figure 8-33 shows a clinical case with the Er,Cr:YSGG laser.

There is general consensus that erbium lasers should be used with protocols below the ablation threshold, preventing any unwanted tissue removal. However, the literature shows that dentin desensitization with subablative energy densities for Er:YAG or CO_2 lasers is temporary. The high temperature of the laser causes dehydration of dentin, which can result in an increased concentration of organic and inorganic constituents within the dentinal tubules and precipitation of these

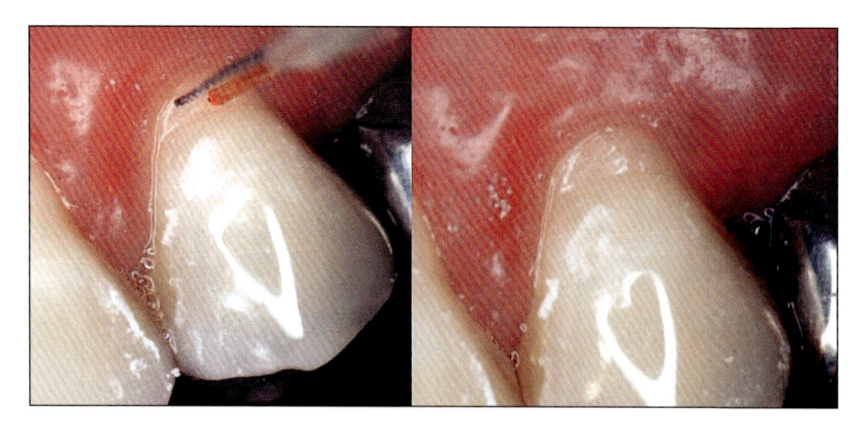

8 Nonrestorative Protocols: Occlusal, Chemical, and Laser Therapies

Fig 8-32 Treatment of a dentin surface with an Er:YAG laser. Protocol: 32.4 mJ/pulse (at the display 80 mJ) at a repetition rate of 2 Hz applied over four irradiations of 20 seconds each, with an interval of 10 seconds between them, 6 mm away from the dentin surface.

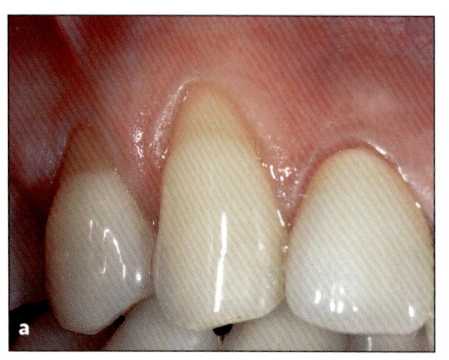

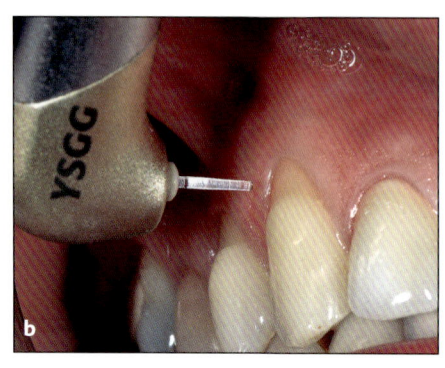

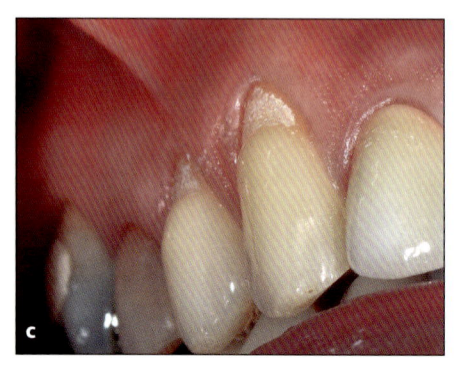

Fig 8-33 *(a)* NCCLs on the maxillary right canine and first premolar. *(b)* Irradiation with an Er,Cr:YSGG laser (0.25 W, 0% water, 10% air, 20 Hz). *(c)* Final view of the irradiated tooth surfaces. (Courtesy of H. Guney Yilmaz, Near East University, Mersin, Turkey.)

Box 8-2 | Step-by-step protocol for treatment of CDH with lasers and chemical desensitizers

1. Differential diagnosis, patient history, and clinical and radiographic examination
2. Evaluation of occlusal contacts and occlusal therapy if needed
3. Observation of parafunctional habits and diet, and education of the patient as to risk factors and how to remove them
4. Recommendation of soft toothbrush, less abrasive dentifrice, and oral hygiene instructions
5. Irradiation with low-power laser (three sessions with interval of 72 hours) if CDH still persists after prior steps
6. After the third session of low-power laser, irradiation with a high-power laser in conjunction with a desensitizing agent

substances in the oral entrance of tubules, thereby restricting the movement of dentinal fluid and causing desensitization.[178] Pain relief is temporary and tends to return after rehydration of the dentin. Further studies should be undertaken to evaluate the dentin desensitization achieved with high-power lasers using subablative energy.

A major concern with the use of high-power lasers for dentin desensitization is the appropriate use of protocols that avoid increases in temperature that can cause irreversible damage to the dental pulp. According to the classic work of Zach and Cohen,[179] temperature increases over 5.6°C are critical and could compromise the vitality of teeth. It is therefore critical that recommended protocols and parameters be followed.

Combined Protocol

A suggested protocol for treating CDH is a combination of laser therapy and use of desensitizing agents. This approach would cover the two strategies of CDH treatment: physical blockage of dentinal tubules and desensitization.[113,114] Box 8-2 illustrates this protocol.

Clinical "masking" of CDH with desensitizing agents should be avoided because it can hide improved results from biocorrosion reduction or occlusal therapy to control and resolve effects from pathologic cervical stress concentration. A change in dietary habits away from acidic foods is essential to the resolution of CDH and NCCL development, and the elimination of gastric reflux conditions and the achievement of appropriate oral hygiene

Fig 8-34 Enamel crack protective covering procedure using an adhesive system. *(a)* Enamel crack present in the maxillary left second premolar. *(b)* Application of 37% phosphoric acid gel. *(c)* Conditioned surface. *(d)* View of the tooth after application of the adhesive. The authors also suggest the use of chemical desensitizers for cervical microfractures.

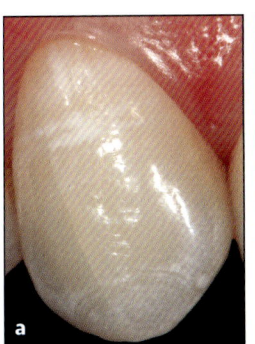

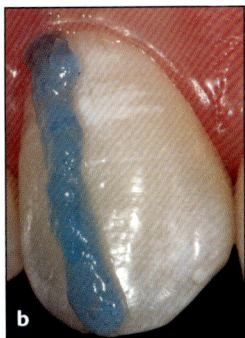

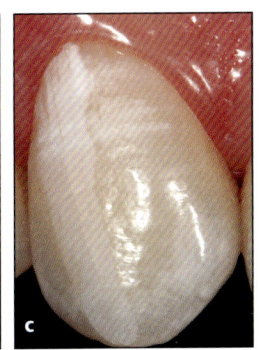

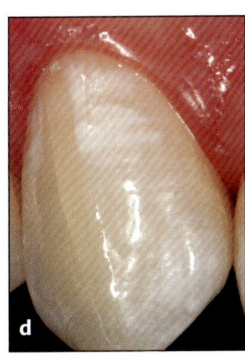

techniques are important to the success of any therapy. Occlusal diagnosis and minimal occlusal modification are preferred over more major therapies. However, considering their effectiveness and simplicity, laser treatment and chemical desensitizers are conservative options for the treatment of CDH with a high margin of safety according to current scientific evidence.

Considerations for Tooth Whitening

Tooth whitening is one of the most widespread techniques in esthetic dentistry and is often performed alongside restorative treatment at the patient's request. Tooth whitening essentially comprises an oxidation-reduction reaction of peroxide that breaks the long molecular chains of tooth pigment, thereby reducing its light absorption and reflection and causing the perception of whiter teeth.[180] There are many methods and approaches to tooth whitening, and these can be found elsewhere. What is relevant to our discussion is the postoperative sensitivity caused by tooth whitening.

Tooth sensitivity is the most common side effect of bleaching treatment. The hypothesis presented for postbleaching sensitivity is that the peroxide penetrates into tooth structure, causing direct neuronal activation of pain receptors. For patients with CDH or NCCLs, defects in the enamel as well as areas of exposed dentin resulting from occlusal stress or biocorrosion allow the diffusion of peroxide further into the tooth, increasing the risks of transient pain and postoperative discomfort. Therapies for CDH can reduce this pain by lowering the permeability of dentin or reducing the neural response triggered by traditional stimuli,[181–183] but patients with CDH or NCCLs should not undergo tooth whitening procedures without first controlling the etiologic factors. Therapeutic interventions include direct sealing of the dentinal tubules or enamel cracks by dental adhesives or derivatives (Fig 8-34), depolarizing agents, desensitizing substances added to whitening toothpastes, rinse solutions, professional application of fluoride varnish, or application of gels to tooth surfaces in trays.[184–186] The clinician must be certain that the application of these products does not render the bleaching agent useless.

Conclusion

Let's review what we have covered in this chapter:
- Etiologic determination is necessary prior to selection of treatment strategies for CDH and NCCLs.
- Preventive management strategies should consider parafunctional habits, occlusal prematurities, periodontal factors, diet, and other oral habits.
- Occlusal therapy can mitigate the development of CDH and NCCLs by correcting occlusal imbalance and removing any occlusal prematurities.
- Chemical desensitizers and occluding agents can be used to prevent further CDH and block its mechanism of action prior to restorative or surgical treatment.
- Neural desensitizing agents prevent repolarization of nerve fibers, and tubule-occluding agents block the dentinal tubules that transmit nociceptive pain responses.
- Low-power lasers are used to reduce pain symptoms of CDH (desensitization) by interfering with the polarity of the Na^+/K^+ pump, thereby blocking transmission of painful stimuli.
- High-power lasers are used to obliterate dentinal tubules by melting and resolidification of the dentin surface. High-power lasers have the potential to damage pulp tissue, so recommended protocols should be followed.
- A suggested protocol for treating CDH is a combination of laser therapy and use of desensitizing agents.
- Tooth whitening should not be performed in patients with CDH and/or NCCLs before the etiologic factors are controlled, and the CDH needs to be treated first.

Acknowledgments

Ana Cecilia Corrêa Aranha would like to thank CNPq (grants #306857/2013-8) for the scholarship and the Special Laboratory of Lasers in Dentistry at the University of São Paulo School of Dentistry.

References

1. Rees JS, Jin LJ, Lam S, Kudanowska I, Vowles R. The prevalence of dentine hypersensitivity in a hospital clinic population in Hong Kong. J Dent 2003;31:453–461.
2. Lee HE, Eakle WS. Possible role of tensile stress in the etiology of cervical erosive lesions of teeth. J Prosthet Dent 1984;53:374–380.
3. Gomes de Oliveira S, Seraidarian PI, Landre J Jr, Oliveira DD, Cavalcanti BN. Tooth displacement due to occlusal contacts: A three-dimensional finite element study. J Oral Rehabil 2006;33:874–880.
4. Caputo AA, Standlee JP. Biomechanics in clinical dentistry. Chicago: Quintessence, 1987.
5. Grippo JO. Abfractions: A new classification of hard tissue lesions of teeth. J Esthet Dent 1991;3:14–19.
6. Grippo JO, Simring M, Coleman TA. Abfraction, abrasion, biocorrosion, and the enigma of noncarious cervical lesions: A 20-year perspective. J Esthet Restor Dent 2012;24:10–23.
7. Coleman TA, Grippo JO, Kinderknecht KE. Cervical dentin hypersensitivity. Part II: Associations with abfractive lesions. Quintessence Int 2000;31:466–473.
8. Coleman TA. Detecting and quantifying cervical dentin hypersensitivity using air indexing combined with the T-scan system. In: Kerstein RB (ed). Computerized Occlusal Analysis Technology Applications in Dental Medicine. Hershey, PA: IGI Global, 2015.
9. Ikeda T. Influence of occlusal overload on tooth sensation and periodontal tissue [in Japanese]. Nihon Hotetsu Shika Gakkai Zasshi 1987;31:675–688.
10. Ikeda T, Nakano M, Bando E, Suzuki A. The effect of light premature occlusal contact on tooth pain threshold in humans. J Oral Rehabil 1998;25:589–595.
11. Riise C, Sheikholeslam A. The influence of experimental interfering occlusal contacts on the postural activity of the anterior temporal and masseter muscles in young adults. J Oral Rehabil 1982;9:419–425.
12. Christensen GJ. Abnormal occlusion conditions: A forgotten part of dentistry. J Am Dent Assoc 1995;126:1667–1668.
13. Christensen GJ. What causes changes in occlusion? Dent Econ 2013;103(7):24–31.
14. Qadeer A, Rabbani G, Zaidi N, Ahmad E, Khan JM, Khan RH. 1-Anilino-8-naphthalene sulfonate (ANS) is not a desirable probe for determining the molten globule state of chymopapain. PLoS One 2012;7(11):e50633.
15. Dawson PE. Functional Occlusion from TMJ to Smile Design. St Louis: Mosby, 2007.
16. Piper M. Functional occlusion. Presented at the Yankee Dental Conference, Boston, 25–29 January 2012.
17. Guichet NF. Biologic laws governing functions of muscles that move the mandible. Part II. Condylar position. J Prosthet Dent 1977;38:35–41.
18. Guichet NF. The Denar system and its application in everyday dentistry. Dent Clin North Am 1979;23:243–257.
19. Williamson EH, Lundquist DO. Anterior guidance: Its effect on electromyographic activity of the temporal and masseter muscles. J Prosthet Dent 1983;49:816–823.
20. Kerstein RB, Wright NR. Electromyographic and computer analyses of patients suffering from chronic myofascial pain-dysfunction syndrome: Before and after treatment with immediate complete anterior guidance development. J Prosthet Dent 1991;66:677–686.
21. Kerstein RB. Disocclusion time-reduction therapy with immediate complete anterior guidance development to treat chronic myofascial pain-dysfunction syndrome. Quintessence Int 1992;23:735–747.
22. Kerstein RB, Chapman R, Klein M. A comparison of ICAGD (immediate complete anterior guidance development) to mock ICAGD for symptom reductions in chronic myofascial pain dysfunction patients. Cranio 1997;15:21–37.
23. Kerstein RB, Radke J. Masseter and temporalis excursive hyperactivity decreased by measured anterior guidance development. Cranio 2012;30:243–254.
24. Kerstein RB. Disclusion time measurement studies: A comparison of disclusion time between chronic myofascial pain dysfunction patients and nonpatients: A population analysis. J Prosthet Dent 1994;72:473–480.
25. Kornfeld B. Preliminary report of clinical observations of cervical erosions, a suggested analysis of the cause and treatment for its relief. Dent Items Interest 1932;(54):905–909.
26. Coleman TA, Grippo JO, Kinderknecht KE. Cervical dentin hypersensitivity. Part III: Resolution following occlusal equilibration. Quintessence Int 2003;34:427–434.
27. Guichet NF. Occlusion. In: Howat AP, Capp NJ, Barrett NVJ (eds). A Colour Atlas of Occlusion and Malocclusion. St Louis: Mosby, 1990.
28. Guichet NE. Occlusion: A Teaching Manual. Anaheim, CA: Denar, 1977.
29. Okeson JP. Management of Temporomandibular Disorders and Occlusion. St Louis: Mosby, 2012.
30. Shiau HJ. Dentin hypersensitivity. J Evid Based Dent Pract 2012;12(suppl 3):220–228.
31. Davari AR, Ataei E, Assarzadeh H. Dentin hypersensitivity: Etiology, diagnosis and treatment; A literature review. J Dent (Shiraz) 2013;14(3):136–145.
32. Greenhill JD, Pashley DH. The effects of desensitizing agents on the hydraulic conductance of human dentin in vitro. J Dent Res 1981;60:686–698.
33. Pashley DH. Smear layer: Physiological considerations. Oper Dent Suppl 1984;3:13–29.
34. Sandoval E, Shannon IL. Stannous fluoride and dentin solubility. Tex Rep Biol Med 1969;27:111–116.
35. Rimondini L, Palazzo B, Iafisco M, Canegallo F. The remineralizing effect of a carbonate hydroxyapatite microparticles on dentine on dentine. Mater Sci Forum 2007;539:602–605.
36. Yuan P, Shen X, Liu J, et al. Effects of dentifrice containing hydroxyapatite on dentinal tubule occlusion and aqueous hexavalent chromium cations sorption: A preliminary study. PLoS One 2012;7(12):e45283.
37. Blitzer B. A consideration of the possible causes of dental hypersensitivity: Treatment by a strontium-ion dentifrice. Periodontics 1967;5:318–321.
38. Burwell AK, Litkowski LJ, Greenspan DC. Calcium sodium phosphosilicate (NovaMin): Remineralization potential. Adv Dent Res 2009;21:35–39.
39. Cohen S, Schiff T, Mccool J, Volpe A, Petrone ME. Anticalculus efficacy of a dentifrice containing potassium nitrate, soluble pyrophosphate, PVM/MA copolymer, and sodium fluoride in a silica base: A twelve-week clinical study. J Clin Dent 1994;5(special issue):93–96.
40. Petrou I, Heu R, Stranick M, et al. A breakthrough therapy for dentin hypersensitivity: How dental products containing 8% arginine and calcium carbonate work to deliver effective relief of sensitive teeth. J Clin Dent 2009;20:23–31.
41. Pradeep AR, Sharma A. Comparison of clinical efficacy of a dentifrice containing calcium sodium phosphosilicate to a dentifrice containing potassium nitrate and to a placebo on dentinal hypersensitivity: A randomized clinical trial. J Periodontol 2010;81:1167–1173.
42. Reynolds EC. Anticariogenic complexes of amorphous calcium phosphate stabilized by casein phosphopeptides: A review. Spec Care Dentist 1998;18:8–16.
43. Guyton AC, Hall JE. Textbook of Medical Physiology, ed 11. Philadelphia: Saunders, 2006.
44. Orchardson R, Gillam DG. Managing dentin hypersensitivity. J Am Dent Assoc 2006;137:990–998.
45. Borges A, Barcellos D, Gomes C. Dentin hypersensitivity—Etiology, treatment possibilities and other related factors: A literature review. World J Dent 2012;3:60–67.
46. Addy M. Dentine hypersensitivity: Definition, prevalence, distribution and etiology. In: Addy M, Embery G, Edgar WM, Orchardson R (eds). Tooth Wear and Sensitivity: Clinical Advances in Restorative Dentistry. London: Martin Dunitz, 2000:239–248.
47. Kishore A, Mehrotra KK, Saimbi CS. Effectiveness of desensitizing agents. J Endod 2002;28:34–35.

48. Frechoso SC, Menendez M, Guisasola C, Arregui I, Tejerina JM, Sicilia A. Evaluation of the efficacy of two potassium nitrate bioadhesive gels (5% and 10%) in the treatment of dentine hypersensitivity. A randomised clinical trial. J Clin Periodontol 2003;30:315–320.
49. Hodosh M, Hodosh SH, Hodosh AJ. KNO_3/benzocaine/tetracaine gel use for maintenance visit pain control. Gen Dent 2007;55:312–315.
50. Craig GG, Knight GM, McIntyre JM. Clinical evaluation of diamine silver fluoride/potassium iodide as a dentine desensitizing agent. A pilot study. Aust Dent J 2012;57:308–311.
51. Sharma S, Shetty NJ, Uppoor A. Evaluation of the clinical efficacy of potassium nitrate desensitizing mouthwash and a toothpaste in the treatment of dentinal hypersensitivity. J Clin Exp Dent 2012;4:e28–e33.
52. Cuenin MF, Scheidt MJ, O'Neal RB, et al. An in vivo study of dentin sensitivity: The relation of dentin sensitivity and the patency of dentin tubules. J Periodontol 1991;62:668–673.
53. Pashley DH, O'Meara JA, Kepler EE, Galloway SE, Thompson SM, Stewart FP. Dentin permeability. Effects of desensitizing dentifrices in vitro. J Periodontol 1984;55:522–525.
54. Cunha-Cruz J, Stout JR, Heaton LJ, Wataha JC, Northwest P. Dentin hypersensitivity and oxalates: A systematic review. J Dent Res 2011;90:304–310.
55. Morris MF, Davis RD, Richardson BW. Clinical efficacy of two dentin desensitizing agents. Am J Dent 1999;12:72–76.
56. Pillon FL, Romani IG, Schmidt ER. Effect of a 3% potassium oxalate topical application on dentinal hypersensitivity after subgingival scaling and root planing. J Periodontol 2004;75:1461–1464.
57. Talesara K, Kulloli A, Shetty S, Kathariya R. Evaluation of potassium binoxalate gel and Nd:YAG laser in the management of dentinal hypersensitivity: A split-mouth clinical and ESEM study. Lasers Med Sci 2014;29:61–68.
58. Calabria M, Porfirio R, Fernandes S, et al. Comparative in vitro effect of TiF_4 to NaF and potassium oxalate on reduction of dentin hydraulic conductance. Oper Dent 2014;39:427–432.
59. Taha T, Clarkson BH (eds). Clinician's Guide to the Diagnosis and Management of Tooth Sensitivity. Berlin: Springer, 2014.
60. Gutentag H. The effect of strontium chloride on peripheral nerve in comparison to the action of "stabilizer" and "labilizer" compounds. Penn Dent J (Phila) 1965;68(2):37–43.
61. Uchida A, Wakano Y, Fukuyama O, Miki T, Iwayama Y, Okada H. Controlled clinical evaluation of a 10% strontium chloride dentifrice in treatment of dentin hypersensitivity following periodontal surgery. J Periodontol 1980;51:578–581.
62. Miller S, Truong T, Heu R, Stranick M, Bouchard D, Gaffar A. Recent advances in stannous fluoride technology: Antibacterial efficacy and mechanism of action towards hypersensitivity. Int Dent J 1994;44(suppl 1):83–98.
63. Gedalia I, Brayer L, Kalter N, Richter M, Stabholz A. The effect of fluoride and strontium application on dentin: In vivo and in vitro studies. J Periodontol 1978;49:269–272.
64. Kobler A, Kub O, Schaller HG, Gernhardt CR. Clinical effectiveness of a strontium chloride- containing desensitizing agent over 6 months: A randomized, double-blind, placebo-controlled study. Quintessence Int 2008;39:321–325.
65. Rosenthal WM [inventor]. Block Drug Co, assignee. Strontium in toothpaste. US patent 3122483. 21 July 1960.
66. Davies M, Paice EM, Jones SB, Leary S, Curtis AR, West NX. Efficacy of desensitizing dentifrices to occlude dentinal tubules. Eur J Oral Sci 2011;119:497–503.
67. Bekes K, Schmelz M, Schaller HG, Gernhardt CR. The influence of application of different desensitisers on root dentine demineralisation in situ. Int Dent J 2009;59:121–126.
68. Olley RC, Pilecki P, Hughes N, et al. An in situ study investigating dentine tubule occlusion of dentifrices following acid challenge. J Dent 2012;40:585–593.
69. Pinto SC, Silveira CM, Pochapski MT, Pilatt GL, Santos FA. Effect of desensitizing toothpastes on dentin. Braz Oral Res 2012;26:410–417.
70. Aranha AC, Pimenta LA, Marchi GM. Clinical evaluation of desensitizing treatments for cervical dentin hypersensitivity. Braz Oral Res 2009;23:333–339.
71. Arrais CA, Chan DC, Giannini M. Effects of desensitizing agents on dentinal tubule occlusion. J Appl Oral Sci 2004;12:144–148.
72. Brahmbhatt N, Bhavsar N, Sahayata V, Acharya A, Kshatriya P. A double blind controlled trial comparing three treatment modalities for dentin hypersensitivity. Med Oral Patol Oral Cir Bucal 2012;17:e483–e490.
73. Davidson DF, Suzuki M. The Gluma bonding system: A clinical evaluation of its various components for the treatment of hypersensitive root dentin. J Can Dent Assoc 1997;63:38–41.
74. Ishihata H, Finger WJ, Kanehira M, Shimauchi H, Komatsu M. In vitro dentin permeability after application of Gluma(R) desensitizer as aqueous solution or aqueous fumed silica dispersion. J Appl Oral Sci 2011;19:147–153.
75. Joshi S, Gowda AS, Joshi C. Comparative evaluation of NovaMin desensitizer and Gluma desensitizer on dentinal tubule occlusion: A scanning electron microscopic study. J Periodontal Implant Sci 2013;43:269–275.
76. Samuel SR, Khatri SG, Acharya S. Clinical Evaluation of self and professionally applied desensitizing agents in relieving dentin hypersensitivity after a single topical application: A randomized controlled trial. J Clin Exp Dent 2014;6:e339–e343.
77. Dondi dall'Orologio G, Lorenzi R, Anselmi M, Opisso V. Dentin desensitizing effects of Gluma Alternate, Health-Dent Desensitizer and Scotchbond Multi-Purpose. Am J Dent 1999;12:103–106.
78. Vora J, Mehta D, Meena N, Sushma G, Finger WJ, Kanehira M. Effects of two topical desensitizing agents and placebo on dentin hypersensitivity. Am J Dent 2012;25:293–298.
79. Sethna GD, Prabhuji ML, Karthikeyan BV. Comparison of two different forms of varnishes in the treatment of dentine hypersensitivity: A subject-blind randomised clinical study. Oral Health Prev Dent 2011;9:143–150.
80. Ritter AV. Fluoride varnishes. J Esthet Restor Dent 2003;15:256.
81. Camilotti V, Zilly J, Busato Pdo M, Nassar CA, Nassar PO. Desensitizing treatments for dentin hypersensitivity: A randomized, split-mouth clinical trial. Braz Oral Res 2012;26:263–268.
82. Lochaiwatana Y, Poolthong S, Hirata I, Okazaki M, Swasdison S, Vongsavan N. The synthesis and characterization of a novel potassium chloride-fluoridated hydroxyapatite varnish for treating dentin hypersensitivity. Dent Mater J 2015;34:31–40.
83. Grippo JO. Biocorrosion vs. erosion: The 21st century and a time to change. Compend Contin Educ Dent 2012;33(2):e33–e37.
84. Orchardson R, Gillam DG. Managing dentin hypersensitivity. J Am Dent Assoc 2006;137:990–998.
85. Hooper S, Seong J, Macdonald E, et al. A randomised in situ trial, measuring the anti-erosive properties of a stannous-containing sodium fluoride dentifrice compared with a sodium fluoride/potassium nitrate dentifrice. Int Dent J 2014;64(suppl 1):35–42.
86. Miller JT, Shannon IL, Kilgore WG, Bookman JE. Use of a water-free stannous fluoride-containing gel in the control of dental hypersensitivity. J Periodontol 1969;40:490–491.
87. Korbmacher-Steiner HM, Schilling AF, Huck LG, Kahl-Nieke B, Amling M. Laboratory evaluation of toothbrush/toothpaste abrasion resistance after smooth enamel surface sealing. Clin Oral Investig 2013;17:765–774.
88. Anusavice KJ, Shen C, Rawls HR. Phillips' Science of Dental Materials. Philadelphia: Saunders, 2012.
89. Sohn S, Yi K, Son HH, Chang J. Caries-preventive activity of fluoride-containing resin-based desensitizers. Oper Dent 2012;37:306–315.
90. Zhou SL, Zhou J, Watanabe S, Watanabe K, Wen LY, Xuan K. In vitro study of the effects of fluoride-releasing dental materials on remineralization in an enamel erosion model. J Dent 2012;40:255–263.
91. Azarpazhooh A, Limeback H. Clinical efficacy of casein derivatives: A systematic review of the literature. J Am Dent Assoc 2008;139:915–924.
92. Geiger S, Matalon S, Blasbalg J, Tung M, Eichmiller FC. The clinical effect of amorphous calcium phosphate (ACP) on root surface hypersensitivity. Oper Dent 2003;28:496–500.
93. Kowalczyk A, Botulinski B, Jaworska M, Kierklo A, Pawinska M, Dabrowska E. Evaluation of the product based on Recaldent technology in the treatment of dentin hypersensitivity. Adv Med Sci 2006;51(suppl 1):40–42.
94. Park YK, Koo MH, Abreu JA, Ikegaki M, Cury JA, Rosalen PL. Antimicrobial activity of propolis on oral microorganisms. Curr Microbiol 1998;36:24–28.
95. Torwane NA, Hongal S, Goel P, et al. Effect of two desensitizing agents in reducing dentin hypersensitivity: An in-vivo comparative clinical trial. J Clin Diagn Res 2013;7:2042–2046.

96. Acharya AB, Surve SM, Thakur SL. A clinical study of the effect of calcium sodium phosphosilicate on dentin hypersensitivity. J Clin Exp Dent 2013;5:e18–e22.
97. Gillam DG, Tang JY, Mordan NJ, Newman HN. The effects of a novel Bioglass dentifrice on dentine sensitivity: A scanning electron microscopy investigation. J Oral Rehabil 2002;29:305–313.
98. Neuhaus KW, Milleman JL, Milleman KR, et al. Effectiveness of a calcium sodium phosphosilicate-containing prophylaxis paste in reducing dentine hypersensitivity immediately and 4 weeks after a single application: A double-blind randomized controlled trial. J Clin Periodontol 2013;40:349–357.
99. Joshi S, Gowda AS, Joshi C. Comparative evaluation of NovaMin desensitizer and Gluma desensitizer on dentinal tubule occlusion: A scanning electron microscopic study. J Periodontal Implant Sci 2013;43:269–275.
100. Jones SB, Parkinson CR, Jeffery P, et al. A randomised clinical trial investigating calcium sodium phosphosilicate as a dentine mineralising agent in the oral environment. J Dent 2015;43:757–764.
101. Wang Z, Jiang T, Sauro S, et al. The dentine remineralization activity of a desensitizing bioactive glass-containing toothpaste: An in vitro study. Aust Dent J 2011;56:372–381.
102. Neuhaus KW, Milleman JL, Milleman KR, et al. Effectiveness of a calcium sodium phosphosilicate-containing prophylaxis paste in reducing dentine hypersensitivity immediately and 4 weeks after a single application: A double-blind randomized controlled trial. J Clin Periodontol 2013;40:349–357.
103. Yan B, Yi J, Li Y, Chen Y, Shi Z. Arginine-containing toothpastes for dentin hypersensitivity: Systematic review and meta-analysis. Quintessence Int 2013;44:709–723.
104. Uraz A, Erol-Simsek O, Pehlivan S, Suludere Z, Bal B. The efficacy of 8% Arginine-CaCO3 applications on dentine hypersensitivity following periodontal therapy: A clinical and scanning electron microscopic study. Med Oral Patol Oral Cir Bucal 2013;18:e298–e305.
105. Shiau HJ. Dentin hypersensitivity. J Evid Based Dent Pract 2012;12(suppl 3):220–228.
106. Ayad F, Ayad N, Zhang YP, Devizio W, Cummins D, Mateo LR. Comparing the efficacy in reducing dentin hypersensitivity of a new toothpaste containing 8.0% arginine, calcium carbonate, and 1450 ppm fluoride to a commercial sensitive toothpaste containing 2% potassium ion: An eight-week clinical study on Canadian adults. J Clin Dent 2009;20:10–16.
107. Docimo R, Montesani L, Maturo P, et al. Comparing the efficacy in reducing dentin hypersensitivity of a new toothpaste containing 8.0% arginine, calcium carbonate, and 1450 ppm fluoride to a benchmark commercial desensitizing toothpaste containing 2% potassium ion: An eight-week clinical study in Rome, Italy. J Clin Dent 2009;20:137–143.
108. Elias Boneta AR, Galan Salas RM, Mateo LR, et al. Efficacy of a mouthwash containing 0.8% arginine, PVM/MA copolymer, pyrophosphates, and 0.05% sodium fluoride compared to a commercial mouthwash containing 2.4% potassium nitrate and 0.022% sodium fluoride and a control mouthwash containing 0.05% sodium fluoride on dentine hypersensitivity: A six-week randomized clinical study. J Dent 2013;41(suppl 1):S34–S41.
109. Hu D, Stewart B, Mello S, et al. Efficacy of a mouthwash containing 0.8% arginine, PVM/MA copolymer, pyrophosphates, and 0.05% sodium fluoride compared to a negative control mouthwash on dentin hypersensitivity reduction. A randomized clinical trial. J Dent 2013;41(suppl 1):S26–S33.
110. Sharma D, Mcguire JA, Amini P. Randomized trial of the clinical efficacy of a potassium oxalate-containing mouthrinse in rapid relief of dentin sensitivity. J Clin Dent 2013;24:62–67.
111. Sharma D, Hong CX, Heipp PS. A novel potassium oxalate-containing tooth-desensitising mouthrinse: A comparative in vitro study. J Dent 2013; 41(suppl 4):S18–S27.
112. Sharma D, Hong CX, Heipp PS. A novel potassium oxalate-containing tooth-desensitising mouthrinse: A comparative in vitro study. J Dent 2013; 41(suppl 4):S18–S27.
113. Benetti AR, Franco EB, Franco EJ, Pereira JC. Laser therapy for dentin hypersensitivity: A critical appraisal. J Oral Laser Appl 2004;4:271–278.
114. Kimura Y, Wilder-Smith P, Yonaga K, Matsumoto K. Treatment of dentine hypersensitivity by lasers: A review. J Clin Periodontol 2000;27:715–721.
115. Lin PY, Cheng YW, Chu CY, Chien KL, Lin CP, Tu YK. In-office treatment for dentin hypersensitivity: A systematic review and network meta-analysis. J Clin Periodontol 2013;40:53–64.
116. da Rosa WL, Lund RG, Piva E, da Silva AF. The effectiveness of current dentin desensitizing agents used to treat dental hypersensitivity: A systematic review. Quintessence Int 2013;44:535–546.
117. He S, Wang Y, Li X, Hu D. Effectiveness of laser therapy and topical desensitising agents in treating dentine hypersensitivity: A systematic review. J Oral Rehabil 2011;38:348–358.
118. Sgolastra F, Petrucci A, Gatto R, Monaco A. Effectiveness of laser in dentinal hypersensitivity treatment: A systematic review. J Endod 2011;37:297–303.
119. Sgolastra F, Petrucci A, Severino M, Gatto R, Monaco A. Lasers for the treatment of dentin hypersensitivity: A meta-analysis. J Dent Res 2013;92:492–499.
120. Jokstad A. The effectiveness of lasers to reduce dentinal hypersensitivity remains unclear. J Evid Based Dent Pract 2012;12(3 suppl):231–232.
121. Aranha AC, Pimenta LA, Marchi GM. Clinical evaluation of desensitizing treatments for cervical dentin hypersensitivity. Braz Oral Res 2009;23:333–339.
122. Lopes AL, Aranha AC. Comparative evaluation of the effects of the Nd:YAG laser and a desensitizer agent on the treatment of dentin hypersensitivity. A clinical study. Photomed Laser Surg 2013;31:132–138.
123. Lopes AO, de Paula Eduardo C, Aranha AC. Clinical evaluation of low-power laser and a desensitizing agent on dentin hypersensitivity. Lasers Med Sci 2015;30:823–829.
124. Karu T. Molecular mechanism of the therapeutic effect of low-intensity laser radiation. Lasers Life Sci 1988;2:53–74.
125. Karu T. Photobiology of low-power lasers effects. Heath Phys 1989;56: 691–704.
126. Sun G, Tunér J. Low-level laser therapy in dentistry. Dent Clin North Am 2004;48:1061–1076.
127. Chow R, Arwati P, Laakso L, Bjordal J, Baxter G. Inhibitory effects of laser irradiation on peripheral mammalian nerves and relevance to analgesic effects: A systematic review. Photomed Laser Surg 2011;29:365–381.
128. Tunér J, Hode L. The Laser Therapy Handbook [in English]. Grängesberg: Prima Books AB, 1997.
129. Yu W, Naim JO, McGowan M, Ippolito K, Lanzafame RJ. Photomodulation of oxidative metabolism and electron chain enzymes in rat liver mitochondria. Photochem Photobiol 1997;66:866–871.
130. Gordon MW. The correlation between in vivo mitochondrial changes and tryptophan pyrrolase activity. Arch Biochem Biophys 1960;91:75–82.
131. Wakabayashi H, Hamba M, Matsumoto K, Nakayama T. Eletrophysiological study of irradiation of semiconductor laser on the activity of the trigeminal subnucleues caudal neurons. J Jap Soc Laser Dent 1992;3:65–74.
132. Karu T, Pyatibrat L. Gene expression under laser and light-emitting diodes radiation for modulation of cell adhesion: Possible applications for biotechnology. IUBMB Life 2011;63:747–753.
133. Matsui S, Tsujimoto Y, Matsushima K. Stimulatory effects of hydroxyl radical generation by Ga-Al-As laser irradiation on mineralization ability of human dental pulp cells. Biol Pharm Bull 2007;30:27–31.
134. Ferreira AN, Silveira L, Genovese WJ, et al. Effect of GaAlAs laser on reactional dentinogenesis induction in human teeth. Photomed Laser Surg 2006;24:358–365.
135. Groth EB. Scientific Contribution to the Treatment of Dentin Hypersensitivity with Low Power Laser of Ga-Al-As [thesis in Portuguese]. São Paulo: University of São Paulo, 1993.
136. Noya MS, Bezerra RB, Lopes JL, Pinheiro AL. Clinical evaluation of the immediate effectiveness of GaAlAs laser on the therapy of dentin hypersensitivity. J Appl Oral Sci 2004;12:363–366.
137. Gentile LC, Greghi SL. Clinical evaluation of dentin hypersensitivity treatment with the low intensity gallium-aluminum-arsenide laser – AsGaAl. J Appl Oral Sci 2004;12:267–272.
138. Tengrungsun T, Sangkla W. Comparative study in desensitizing efficacy using the GaAlAs laser and dentin bonding agent. J Dent 2008;36: 392–395.

139. Vieira AH, Passos VF, de Assis JS, Mendonça JS, Santiago SL. Clinical evaluation of a 3% potassium oxalate gel and a GaAlAs laser for the treatment of dentinal hypersensitivity. Photomed Laser Surg 2009;27:807–812.
140. Orhan K, Aksoy U, Can-Karabulut DC, Kalender A. Low-level laser therapy of dentin hypersensitivity: A short-term clinical trial. Lasers Med Sci 2011;26:591–598.
141. Ladalardo TC, Pinheiro A, Campos RA, et al. Laser therapy in the treatment of dentine hypersensitivity. Braz Dent J 2004;15:144–150.
142. Corona SA, Nascimento TN, Catirse AB, Lizarelli RF, Dinelli W, Palma-Dibb RG. Clinical evaluation of low-level laser therapy and fluoride varnish for treating cervical dentinal hypersensitivity. J Oral Rehabil 2003;30:1183–1189.
143. Dilsiz A, Aydin T, Canakci V, Gungormus M. Clinical evaluation of Er:YAG, Nd:YAG, and diode laser therapy for desensitization of teeth with gingival recession. Photomed Laser Surg 2010;28(suppl 2):S11–S17.
144. Dilsiz A, Aydın T, Emrem G. Effects of the combined desensitizing dentifrice and diode laser therapy in the treatment of desensitization of teeth with gingival recession. Photomed Laser Surg 2010;28(suppl 2):S69–S74.
145. Canadian Advisory Board on Dentin Hypersensitivity. Consensus-based recommendations for the diagnosis and management of dentin hypersensitivity. J Can Dent Assoc 2003;69:221–228.
146. Tunar OL, Gürsoy H, Çakar G, Kuru B, Ipci SD, Yılmaz S. Evaluation of the effects of Er:YAG laser and desensitizing paste containing 8% arginine and calcium carbonate, and their combinations on human dentine tubules: A scanning electron microscopic analysis. Photomed Laser Surg 2014;32:540–545.
147. Brännström M. The hydrodynamics of the dental tubule and pulp fluid: Its significance in relation to dentinal sensitivity. Annu Meet Am Inst Oral Biol 1966;23:219.
148. Myers TD, McDaniel JD. The pulsed Nd:YAG dental laser: Review of clinical applications. J Calif Dent Assoc 1991;19:25–30.
149. Gelskey SC, White JM, Pruthi VK. The effectiveness of the Nd:YAG laser in the treatment of dental hypersensitivity. J Can Dent Assoc 1993;59:377–386.
150. Lan WH, Liu HC. Sealing of human dentinal tubules by Nd:YAG laser. J Clin Laser Med Surg 1995;13:329–333.
151. Lan WH, Liu HC. Treatment of dentin hypersensitivity by Nd:YAG laser. J Clin Laser Med Surg 1996;14:89–92.
152. Liu HC, Lin CP, Lan WH. Sealing depth of Nd:YAG laser on human dentinal tubules. J Endod 1997;23:691–693.
153. Gutknecht N, Moritz A, Dercks HW, Lampert F. Treatment of hypersensitive teeth using neodymium: yttrium-aluminum-garnet lasers: A comparison of the use of various settings in an in vivo study. J Clin Laser Med Surg 1997;15:171–174.
154. Lan WH, Liu HC, Lin CP. The combined occluding effect of sodium fluoride varnish and Nd:YAG laser irradiation on human dentinal tubules. J Endod 1999;25:424–426.
155. Yonaga K, Kimura Y, Matsumoto K. Treatment of cervical dentin hypersensitivity by various methods using pulsed Nd:YAG laser. J Clin Laser Med Surg 1999;17:205–210.
156. Lier BB, Rosing CK, Aass AM, Gjermo P. Treatment of dentin hypersensitivity by Nd:YAG laser. J Clin Periodontol 2002;29:501–506.
157. Ciaramicoli MT, Carvalho RC, Eduardo CP. Treatment of cervical dentin hypersensitivity using neodymium:yttrium-aluminum-garnet laser. Clinical evaluation. Lasers Surg Med 2003;33:358–362.
158. De Magalhães MF, Matson E, De Rossi W, Bento Alves J. A morphological in vitro study of the effects of Nd:YAG laser on irradiated cervical dentin. Photomed Laser Surg 2004;22:527–532.
159. Lan WH, Lee BS, Liu HC, Lin CP. Morphologic study of Nd:YAG laser in treatment of dentinal hypersensitivity. J Endod 2004;30:131–134.
160. Aranha AC, Domingues FB, Franco VO, Gutknecht N, Eduardo CP. Effects of Er:YAG and Nd:YAG lasers on dentin permeability in root surfaces: A preliminary in vitro study. Photomed Laser Surg 2005;23:504–508.
161. Naylor F, Aranha AC, Eduardo CP, Arana-Chavez VE, Sobral MA. Micromorphological analysis of dentinal structure after irradiation with Nd:YAG laser and immersion in acidic beverages. Photomed Laser Surg 2006;24:745–752.
162. Folwaczny M, Mehl A, Haffner C, Benz C, Hickel R. Root substance removal with Er:YAG laser radiation at different parameters using a new delivery system. J Periodontol 2000;71:147–155.
163. Wichgers T, Emert R. Dentin hypersensitivity. Gen Dent 1997;37:251–259.
164. Zhang C, Matsumoto K, Kimura Y, Harashima T, Takeda FH, Zhou H. Effects of CO2 laser in treatment of cervical dentinal hypersensitivity. J Endod 1998;24:595–597.
165. Palazon MT, Scaramucci T, Aranha AC, et al. Immediate and short-term effects of in-office desensitizing treatments for dentinal tubule occlusion. Photomed Laser Surg 2013;31:274–282.
166. Orchardson R, Peacock JM, Whitters CJ. Effect of pulsed Nd:YAG laser radiation on action potential conduction in isolated mammalian spinal nerves. Lasers Surg Med 1997;21:142–148.
167. Moritz A, Gutknecht N, Schoop U, et al. The advantage of CO_2 treated dental necks, in comparison with a standard method: Results of an in vivo study. J Clin Laser Med Surg 1996;14:27–32.
168. Moritz A, Schoop U, Goharkhay K, et al. Long-term effects of CO_2 laser irradiation on treatment of hypersensitive dental necks: Results of an in vivo study. J Clin Laser Med Surg 1998;16:211–215.
169. Romano AC, Aranha AC, Lopes da Silveira B, Baldochi SL, Eduardo CP. Evaluation of carbon dioxide laser irradiation associated with calcium hydroxide in the treatment of dentineal hypersensitivity. A preliminary study. Lasers Med Sci 2011;26:35–42.
170. Schwarz F, Arweiler N, Georg T, Reich E. Desensitizing effects of an Er:YAG laser on hypersensitive dentine. J Clin Periodontol 2002;29:211–215.
171. Chan A. Treatment of dentin hypersensitivity with Er:YAG laser. A preliminary study. J Oral Laser Appl 2000;1(suppl 1):9.
172. Watanabe H, Kataoka K, Iwami H, Okagami Y, Ishikawa I. In vitro and in vivo studies on application of erbium:YAG laser for dentine hypersensitivity. International Congress Series 2003:455–457.
173. Birang R, Poursamimi J, Gutknecht N, Lampert F, Mir M. Comparative evaluation of the effects of Nd:YAG and Er:YAG laser in dentine hypersensitivity treatment. Lasers Med Sci 2007;22:21–24.
174. Belal MH, Yassin A. A comparative evaluation of CO_2 and erbium-doped yttrium aluminium garnet laser therapy in the management of dentin hypersensitivity and assessment of mineral content. J Periodontal Implant Sci 2014;44:227–234.
175. Aranha AC, Eduardo CP. In vitro effects of Er,Cr:YSGG laser on dentine hypersensitivity. Dentine permeability and scanning electron microscopy analysis. Lasers Med Sci 2012;27:827–834.
176. Yilmaz HG, Cengiz E, Kurtulmus-Yilmaz S, Leblebicioglu B. Effectiveness of Er,Cr:YSGG laser on dentine hypersensitivity: A controlled clinical trial. J Clin Periodontol 2011;38:341–346.
177. Lee SY, Jung HI, Jung BY, Cho YS, Kwon HK, Kim BI. Desensitizing efficacy of nano-carbonate apatite dentifrice and Er,Cr:YSGG laser: A randomized clinical trial. Photomed Laser Surg 2015;33:9–14.
178. Pashley DH, Stewart FP, Galloway SE. Effects of air-drying in vitro on human dentin permeability. Arch Oral Biol 1984;29:379–383.
179. Zach L, Cohen G. Pulp response to externally applied heat. Oral Surg Oral Med Oral Pathol 1965;19:515–530.
180. Li Y, Greenwall L. Safety issues of tooth whitening using peroxide-based materials. Br Dent J 2013;215:29–34.
181. Haywood VB, Leonard RH, Nelson CF, Brunson WD. Effectiveness, side effects and long-term status of nightguard vital bleaching. J Am Dent Assoc 1994;125:1219–1226.
182. Berman LH. Intrinsic staining and hypoplastic enamel: Etiology and treatment alternatives. Gen Dent 1982;30:484–488.
183. Briso AL, Rahal V, Sundfeld RH, dos Santos PH, Alexandre RS. Effect of sodium ascorbate on dentin bonding after two bleaching techniques. Oper Dent 2014;39:195–203.
184. Palé M, Mayoral JR, Llopis J, Vallès M, Basilio J, Roig M. Evaluation of the effectiveness of an in-office bleaching system and the effect of potassium nitrate as a desensitizing agent. Odontology 2014;102:203–210.
185. Thiesen CH, Rodrigues-Filho R, Prates LHM, Sartori N. The influence of desensitizing dentifrices on pain induced by in-office bleaching. Braz Oral Res 2013;27:517–523.
186. Petersson LG. The role of fluoride in the preventive management of dentin hypersensitivity and root caries. Clin Oral Investig 2013;17(suppl 1):S63–S71.

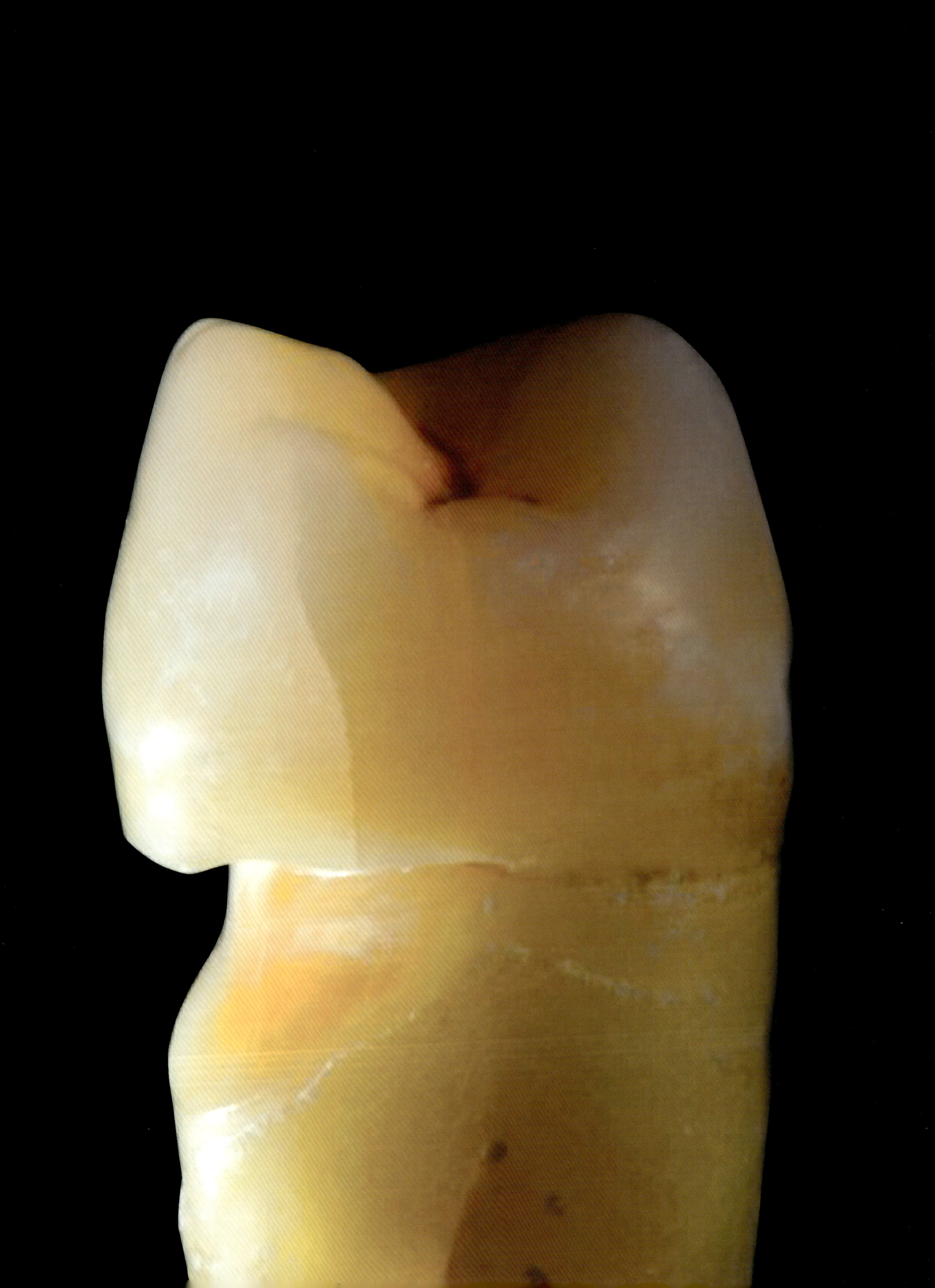

9

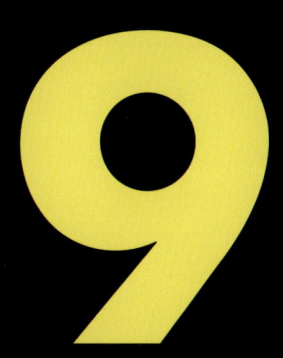

Restorative Protocols: Adhesive Bonding, Materials, and Techniques

Composition of Adhesive Systems

The first report of a successful attempt to bond restorative materials to tooth tissue was described by Buonocore in 1955.[1] Since then, the composition of adhesive systems has evolved dramatically. Currently, adhesive systems available on the market are composed of polymerizable monomers, predominantly methacrylates. This allows for good interaction with resin composite as a direct restorative material, because most composites are also based on methacrylates. However, adhesives must accommodate requirements of hydrophilicity, ionic interaction with the hydroxyapatite component, and more recently, collagen cross-linking. Research efforts have focused on improving adhesion to tooth structure by transforming the bond from a pure micromechanical interlocking to true chemical interactions with the different components of the substrate (ie, enamel or dentin).

Monomers

Traditional methacrylate monomers used in restorative composites are also present in adhesives systems. These cross-linking monomers are used mainly to increase the cohesive strength of the adhesive layer.[2] However, because of their relatively hydrophobic character, these monomers are not completely compatible with moist substrates such as dentin and are not able to penetrate down the water-filled dentinal tubules to form a thick hybrid layer.[3]

Because of the susceptibility of methacrylate monomers to water and enzymatic degradation,[4] other types of polymerizable materials, such as methacrylamides, have recently been introduced in commercial products.[5] Considering that the adhesives are commonly applied to wet dentin, which contains intrinsic moisture and active esterases, polymer degradation can compromise the stability of the bonded interface and thereby the clinical performance of adhesive restorations, not to mention raise toxicity concerns.

Functional monomers are also added to adhesives systems to improve their interaction with the bonding substrate. These functional groups can enhance the wettability of the adhesive, aid with demineralization of the tooth tissue, release fluoride ions, and/or increase the antibacterial character of the adhesive. Hydroxyethyl methacrylate (HEMA) is the hydrophilic monomer most commonly used in dental adhesive formulations. The disadvantage of having such a hydrophilic monomer in the composition is that it accelerates water uptake and hydrolysis of the hybrid layer,[6] which can compromise stability.[7,8]

Monomers containing functional groups derived from phosphoric and carboxylic acids are also commonly added to adhesives to function as self-etch (SE) agents.[9] The phosphoric acid–derived 10-methacryloyloxydecyl dihydrogenphosphate (MDP) is one of most successful monomers developed for this purpose.[10,11] This monomer is not only able to etch and demineralize the tooth substrate, but it can also form strong ionic bonds with the calcium present in the tooth tissue.[10,12]

Certain manufacturers also include polyacrylic acid (the same kind used in glass-ionomer cements) in their adhesive formulations to chelate the hydroxyapatite and to improve hydrogen bonding and the mechanical properties in the hybrid layer.[9]

Solvents

Apart from reducing adhesive viscosity, the addition of organic solvents to etch-and-rinse (ER) adhesive systems allows for their penetration into demineralized dentin. When the adhesive is applied to moist dentin, the solvent acts to displace water from the substrate, facilitating the penetration of hydrophilic monomers.[13] For SE adhesives, the use of water as a solvent is indispensable to ensure ionization of the acidic monomers responsible for substrate etching.[14]

However, water by itself or combined with other solvents is a poor solvent for hydrophobic monomers used in adhesives.[9] Thus, solvent systems containing acetone and ethanol are commonly added to adhesives to overcome this problem. Solvents must be evaporated during bonding because the presence of residual solvent reduces the degree of conversion of the adhesive and can compromise the stability of the bonding interface.[15]

Initiators

Adhesives form a thin, translucent layer on the tooth substrate, which represents the best scenario for the polymerization of resins. Because light transmission is severely impaired through the composites, adhesive systems also contain initiators to ensure the immobilization of the hybrid layer and the bond layer before the application of the restorative resin composite. Camphorquinone is the most commonly used photoinitiator in adhesive systems. This photoinitiator absorbs light over a wide spectrum of light (360 to 510 nm).[16] Additional co-initiators (eg, iodonium salts) have also been added to adhesives to improve the efficiency of polymerization.[17,18]

Other components

Some manufacturers add fillers to their adhesive systems (filled adhesives) to increase the cohesive strength and thickness of the adhesive layer. The real effect of filler addition on the strength of the adhesive layer is still in question.[19,20]

The addition of antibacterial monomers to adhesive systems has also been proposed and adopted by some manufacturers. The quaternary ammonium methacrylate methacryloyloxydecylpyridinium bromide (MDPB) added to dental adhesives has demonstrated antibacterial activity against *Streptococcus mutans*, *Lactobacillus casei*, and *Actinomyces naeslundii*.[21,22] Clinically, adhesives containing MDPB have demonstrated the capacity to inhibit caries lesions around orthodontic brackets.[23] Other components added to dental adhesives to promote antibacterial activity are glutaraldehyde and chlorhexidine. Both have been demonstrated to improve the stability of the bonded interface.[24,25]

Evidence-Based Adhesive Bonding Protocols

The hybrid layer is a mixture of dentin organic matrix, residual hydroxyapatite crystallites, resin monomers, and solvents.[26] Therefore, the hybrid layer stability ultimately depends on the intrinsic resistance of these individual components against degradation.[27-29] Several clinical studies have focused on the effects of modified standard clinical protocols to obtain adhesive interfaces with superior resistance to degradation.[30-51] The protocol described here is based on conclusions from these studies.

1. Isolate the field

Many professionals consider rubber dam to be an essential component of modern adhesive dentistry, and yet studies have found that the use of rubber dam during operative dentistry procedures is not common in private practice.[52,53] Recently, a meta-analysis revealed that the type of field isolation (rubber dam versus cotton rolls/retraction cord isolation) had no influence on the performance of adhesive restorations in noncarious cervical lesions (NCCLs).[31] However, it is imperative that the field is dry, clean, and visible.

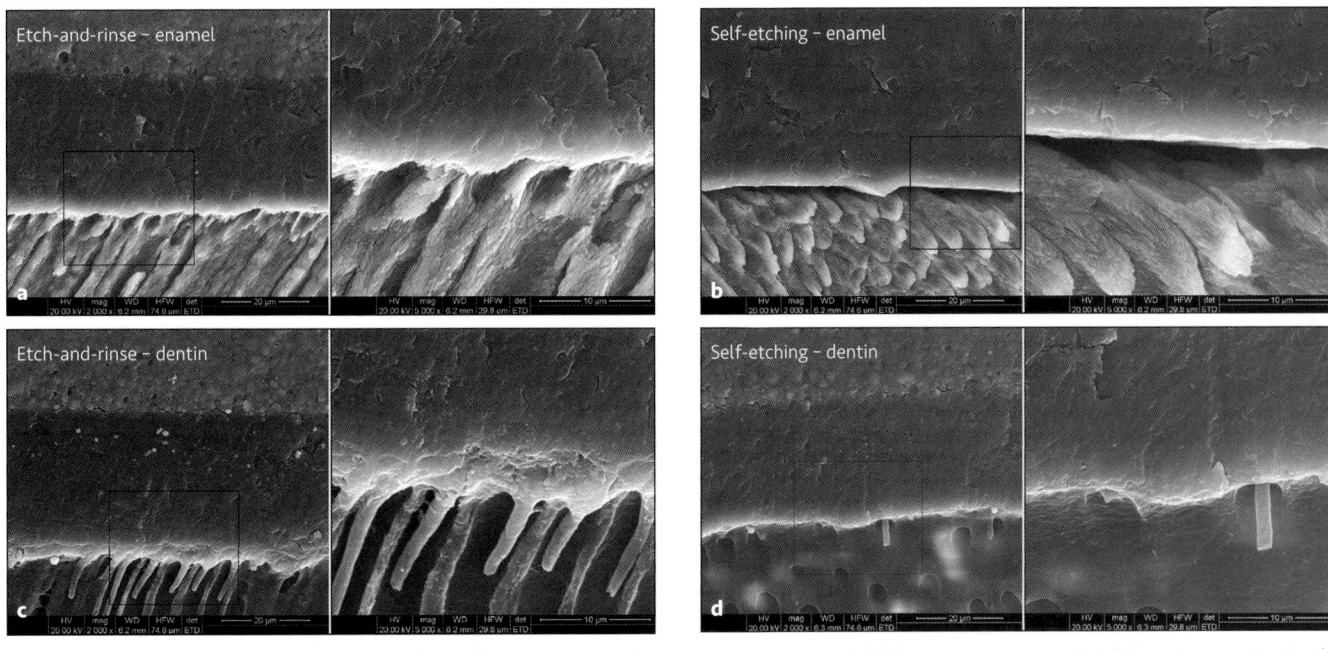

Fig 9-1 Adhesive layers resulting from ER and SE adhesive systems. *(a)* ER system on enamel. *(b)* SE system on enamel. *(c)* ER system on dentin. *(d)* SE system on dentin.

2. Do not perform cavity preparation

Some researchers recommend roughening the superficial sclerotic dentin with a diamond bur to increase the retention rate of adhesive restorations in NCCLs.[31,54–56] However, not all evidence supports this claim; at least two clinical trials showed no significant difference in retention between NCCLs that were roughened versus not roughened.[34,55] Therefore, cavity preparation should be avoided before the application of SE or ER adhesive systems.

3. Select the appropriate adhesive system

Etch-and-rinse adhesives

For ER adhesive systems, the use of 34% to 38% phosphoric acid is recommended, preferably a gel. The application should begin in the enamel (30 seconds) and then move to the dentin (15 seconds). The tooth should then be rinsed with water for 30 seconds. In any given NCCL, areas of total or partial sclerosis and areas of nonsclerosis may be observed. Prolonged etching in areas of sclerotic dentin will not improve bond strength[56,57] and may even lead to increased degradation of the bonded interface.[58,59]

Recent studies have shown evidence of improved bond strengths with the use of benzalkonium-chloride and chlorhexidine.[60–62] These substances are enzymatic inhibitors and thereby help to prevent degradation of the collagen fiber network.[63,64] However, their application is not a simple procedure, and care must be taken to avoid dehydration of the dentin substrate prior to application of the adhesive.[38]

Self-etch adhesives

For SE adhesive systems, two techniques can be used. Selective enamel etching[65,66] involves the application of 34% to 38% phosphoric acid gel to enamel only for 30 seconds followed by rinsing with water for 30 seconds. Although this procedure has become popular among clinicians, it does not always result in an increased retention rate in NCCLs.[30,37,41,42]

An alternative approach for bonding to NCCLs is to apply dentin conditioners such as ethylenediaminetetraacetic acid (EDTA) to the dentin to increase the bonding performance. Pretreatment with EDTA has been shown to improve the resin-dentin bond strength of the SE adhesive to natural and sclerotic dentin.[56,67,68] Furthermore, EDTA also removes the smear layer from the surface,[69,70] which facilitates better interaction between the SE adhesive and sclerotic dentin. A recent clinical study showed that preliminary conditioning with EDTA before application of a one-step SE adhesive significantly improved the retention rates of composite restorations in NCCLs after 18 months of clinical service.[43] With this technique, 17% EDTA should be applied to the dentin for 2 minutes and then rinsed with water for 30 seconds. The tooth should be kept moist.

Figure 9-1 illustrates the adhesive layers resulting from ER and SE systems.

Universal adhesives

There is still some debate whether universal adhesives should be applied to dentin as ER adhesives.[71,72] The available research data suggests that universal adhesives may not be the best choice for etching dentin. If the clinician decides to use a universal adhesive, it should contain MDP.

4. Adhesive application

Several techniques can be used to improve adhesion.

Use of a nonsimplified adhesive or a hydrophobic resin coating

It is always preferable to use the full version of each adhesive strategy (ie, three-step ER or two-step SE adhesive). If simplified adhesives are selected (ie, two-step ER or one-step SE adhesive), the material should be applied with a hydrophobic resin coating.[30,31,73] The use of a hydrophobic coating after the application of simplified adhesive systems leads to a thicker and more uniform adhesive layer with less retained water and solvent and a significant reduction in the fluid flow rate.[74,75] Dentin adhesive systems that utilize the separated non-solvated hydrophobic bonding resin (ie, three-step ER and two-step SE) show a higher degree of polymerization and less permeability to water,[76,77] resulting in a more stable resin-dentin interface.[78]

Multiple coats

It is important to apply multiple coats of simplified ER and SE adhesives in NCCLs to yield a strong adhesive interface[79,80] and make it less prone to degradation over time.[78] For simplified ER and SE adhesives, this technique improves the saturation of the hybrid layer with resin monomers while favoring solvent evaporation. One clinical study observed that multiple adhesive coats significantly improved retention rates for simplified ER and SE adhesives after 18 months of clinical service.[50] Therefore, at least two coats should be applied for 10 to 15 seconds each using a microbrush.

Extending application time prior to polymerization

Extending the application time prior to polymerization can ensure better resin penetration and higher solvent evaporation for simplified ER adhesives.[81,82] For SE adhesives, this protocol was also shown to improve the immediate bonding,[83,84] although data is still lacking on the durability of these adhesive interfaces. Application time may be extended to up to 60 seconds.

Vigorous adhesive application

The gentle application of simplified ER systems limits the diffusion of high-molecular weight resin monomers into the wet demineralized dentin.[85-87] Vigorous application, on the other hand, compresses the collapsed collagen network and, as the pressure is relieved, may draw more of the adhesive solution into this network as it expands.[88,89] This technique can be applied on either wet or dry demineralized dentin[88,90] and has been shown to increase the durability of adhesive interfaces produced with SE adhesives. Excellent results in terms of retention rate were observed when both an ER adhesive[40] and a simplified SE adhesive[51] were vigorously applied in NCCLs. One additional advantage of vigorous application is a significant reduction in marginal discoloration of the enamel margins in the long term.[51] Therefore, vigorous application could be considered a feasible alternative to selective enamel etching.[91]

It is important to note that this technique cannot be performed with a bristle brush applicator. The operator should apply the adhesive using a rigid microbrush applicator with as much manual pressure as possible on the dentin surface.[92] Sonic devices used for adhesive application show promising results[93,94] and may one day standardize the adhesive application procedure, but future clinical evaluation is warranted.

Unlike the previous techniques mentioned, vigorous application of the adhesive system does not prolong the clinical procedure, making it a preferable technique for many clinicians intent on simplifying and accelerating application protocols.

5. Air drying the adhesive

Following the adhesive application, it is necessary to air dry the adhesive to aid solvent evaporation. This is always necessary for simplified adhesives as well as for the second bottle of a three-step ER or the first bottle of a two-step SE adhesive system. Air drying is not recommended for the third bottle of a three-step ER or the second bottle of a two-step SE adhesive system because they do not present solvents.

Most manufacturer instructions recommend 10 to 20 seconds of air drying for solvent evaporation, but complete solvent elimination is technically impossible.[9] Unfortunately, the retention of solvents and/or water during polymerization compromises the integrity of the adhesive interface.[9] Consequently, the mechanical properties of the adhesive are affected,[95] which ultimately hampers adhesive performance.[96-98]

There is no consensus in the literature regarding the appropriate air-drying time for solvent evaporation,[99-103] and no clinical studies have evaluated this variable in NCCLs. Therefore, it is recommended to follow the manufacturer instructions and use other techniques to aid in solvent evaporation (ie, vigorous application of the adhesive and extended application time). Suction drying with a suction tip has been evaluated as an alternative to the air syringe for solvent evaporation,[104,105] but more studies are warranted to evaluate the efficacy of this technique on simplified adhesive systems.

6. Light curing

As the very last step, it is necessary to cure the adhesive system before applying the resin composite. One simple way to maximize the suboptimal polymerization of adhesive systems is to extend the curing time.[76,77] This technique appears to be a possible means for improving the immediate performance of these adhesives,[106-109] although it has not been evaluated in NCCLs. The higher energy density produced by the longer exposure time enhances the formation of free radicals, which initiate polymerization.[110] In addition, the heat produced by light-curing units[111,112] likely increases solvent evaporation rates.[107] However, recent in vitro studies have demonstrated that prolonging the exposure time during light curing may only slow down the degradation rate of the adhesive interface for two-step ER[107] and one-step SE adhesives.[109]

It is important to note that several light-emitting diode (LED) curing lights present narrow wavelength distribution with a single-wave emission around 468 nm, which corresponds to the maximum absorption peak of camphorquinone, so adhesives containing alternative initiators may not be efficiently light cured by some LED devices. Furthermore, the use of solvents can modify the absorption peak of photoinitiators (like camphorquinone) and thereby reduce the polymerization of the adhesive. A simple tip for the clinician is to check if the device is able to polymerize one adhesive drop over a glass plate.

The authors recommend light curing the adhesive system for at least 40 seconds at a minimum of 600 mw/cm^2.

Composition of Composite Resins

Composite resins have evolved significantly since the materials were first introduced to dentistry more than 50 years ago. These materials became increasingly popular because they have good mechanical strength, polymerization advantages during placement, and good esthetics, which together result in excellent clinical results.[113,114] Until recently, the most important changes to the composition of composite resins related to reducing the particle size of fillers to produce materials that were more easily or effectively polished and produced greater wear resistance. Current changes in formulation have been focused on the polymeric matrix of the material, principally to develop systems with reduced polymerization shrinkage. Reduced polymerization shrinkage stress allows for greater adhesive capability to tooth structure.[115] Composite materials are composed of an organic matrix, reinforcing fillers, silane coupling agent, and chemical agents that promote or modulate the polymerization reaction.

Monomers

The monomers used in composite resins are key to understanding their physicochemical properties. The bis-GMA monomer (bisphenol glycidyl methacrylate) forms the basis of current composite resins.[116-119] The presence of two aromatic rings in the structure introduces high molecular weight and rigidity for polymeric reactivity. It also yields a high viscosity characteristic of the presence of intermolecular hydrogen bonds between hydroxyl groups. Because of the low reactive mobility of this monomer, arrays with high concentration of bis-GMA tend to have a low degree of conversion and volumetric shrinkage.[114,119-121] To increase the degree of composite conversion, other monomers with lower molecular weight are added to increase the viscosity. TEGDMA (triethylene glycol dimethacrylate) is most frequently used in combination with bis-GMA because together they yield a greater flexibility that provides increased mobility of the reaction and a greater degree of conversion. The lower–molecular weight monomer, however, is associated with greater volumetric shrinkage.[122]

The monomer UDMA (urethane dimethacrylate), when combined with bis-EMA (ethoxylated bisphenol A dimethacrylate), was found to produce high conversion with low volumetric shrinkage.[110] Both have high molecular weight and low viscosity. To minimize the problem of low viscosity incorporation, monomer diluents are commonly added; however, diluents change the matrix properties by increasing water sorption and polymerization contractility.[114,123] Some composite resins include modified monomers developed to reduce this shrinkage.[115]

The latest trend has been toward the development of flowable composites containing adhesive monomers. These formulations are based on traditional methacrylate systems but incorporate acidic monomers typically found in dentin bonding agents, such as glycerolphosphate dimethacrylate (GPDM), which may be capable of generating adhesion through mechanical and biochemical interactions with tooth structure. These materials are currently recommended as liners and for small restorations.[115]

Fillers

The fillers in composites aim to improve the mechanical properties and wear resistance and reduce the polymerization shrinkage. The particles generally include glass, quartz, or some other form of silica.[123] There are several theories about the role of filler particles in wear resistance, mechanical properties, and degree of conversion for a composite. Research has evaluated the microstructure of the composite with respect to arrangement, size, geometry, and volumetric fraction.[119,124,125]

Silane

The bonding agent silane is applied by manufacturers to inorganic fillers before being mixed into the matrix. It is used to increase the strength of the composite by means of covalent bonds between different fillers and monomers. The silanization between organic and inorganic phases plays an important role depending on process quality, mechanical properties, polymerization strain, and durability of composites when subjected to physicochemical oral environment conditions. The silane hydrolysis process is well studied, and it is expected that the binding matrix decreases in strength over time.[126,127]

Other agents

Accelerators and initiators are responsible for composite polymerization, and according to the material used, the activation mode may be chemical (self-curing), physical (photocuring), or both (dual-curing). Most commercial composites include camphorquinone as a photoinitiator of reactivity, which is activated by blue light at a peak range of 468 nm. Both self-curing and photocuring agents are stable with the organic matrix at room temperature and in the absence of light.[125,127,128] Some commercial formulations have included other photoinitiators that are potentially more color stable.[115]

Classification

Different types of composite materials are distinguished by their consistency. Flowable composites are typically characterized by a lower viscosity due to reduced filler content or the addition of other modifying agents that reduce the surface tension to improve fluidity. Packable composites achieve their thicker consistency by modifying the size distribution of filler particles or adding other components such as fibers. Both of these composites maintain enough filler content to ensure good mechanical properties and low polymerization shrinkage.[115]

Within each type of composite, materials are further distinguished by the characteristics of their reinforcing fillers and, in particular, their size. Composites are classified as "conventional" or "macrofilled" when the average particle size exceeds 1 μm. Macrofilled composites have greater compressive strength but are difficult to polish and cannot retain surface smoothness. "Microfilled" composites, on the other hand, have particle sizes less than 1 μm. Microfilled composites are polishable but generally weak due to their relatively low filler content. Therefore, hybrid composites with an average particle size of 0.4 to 1.0 μm and a filler volume of 50% to 70% were developed to produce adequate strength with enhanced polishability and esthetics. These materials are generally considered to be universal composites because they can be used for most anterior and posterior applications based on their combination of strength and polishing capabilities.

The most recent innovation is nanofilled composites containing only nanoscale particles (particle size of 5 to 75 nm).[124,125] Most manufacturers have modified formulations of their microhybrids to include more nanoparticles because nanofilled and nanohybrid materials currently represent the state of the art in filler formulation.

Composites for NCCLs

Composite materials are widely used to restore NCCLs because they do not require the excessive removal of sound tooth structure. The high modulus of elasticity of many direct placement composite restorative materials more closely replicates that of dentin to offer comparable behavior in response to occlusal loading. Composite resins and adhesive systems are continually being developed with the purpose of improving retention to the dental structure and simplifying clinical procedures. (See Table 2 in the Appendix for scientific data on their longevity.) Micromechanical retention, preservation of tooth structure, good esthetics, and functional features are some aspects to consider in choosing the appropriate material.[128–132]

Hybrid composite resins

In general, hybrid composite resins have been the material of choice for NCCLs because of their superior esthetics, adequate strength, and versatility.[115] However, difficulties in isolation, difficulties in adhesion to dentin margins, and polymerization shrinkage stress of these composite resins make the clinical outcome sensitive to the operator's technique.[132,133] Incremental placement of composite resins reduces the effects from shrinkage, but the time it takes to complete this protocol increases the risk of problems with isolation.

It has been proposed that the filler content of composite resins affects the clinical performance of cervical restorations. For example, compared with microhybrid composites, microfilled composites have a lower elastic modulus that allows them to flex with the tooth during function, reducing failure of the bonded interface and dislodgement of the restoration.[115,134]

Flowable composite resins

Flowable composite resins were created by retaining the same particle sizes as traditional hybrid composites but reducing the filler content, thereby reducing the viscosity of the material.[135] This flowability is regarded as a desirable handling property that allows the material to be injected through small-gauge dispensers, thus simplifying the placement procedure and broadening the range of applications suggested by manufacturers. However, because little is currently known about the long-term retention rates of these materials, they cannot be viewed as replacements for microfilled or hybrid resins. Furthermore, some concern exists regarding their inferior mechanical properties compared with traditional hybrid composites. They may shrink considerably more than traditional composites, and because of their lower filler content, they can be expected to be less rigid.[136]

Although recently developed flowable resin composites have more than 80% filler content by weight, their modulus of elasticity is lower than that of hybrid and microfilled composite resins.[135,136] In theory, then, flowable composites could flex more than microhybrids after curing, allowing for greater relaxation of tensions imposed at the tooth-resin interface by shrinkage during polymerization.[134] However, flowable composite resins showed more microleakage than hybrid composite resins under thermocycling.[135,137] Their use is therefore discouraged in high-stress locations for restorative dentistry, such as NCCLs.

Packable composite resins

Packable esthetic composite resins have been introduced and marketed by dental manufacturers.[134–138] These materials are recommended for use in stress-bearing areas as a replacement for amalgam. Improved condensation properties and contact point tightness make these materials a good choice for posterior restorations.[133,138,139] Esthetic restorative composites have also been developed to mimic the color, reflectance, and translucency exhibited by natural tooth structure.[135,138–140] The high flexural strength, low abrasion, and low polymerization shrinkage of these packable composite resins are attributed to a high nanofiller content.[138,139,141]

Bulk-fill composite resins

The newly developed bulk-fill composite resins claim to offer single increment thicknesses ranging from 4 to 6 mm instead of the 2-mm thickness commonly achieved with conventional hybrid composites.[138,139] Advantages of a thicker increment of material include an increased depth of cure and low shrinkage stress, which are primarily related to modifications in filler content. An ideal bulk-fill composite would be one that could be placed into a preparation with a high C-factor or shrinkage design while maintaining a high degree of cure throughout.[135,138,139] Reduced polymerization stress should result in decreased internal and external marginal gap formation compared with incrementally placed composites, but the potential for internal marginal gap formation still exists with bulk placement. The proportion of gaps relative to the use of conventional 2-mm increments has yet to be determined. If the bulk-fill restorative materials are to provide a true clinical advantage, they require high depths of cure while simultaneously demonstrating a decrease in internal stress and subsequently a decreased incidence of internal gap formation.[137–139]

There is currently a growing trend toward the use of bulk-fill composites among practitioners because of a perceived cost savings stemming from reduced chair time required for placement. This reduced chair time also reduces the risk of soft tissue damage from resin toxicity. However, the clinical performance of these composites is still in question.[138–141] The mechanical properties of bulk-fill composites are similar to those of flowable materials and inferior to those of nanohybrid composites. Because flowable materials are not recommended to represent restoration bulk, it is questionable as to whether bulk-fill composites should be used for this purpose.[138,139,141,142] Nonetheless, these materials do have good hardness, flexural strength, and elastic modulus because of their high filler content. Furthermore, some have shown mechanical properties equivalent to those of conventional composites.[138,139]

Glass-Ionomer Cements

A glass ionomer (GI) is composed of an ion-leachable glass powder and a polyacid liquid that, when mixed, form a solid mass upon setting. The powder in an aluminosilicate glass is prepared by sintering mixtures of silica (SiO_2), alumina (Al_2O_3), fluorite (CaF_2), and aluminum phosphate ($AlPO_4$) at 1,100°C to 1,500°C. The liquid component is a combination of tartaric, maleic, and itaconic acids; polyacrylic acid is also present in some commercial preparations.[143,144] The ionic bond between the carboxyl groups of the polyalkenoic acid and the hydroxyapatite in enamel or dentin is responsible for the chemical bonding of GIs. Although resin-modified GIs have better adhesion to tooth structure than most composite resins, in vitro study of this material has found lower bond strengths due to low cohesion.[129,145] Poor esthetic longevity and low wear resistance against abrasion have limited the use of GIs for restoring NCCLs.[131,146]

Restorative Protocols: Adhesive Bonding, Materials, and Techniques

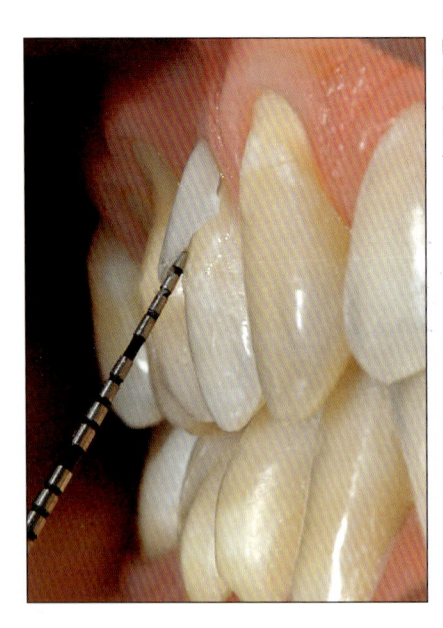

Fig 9-2 Ceramic fragment being placed to cover an NCCL with gingival recession. (Courtesy of the NCCL Research Group, Uberlândia, Brazil.)

Composition of Ceramics

Dental ceramics are inorganic nonmetallic structures consisting of oxygen (O) and one or more metallic or semimetallic elements such as aluminum (Al), boron (B), calcium (Ca), cerium (Ce), lithium (Li), magnesium (Mg), phosphorus (P), potassium (K), silicon (Si), sodium (Na), titanium (Ti), and/or zirconium (Zr).[147] Dental ceramics are similar to tooth enamel in their color stability, excellent surface smoothness, abrasion resistance, and low accumulation of plaque. These qualities make dental ceramics a good choice for NCCL restoration.

The ceramics used in the restoration of NCCLs can be characterized by a glass portion and a crystalline matrix. (There are some glass-free dental ceramics, but they are not indicated for cervical restoration.) The glass portion of the ceramic, constituting Si^{4+}, O^-, and K^+, is responsible for the optical properties of the material, especially the translucency often associated with a natural appearance. This crystalline phase also gives the ceramic its mechanical strength. As a general rule, the more crystals present, the greater the opacity and strength.[148] The metal oxides reinforce the glassy phase and can influence the color of the porcelain.

Ceramic materials have several characteristics that justify their use in NCCL restoration: They do not conduct electricity or heat, they cannot be degraded by abrasion or intraoral chemical substances, they have great smoothness, and they have excellent polishability[149,150] due to glazing.[151] Moreover, the lack of cytotoxicity or hydrolytic degradation and consequent lack of byproduct release over time favors periodontal health.[149,150]

Although their cost is high compared with composite resins, dental ceramics are particularly good choices for the restoration of NCCLs associated with gingival recession because of their gingival tissue biocompatibility. In these instances, restoration of the lesion is indicated prior to periodontal root coverage procedures.[152] Because root coverage in teeth with restored NCCLs promotes intimate contact between the gingival tissue and the restorative material[153] (ie, the restoration will be partly covered by the gingival graft), ceramics are a good choice because they do not adversely affect periodontal health[154,155] (Fig 9-2).

Glass-Ceramics

Crystalline ceramics can be classified into glass-ceramics (feldspathic, leucite, and lithium disilicate), which are predominantly composed of amorphous glass (Fig 9-3), and polycrystalline ceramics (alumina, spinel, zirconia), which are predominantly composed of crystalline particles and have little to no amorphous glass (Fig 9-4). This discussion focuses on glass-ceramics and their application as ceramic fragments to restore NCCLs.

Feldspathic ceramics provide the greatest natural tooth mimicry and were the first used in dentistry. They are a mixture of potassium feldspar or sodium feldspar with quartz. The feldspar is heated to temperatures between 1,200°C to 1,250°C to promote the incongruous merger, and this reaction forms an amorphous structure (liquid glass) and a leucite crystal phase.[156] The molten mass after cooling maintains the glassy state. Metal oxides are added to act as pigments for the porcelain.[148,157]

Feldspathic porcelain has a translucency and a coefficient of thermal expansion similar to those of tooth structure, is resistant to compression and hydrolytic degradation promoted by oral fluids, and does not have corrosive potential. In addition, surface treatments by acid etching improve its adhesive potential (Fig 9-5). However, it has low tensile and flexural strength.[158,159] The manual fabrication (ie, layering) of this material may also lead to internal defects (porosities) that compromise its integrity (Fig 9-6). These pores allow for stress concentration, which can result in catastrophic failure of the porcelain.[160,161]

Ceramic reinforced by leucite

Glass-ceramics are reinforced by the addition of approximately 55% by weight leucite crystals. Leucite crystals embedded in feldspathic ceramic promote an increase in mechanical strength and offer durability in restoring root surface lesions.[160,162] Even with the addition of reinforcing particles, these glass-ceramics can mimic natural tooth coloration (Fig 9-7).

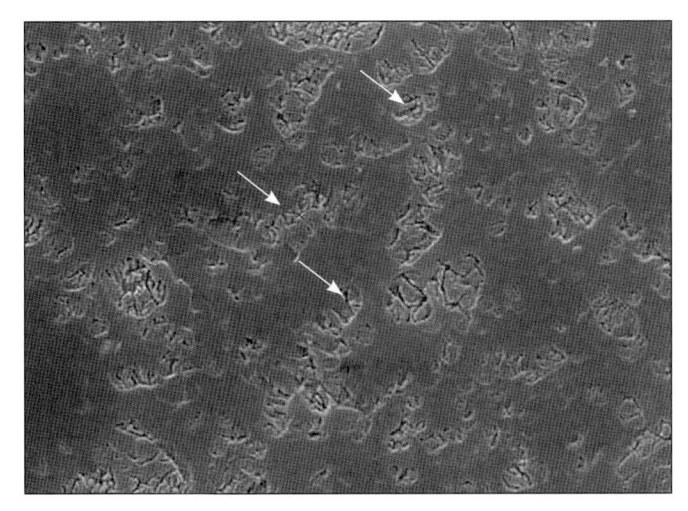

Fig 9-3 Predominantly glass structure with leucite crystals *(arrows)*. (Courtesy of Dr Lucas Zago Naves, Uberlândia, Brazil.)

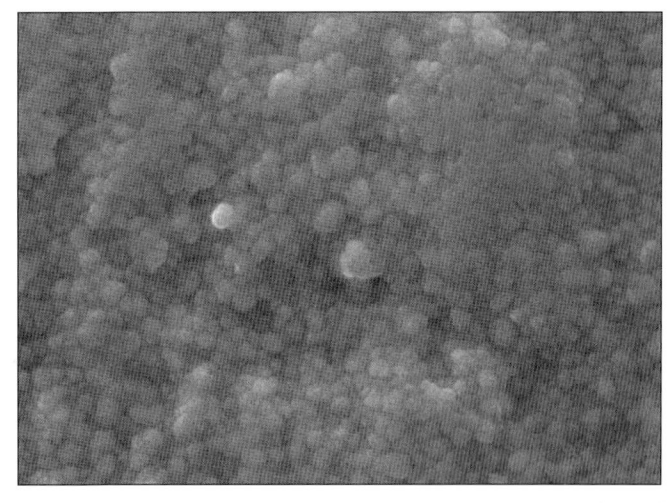

Fig 9-4 Structure of a ceramic polycrystalline zirconia base. Note the lack of a crystalline phase. (Courtesy of Dr Lucas Zago Naves, Uberlândia, Brazil.)

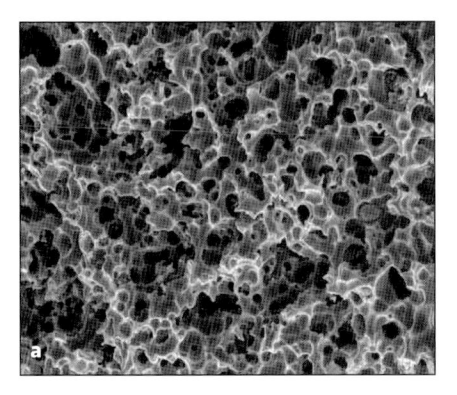

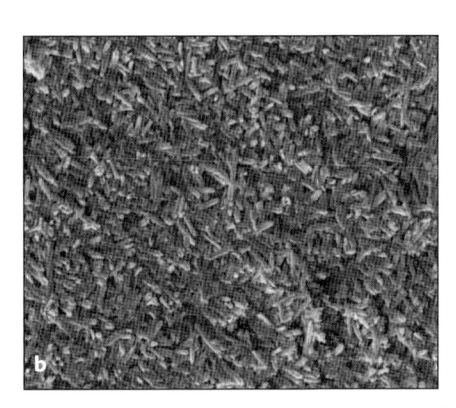

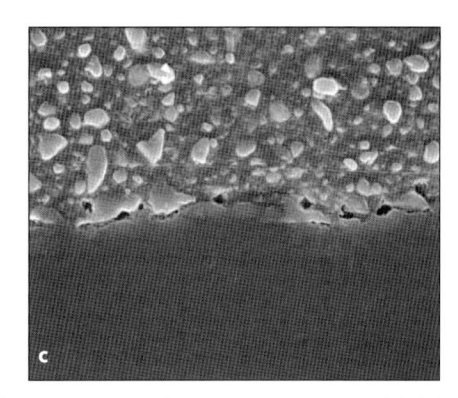

Fig 9-5 Surface treatments by acid etching (hydrofluoric acid 10%) in ceramic-reinforced leucite *(a)* and ceramic-reinforced lithium disilicate *(b)*. *(c)* Interface between glass-ceramic and resin cement. (Courtesy of Dr Lucas Zago Naves, Uberlândia, Brazil.)

Fig 9-6 The internal defects (porosities) present in feldspathic porcelain *(arrows)*. (Courtesy of Dr Lucas Zago Naves, Uberlândia, Brazil.)

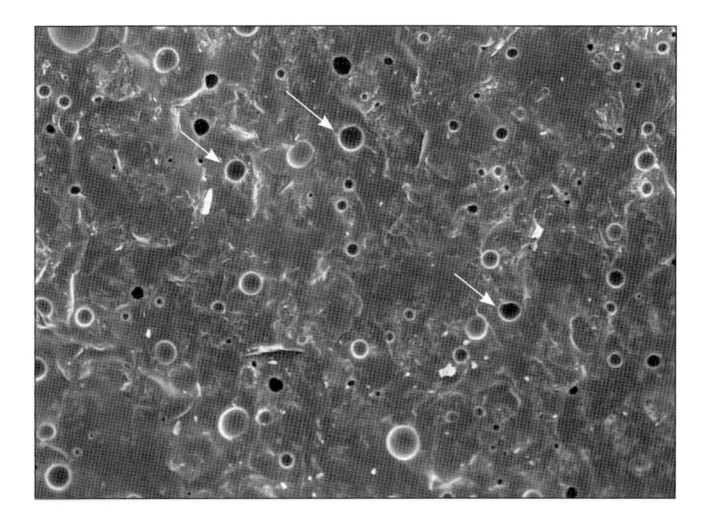

Ceramic reinforced by lithium disilicate

Glass-ceramics reinforced with lithium disilicate have about 60% to 65% lithium disilicate crystals by weight in the crystalline phase with flexural strength of 300 to 400 MPa, up to seven times greater than conventional feldspathic porcelain.[163] The high strength and fracture toughness of these glass-ceramics (eg, IPS Empress 2, Ivoclar Vivadent) are attributed to fine lithium disilicate crystals interlocking in their microstructure, thereby preventing crack initiation.[164] These glass-ceramics have less translucency than feldspathic ceramics but still provide an adequate esthetic result.[165] They are therefore indicated to restore NCCLs.[166]

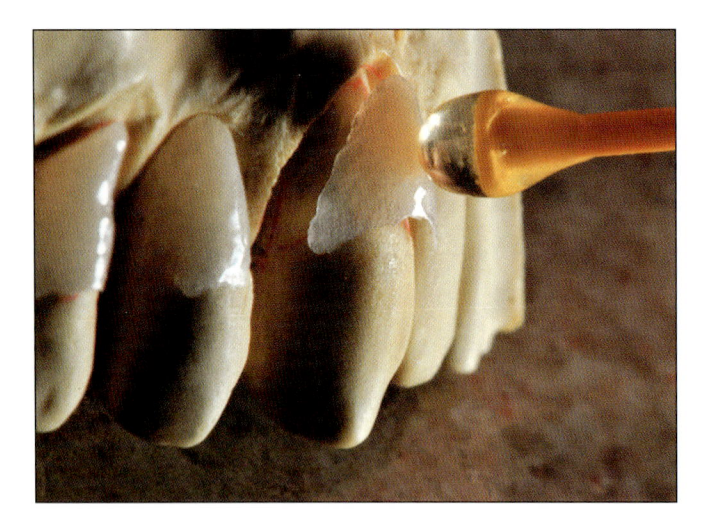

9 Restorative Protocols: Adhesive Bonding, Materials, and Techniques

Fig 9-7 Note the different chromatic aspects of a ceramic fragment to mimic natural tooth structure.

Ceramic Fragments in NCCLs

Following cementation of ceramic fragments, the cementation margin must be polished to reduce buildup of plaque.[167] Plaque accumulation due to the presence of residual cement, poor personal oral hygiene, and high abrasion resistance of common cements results in gingival inflammation and subsequent gingival recession. Maintaining a satisfactory patient oral hygiene pattern after cementation is therefore critical to periodontal health and the success of any restorative procedure. However, the cementation medium and process themselves are also critical. The efficiency of the curing light must be monitored, and the depth of photoactivation must be controlled to ensure proper polymerization.[168] An advantage of ceramics is that they have less polymerization shrinkage than composite resins[169,170] when a thin layer of cement is applied.[171,172]

Light-Curing Units

When using photoactive materials that require polymerization, such as composite resins or cements used to place ceramic fragments, success depends on the efficiency of the light-curing unit and the depth of cure. Most professionals use quartz tungsten halogen (QTH) or LED light-curing units. QTH light-curing units have been used in dentistry for many years to polymerize composite resins.[173] This device consists of a tungsten filament lamp (bulb and reflector), filter, cooling system, and optical fibers for transmission of light to the exposure tip. Over time, the high heat production causes degradation of the bulb and reflector, which induces a loss of effectiveness of the light-curing unit.[174]

Unlike QTH systems, LED lamps have a lifetime of several thousands of hours without significant intensity loss.[175] With a light intensity of 1,200 mW/cm^2, LED lamps currently used in clinical practice promote good polymerization of composite, and the heat generated is of only minor clinical concern for the gingival and pulpal tissues.[176]

In cementing a ceramic fragment, adequate polymerization of cement requires that the light passes through the ceramic. Light is absorbed as it passes through the ceramic, so it may reach the cement with insufficient intensity to polymerize.[177] This can be remedied by extending the light curing times of LED units with high irradiances. Both factors increase the energy dose that reaches the cement for adequate polymerization. Similarly, a composite must receive approximately 16 mJ/cm^2 for polymerization of a 2-mm thickness. This dose is dependent on the activation time and light intensity reaching the composite resin. For example, a light-curing unit with an irradiance value of 400 mW/cm^2 will take 40 seconds to polymerize 2 mm of composite (activation time × irradiance = energy dose, so 40 s × 400 mW/cm^2 = 16 mJ/cm^2). A short curing time with high-intensity LEDs may influence the bulk properties of the material, resulting in lower curing depth, increased residual monomer content, and lower hardness values.[178–181]

In NCCL restorations, this becomes even more critical because the premature degradation of the margin[181] and higher cytotoxicity of the resin-based materials compromise their clinical performance.[182] In addition, the thickness and shade of the ceramic,[177,183] color of the composite resin,[184] color of the cement,[185] and increment volume[186,187] can all affect the success of polymerization. When any of these factors interferes with polymerization (eg, dark or opaque colors hinder the penetration of light), high-intensity LEDs are indicated. In addition, radiometers are important for the clinician to routinely check for performance losses of any light-curing units used in the office.[176]

Fig 9-8 *(a)* In irregular and deep cavities, increments should be placed in three stages to reduce the C-factor in a Class V lesion. The first and second layers should be placed on the opposite walls of the cavity, and the third increment should cover the first two increments and rebuild the buccal contour. *(b)* In shallow cavities, two layers can rebuild the facial contour.

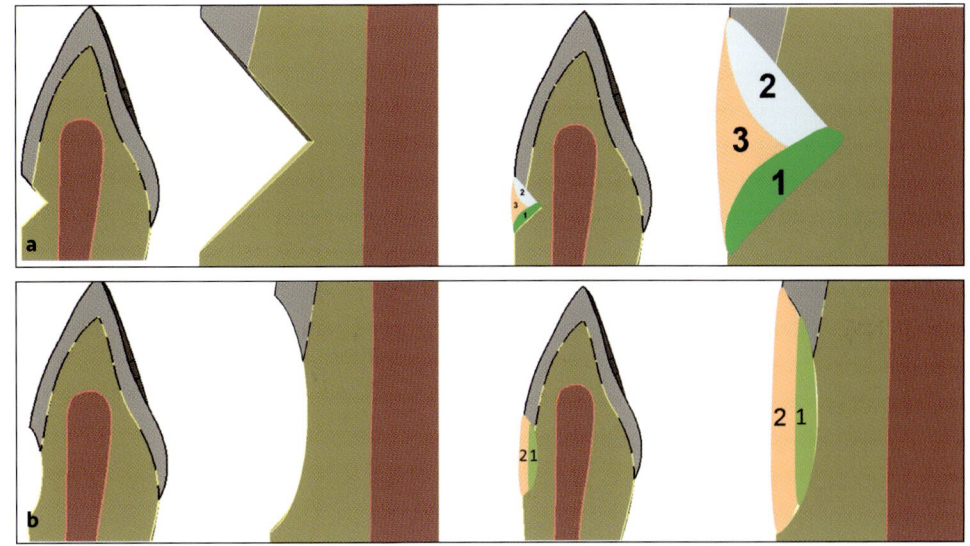

Direct Technique with Composite Resin Restorations

The loss of dental structure in NCCLs involves not only bone loss and gingival recession but also a complete change in the biomechanics of the dental components affected by this pathology. These lesions must be restored in order to prevent further progression and loss of tooth structure. The direct technique for adhesive Class V restorations is a simple, affordable, and universally used protocol for reproducing the esthetics and function of a natural tooth. Glass-ionomer cements[188] and composite resins[189,190] are the most common materials used to restore the lost enamel and dentin at the cervical region, but composite resins have been shown to most closely mimic the biomechanical behavior of sound tooth structure.[166] When restoring NCCLs, it is extremely important to layer the composite resin to reduce the C-factor (Fig 9-8).

Step-By-Step Direct Technique

This section presents the step-by-step placement of direct restorations using composite resin in two case reports.

Case 1

A 39-year-old patient presented with complaints of tooth sensitivity to air exposure and cold drinks. Several NCCLs were identified upon clinical and radiographic examination. The proposed treatment included sealing and restoring these areas and referring the patient for orthodontic evaluation (Fig 9-9).

Case 2

A 57-year-old patient presented with an irregular NCCL in the mandibular right second premolar, which was restored in three layers using a nanohybrid composite resin (Fig 9-10).

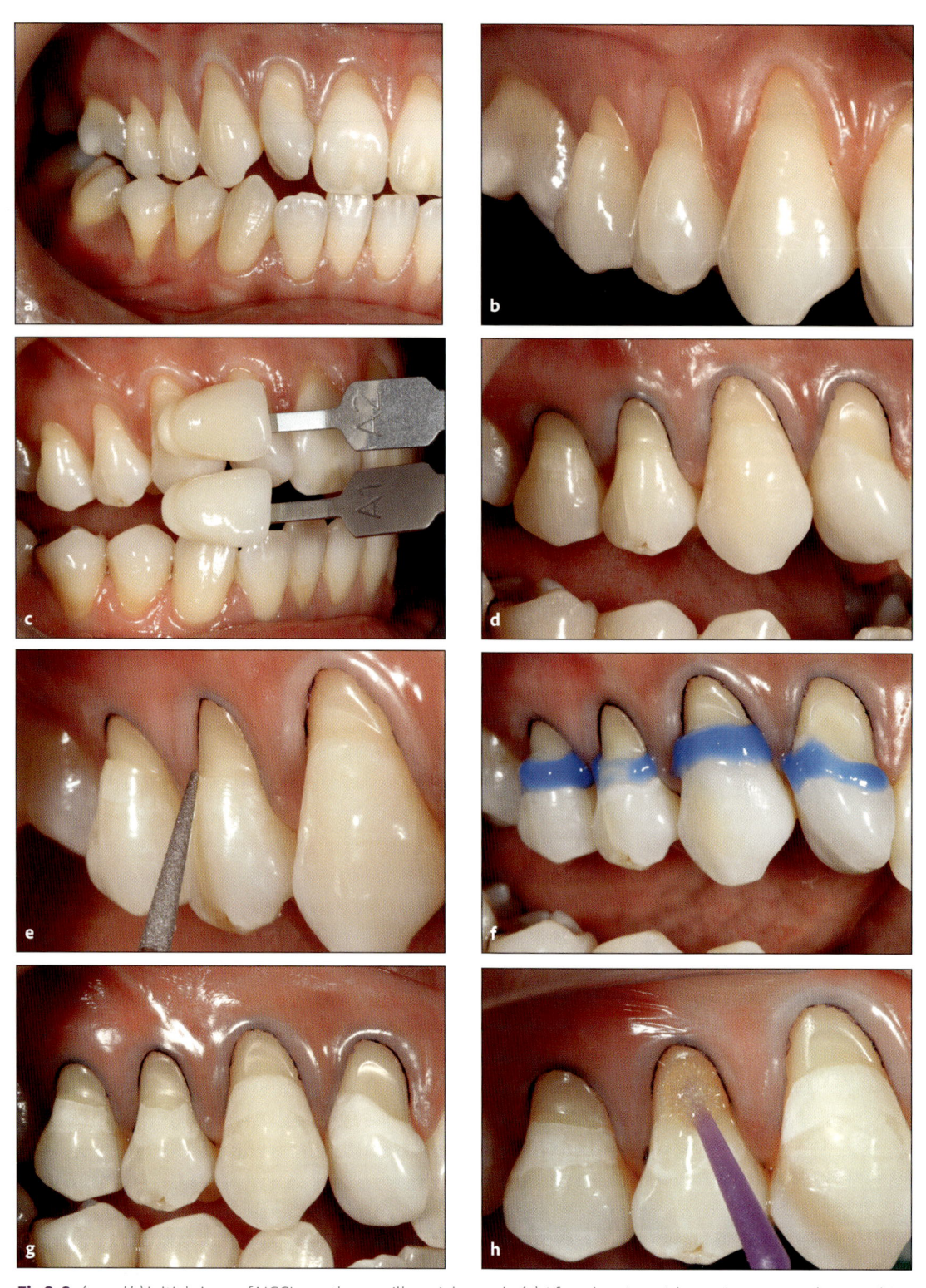

9 Restorative Protocols: Adhesive Bonding, Materials, and Techniques

Fig 9-9 *(a and b)* Initial views of NCCLs on the maxillary right teeth. *(c)* After cleaning with pumice paste, color matching was performed. *(d)* Retraction cord (#000) was inserted inside the gingival sulcus to eliminate crevicular fluid during the restoration. *(e)* Forty-five-degree bevels were placed on the enamel margins of each lesion with a fine diamond bur to mask the tooth-restoration interface. *(f)* Etching of the enamel margins with 37% phosphoric acid for 30 seconds. *(g)* View of demineralized enamel after rinsing with water and air drying. *(h)* Application of the primer from a self-etching adhesive system to the dentin for 20 seconds. →

Direct Technique with Composite Resin Restorations

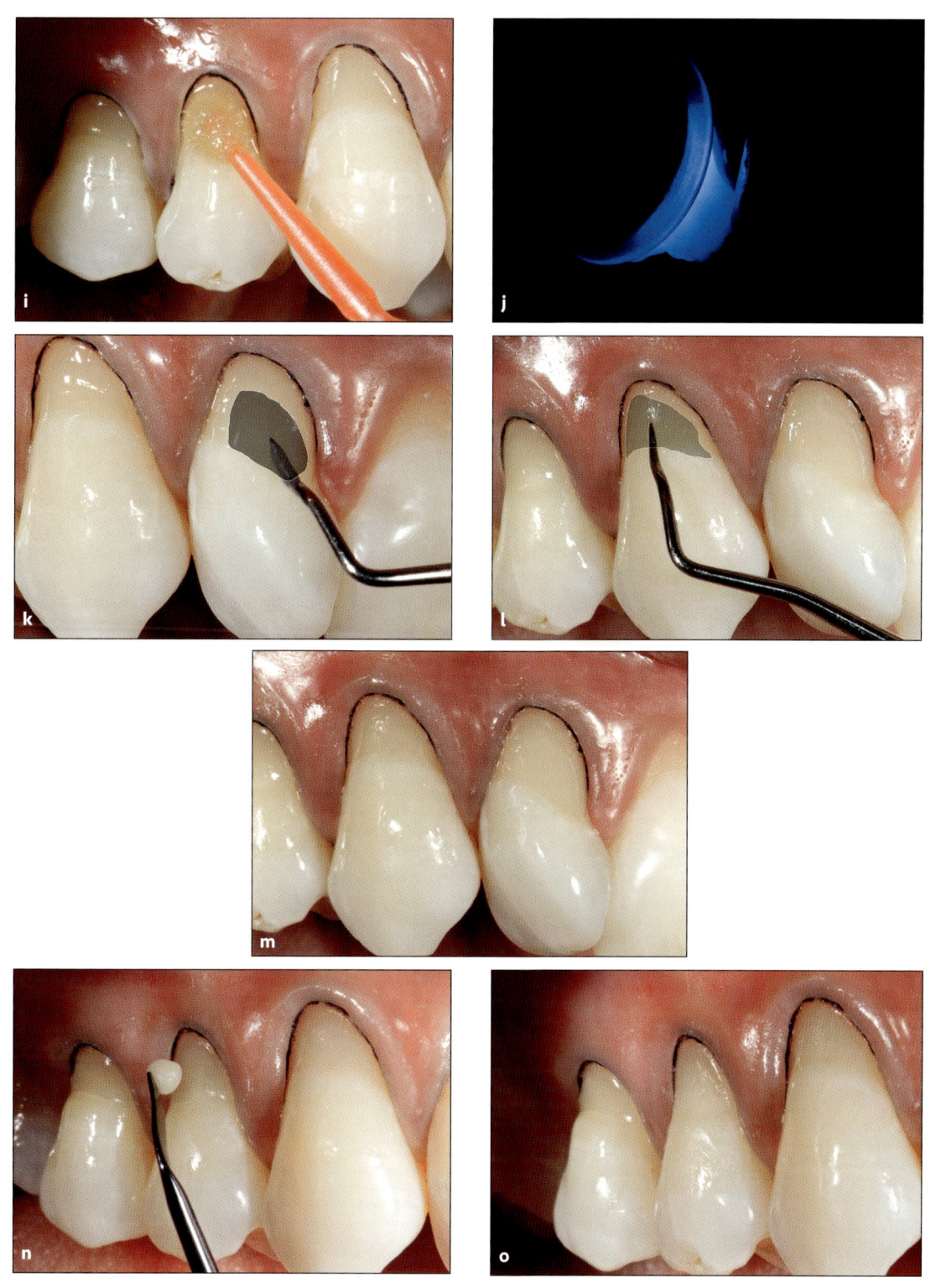

Fig 9-9 *(cont)* *(i)* Application of the adhesive from a self-etching adhesive system on the enamel and dentin. *(j)* Light curing of the adhesive. *(k)* The maxillary right lateral incisor was restored with a nanofilled flowable composite resin in one layer and light cured for 40 seconds. *(l)* The maxillary right canine was restored with the same nanofilled flowable composite resin in one layer and light cured for 40 seconds. *(m)* View after restoration of the lateral incisor and canine. *(n and o)* The maxillary right first premolar was then restored, beginning with a layer of an opaque nanofilled composite resin. →

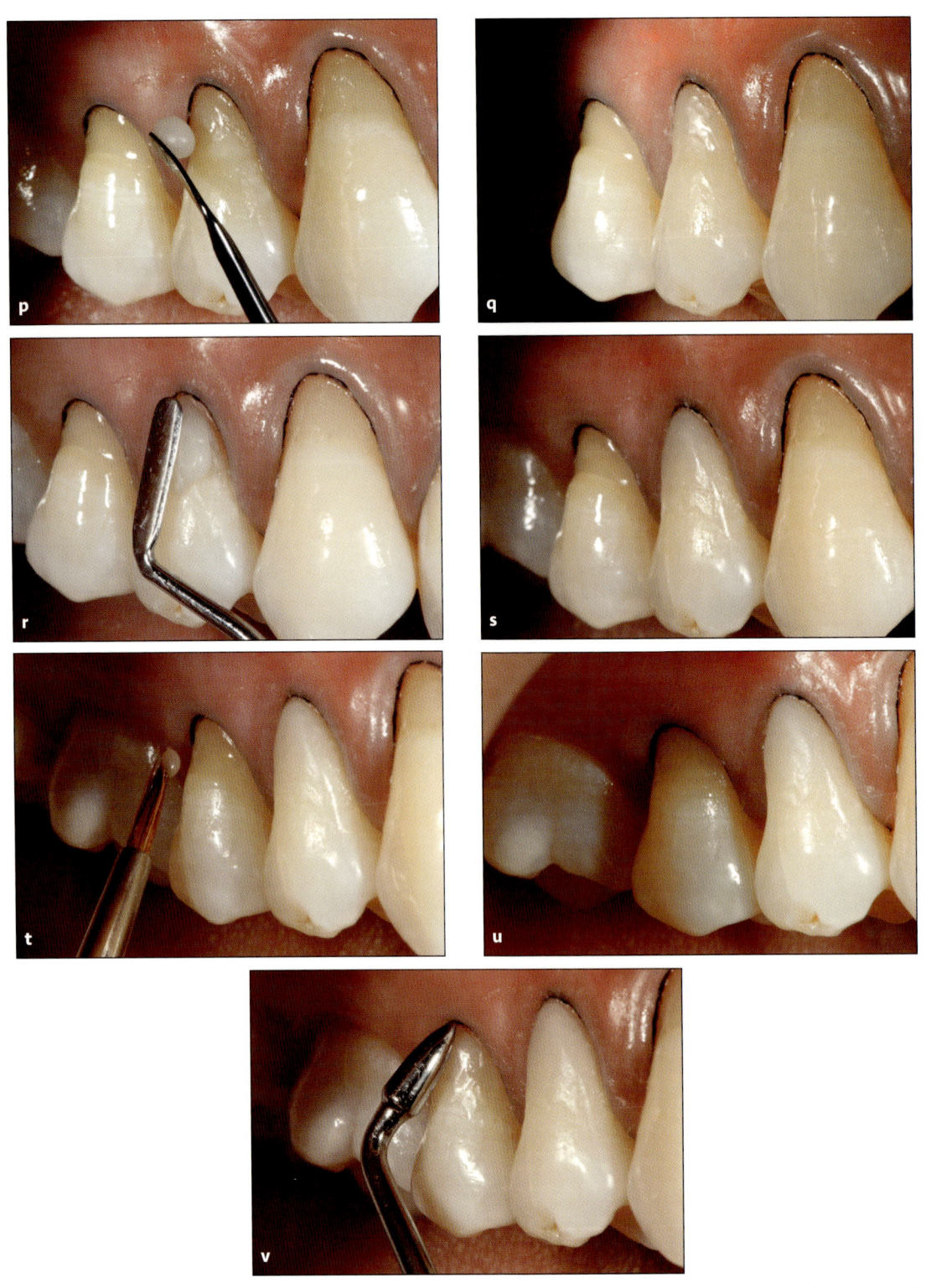

9 Restorative Protocols: Adhesive Bonding, Materials, and Techniques

Fig 9-9 *(cont)* *(p and q)* A second layer of a medium opaque nanofilled composite resin was applied to the dentinoenamel junction. *(r and s)* A third layer of a translucent nanofilled composite resin was applied to the restoration. Note the correct anatomical volume of the cervical region. *(t and u)* The maxillary right second premolar was then restored, beginning with insertion of a nanofilled flowable composite resin at the dentinoenamel junction to improve the adaptation of the next layer. *(v)* Application of a layer of medium opaque nanofilled composite resin.

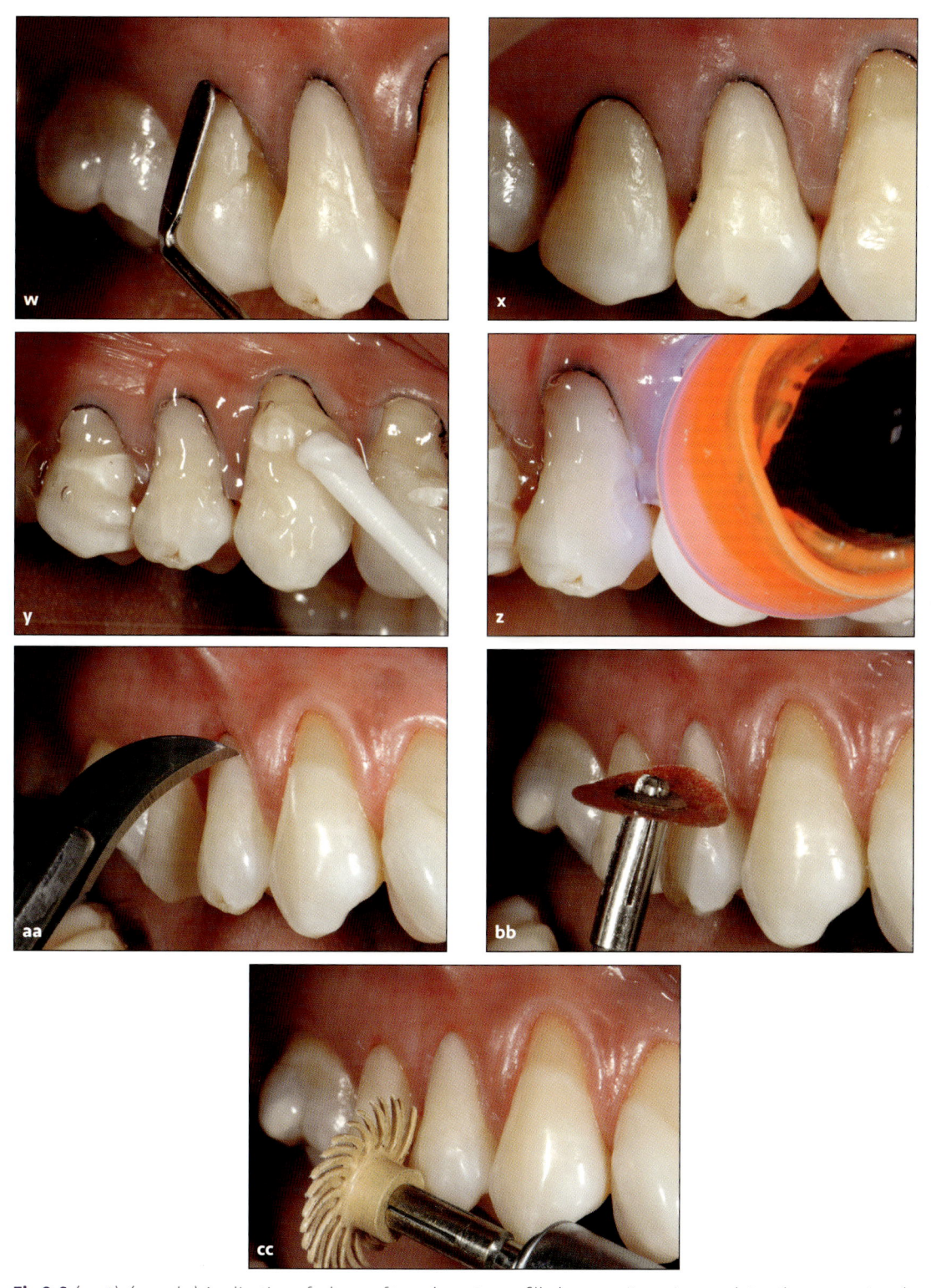

Direct Technique with Composite Resin Restorations

Fig 9-9 *(cont)* *(w and x)* Application of a layer of translucent nanofilled composite resin completes the restoration. *(y and z)* A hydrosoluble gel was applied to each tooth and light cured for 40 seconds. *(aa)* After removal of the retraction cord, any excess composite resin was removed with a scalpel blade #12. *(bb)* Finishing of the restorations with a finishing disc. *(cc)* The proximal regions were finished with a spiral wheel.

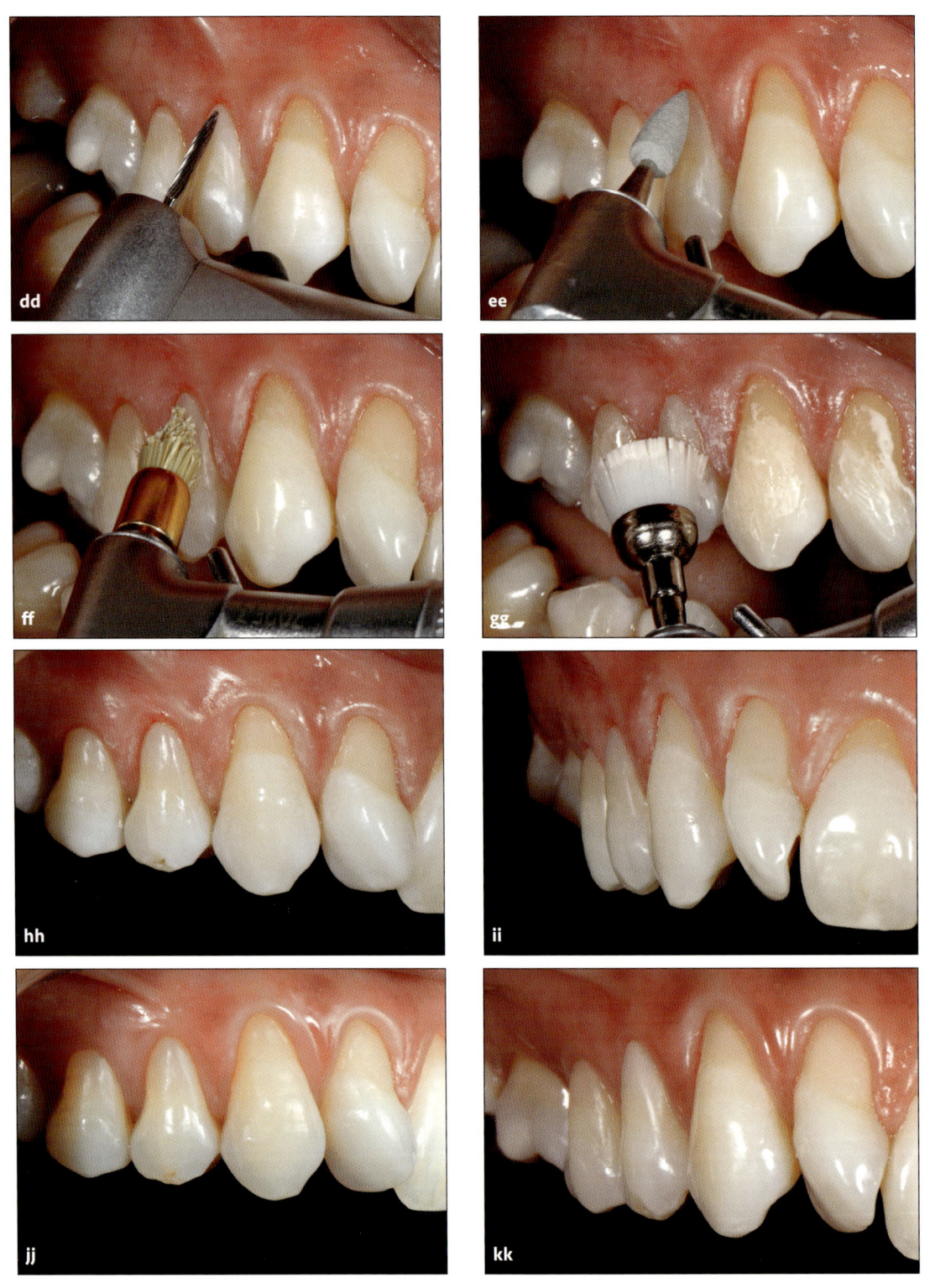

9 Restorative Protocols: Adhesive Bonding, Materials, and Techniques

Fig 9-9 *(cont)* *(dd and ee)* Further finishing was performed with a multilaminated carbide bur and silicone points. *(ff and gg)* Polishing of the restoration was performed with a silicon carbide–impregnated brush and a Robson brush with diamond paste. *(hh and ii)* Final views. *(jj and kk)* Views after 21 days. Note the soft tissue healing.

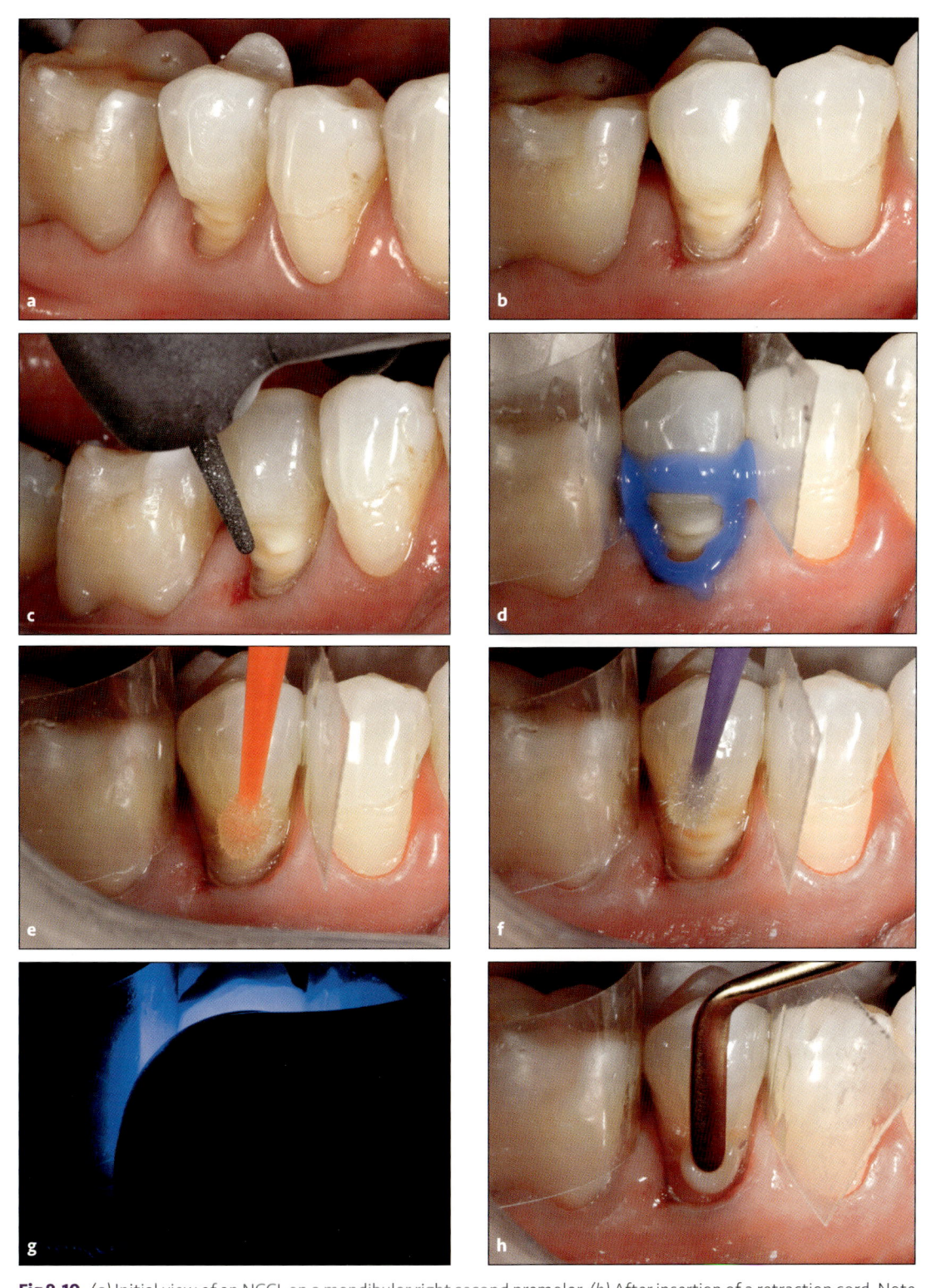

Fig 9-10 *(a)* Initial view of an NCCL on a mandibular right second premolar. *(b)* After insertion of a retraction cord. Note the slight gingival injury resulting from the isolation procedure. *(c)* A 45-degree bevel is placed in the dentinoenamel junction. *(d)* Enamel etching with 37% phosphoric acid for 30 seconds. *(e)* Application of the primer from a self-etching adhesive system. *(f)* After surface air drying, the hydrophobic part of the adhesive was applied. *(g)* The adhesive was light cured for 20 seconds. *(h)* Application of the first layer of the restoration, an opaque nanohybrid filled composite resin with high saturation. →

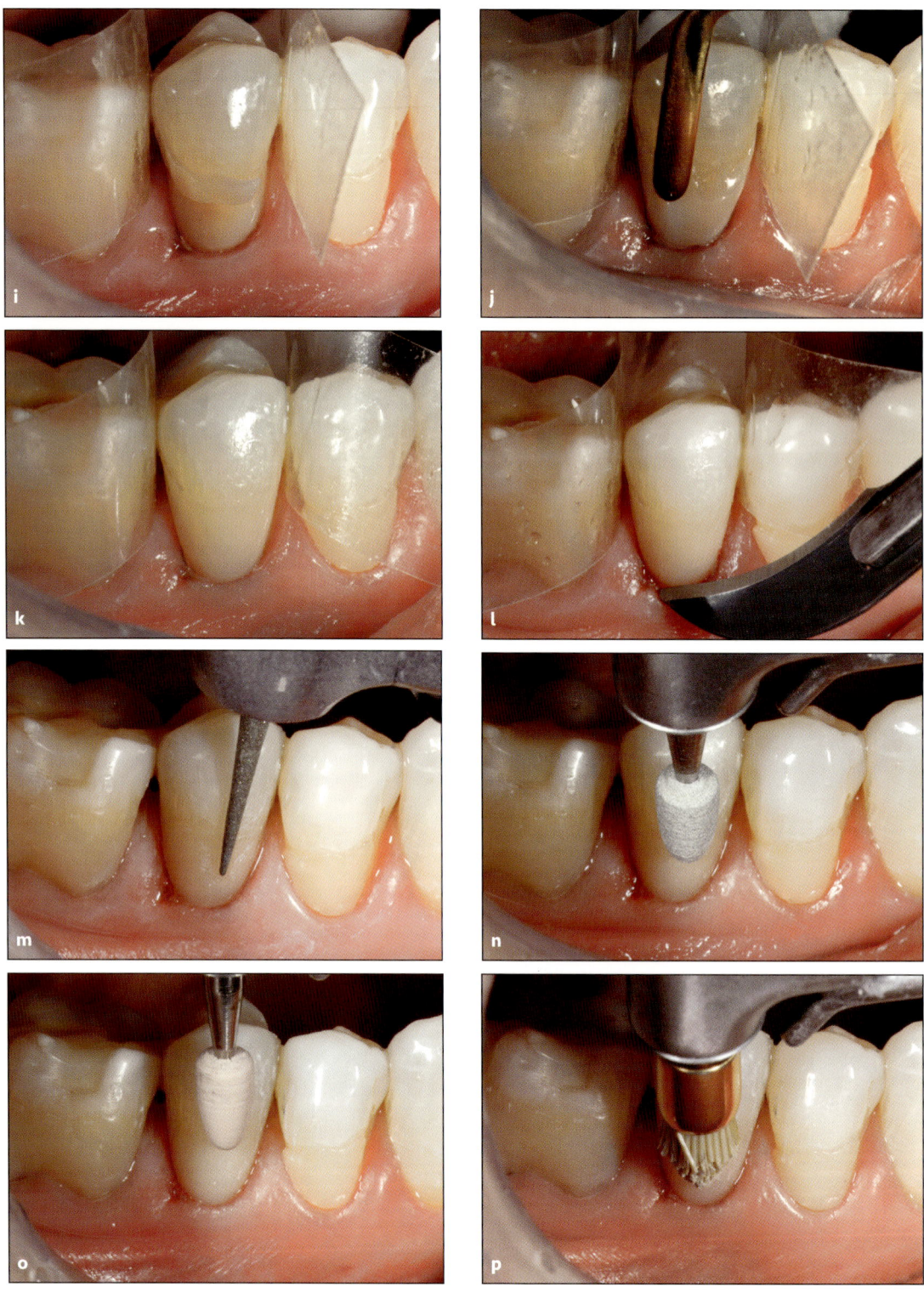

9 Restorative Protocols: Adhesive Bonding, Materials, and Techniques

Fig 9-10 *(cont)* *(i)* Application of a medium translucent nanohybrid composite resin over the tooth-restorative interface. *(j)* Application of the last layer of the restoration, a translucent nanohybrid composite resin. *(k)* Completed composite restoration. *(l)* After removal of the retraction cord, any subgingival excess composite resin was removed with a scalpel blade #12. *(m)* Finishing of the shape and surface with a fine diamond bur. *(n and o)* Finishing and polishing with abrasive silicone points. *(p)* Polishing with a silicon carbide–impregnated brush.

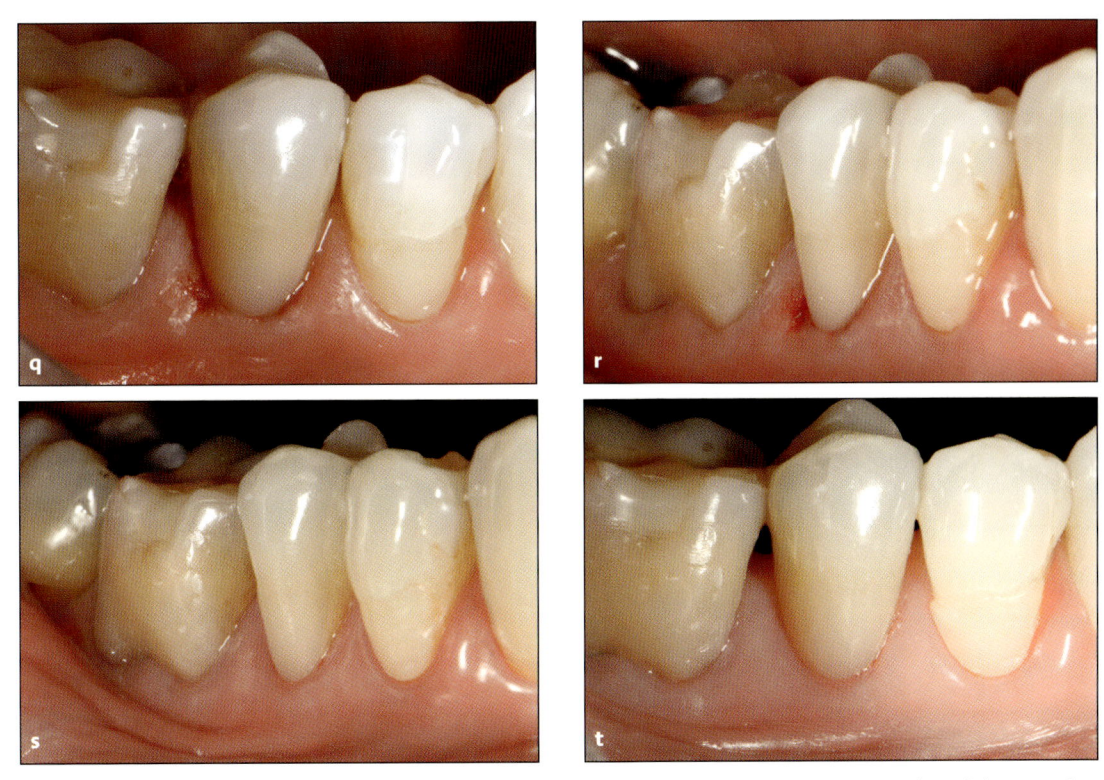

Fig 9-10 *(cont)* *(q and r)* Final views of the mandibular right second premolar NCCL restoration. *(s and t)* Views after 30 days.

Newton Fahl's Direct-Indirect Class V Technique with Composite Resins

Composite resins are the material of choice for restoring NCCLs because they present enhanced color stability, anatomical form, surface texture, and marginal integrity with less marginal discoloration and fewer problems associated with restoration detachment compared with other tooth-colored restoratives.[191,192] In addition to their excellent physical and optical properties, composites can easily be manipulated, inserted, sculpted, and light activated prior to finishing and polishing. To date, the direct approach has been the principal method for restoring both carious and noncarious cervical lesions[193] (see previous section). However, this approach presents several challenges and difficulties:

- Access to difficult-to-reach areas
- Field control
- Composite handling
- Stress caused by polymerization shrinkage on the tooth
- Gingival margin finishing
- Restoration marginal adaptation
- Periodontal health maintenance
- Patient comfort

The novel direct-indirect Class V restoration technique overcomes these challenges to optimize the treatment of NCCLs (see Table 9-1). However, it is important to emphasize that the literature is still scarce in relation to clinical studies that prove the advantages and disadvantages of this technique when compared with direct restorations.

9 Restorative Protocols: Adhesive Bonding, Materials, and Techniques

Table 9-1 Comparison between direct and direct-indirect Class V restorations

Criterion	Direct	Direct-indirect
Access to difficult-to-reach areas	Difficult	Easy
Field control	Rubber dam or modified isolation	Modified isolation
Composite handling	Totally intraoral	Intraoral and extraoral
Stress caused by polymerization shrinkage on the tooth	High	Low
Gingival margin finishing	Done with burs, discs, and rubber rotaries	Done with discs
Restoration marginal adaptation	Difficult to achieve	Excellent
Periodontal health	Depends on quality of gingival margins	Excellent
Patient comfort	Low	High

The Direct-Indirect Technique

By definition, the *direct-indirect technique* is one in which the composite resin is directly applied and sculpted onto the tooth surface before acid etching and adhesive application. It is then light activated, removed, and finished extraorally prior to indirect adhesive cementation. The advantages of this semidirect technique have been discussed extensively in the literature.[194-197] The technique's greatest benefits include the ability to subject chairside-fabricated anterior or posterior restorations to additional light curing and heat-tempering processing, which enhances the physical properties and clinical behavior of the finished composite restorations due to increased conversion of the monomer.[198-201] Especially in the case of direct-indirect composite resin veneers, the benefits go beyond improved physical properties because the technique facilitates greater operator control over the final anatomical and color outcome, rendering the direct-indirect technique an optimal restorative choice and paramount in providing enhanced clinical results over the direct veneering technique.[196]

The Direct-Indirect Class V Restoration

The direct-indirect Class V restoration naturally developed from the direct-indirect veneer technique, as it is essentially a semiveneer covering the cervical and possibly the middle third of the clinical crown, depending on the size of the lesion. Similarly to the veneer technique, the composite resin is applied and adapted to the cervical lesion, light cured, removed, finished, polished, and cemented. Because NCCLs are predominantly V-shaped and deep, and considering that these restorations are cemented, direct-indirect Class V restorations could instead be termed *Class V composite inlays*. The advantages of the direct-indirect Class V restoration over direct restorations are presented in Table 9-1 and discussed in the following sections.

Access to difficult-to-reach areas

Canines and premolars present no major challenge to the direct approach because they are frequently easy to reach and restore. However, molars present greater operative difficulty even to a moderately skilled operator because they are frequently inaccessible due to tooth position in relation to soft and hard tissues. Cavity preparation, material placement, and contouring in those areas can be extremely difficult, and the challenge of direct instrumentation frequently culminates in a burdensome and unsuccessful attempt. The direct-indirect approach successfully bypasses these concerns because the composite is applied in larger increments and pressed over the cervical lesion and beyond the gingival margin without much need for precise contour. The operator primarily uses a finger and finally contouring instruments to achieve a gross anatomical shape, which will subsequently be precisely refined extraorally after light activation and restoration removal from the cavity.

Field control

The traditional approach for restoring Class V lesions requires absolute field control (ie, rubber dam and clamps), as it provides the operator prolonged working time without the need to worry about contamination. This method is especially valuable in the mandible and in situations of inadequate periodontal health. For periodontally healthy patients and in cases where margins are not too subgingival, modified rubber dam techniques and retraction cords can also be alternatively indicated, as they are a simpler, effective way of field control. With the direct-indirect Class V technique, the use of conventional rubber dam and clamps is unnecessary, and alternative field control measures are indicated. Because the Class V inlays are adhesively cemented, they therefore reduce the risk of contaminating the tooth adhesive interface with oral cavity moisture and fluids. The level of field control varies by case and determines whether multiple inlays can be luted one by one or all in a single step.

Composite handling

With the direct approach, composite resin handling may vary from quite easy to extremely difficult, depending on lesion location and effectiveness of the selected field control technique. In easy-to-reach areas, the operator has prolonged working time, and the composite application, contouring, light curing, finishing, and polishing becomes stress free. It is when hard-to-reach areas are restored that the direct-indirect technique presents one of its greatest benefits. The operator is relieved of the concern about precise intraoral contouring because the completion of almost all finishing and polishing is carried out extraorally. However, the direct-indirect technique poses the challenge of handling a composite inlay of minuscule proportions during finishing and polishing, which may require the completion of several cases until the operator reaches his or her comfort zone.

Stress caused by polymerization shrinkage on the tooth

The shrinkage stress exerted on teeth with Class V restorations is influenced by composite resin quantity, cavity geometry, and C-factor.[202,203] Although layering techniques have been suggested to minimize the undesired effects of composite shrinkage (ie, postoperative sensitivity, microleakage),[204-206] divergent findings have been reported regarding the efficacy of incremental layering versus bulk filling.[207-209] Bulk filling NCCLs, however, is a more approachable technique to many operators because it frequently includes use of a single shade, thus minimizing the number of steps and reducing operative time. Incremental layering or bulk filling may be indicated for both the direct and direct-indirect Class V approaches depending on cavity/lesion size and depth. When superior esthetics is of concern, composites of varying chroma and opacity may be used in more than one layer to create more lifelike results. Because the Class V direct-indirect technique recommends extraoral supplemental light curing of the inlay, the bulk-fill technique should be indicated whenever possible. The additional extraoral light curing counteracts problems associated with insufficient curing at the bottom of thicker inlay restorations.

Gingival margin finishing

The marginal finishing for direct-indirect Class V restorations emulates the finishing for relined provisional margins. After the composite is pressed over the cervical margin of the lesion and extended over the free gingival margin, it is light cured and removed from the mouth. A pencil is used to outline the margins for accurate visualization, and finishing is completed with discs. The use of magnification (eg, loupes or a microscope), in association with the sequential use of discs of varying grits, permits finishing the margins to the ideal contour and polish. Unlike the direct-indirect method, finishing direct Class V cervical margins intraorally is an arduous procedure with usually far-from-ideal outcomes, especially in subgingival margins in difficult-to-reach areas. Flashes and overhangs, rough gingival margins, and nicking the cementum are only a few of the probable problems arising from direct finishing as a result of deficient access and instrumentation of the margins.

Restoration marginal adaptation

The conventional technique involves contouring instruments and brushes as the mechanism for adaptation of the composite to the cervical margin of an NCCL. Marginal sealing, integrity, and tightness of the tooth-composite interface depend on correct material placement and the execution of proper adhesive protocols.[210] In simpler clinical scenarios, achieving a tight marginal seal is frequently feasible with often-satisfactory results. However, in more difficult cases adaptation problems are likely to occur. Haller et al investigated in vitro the marginal seal of cervical composite inlays in comparison with conventional Class V restorations,[211] and the results showed better performance of the inlays regarding microleakage. In the study, the inlays were further subjected to additional light curing and heat tempering, which made the bonded inlays more resistant to thermal stress, probably by relaxing material stress and enhancing bond stability. Clinically, the direct-indirect Class V restoration combines the benefits of stress reduction through the material application and polymerization methods employed, providing a superior marginal adaptation.

Periodontal health

The effects of subgingival restorations on periodontal health have been widely investigated. Problems associated with restorative material type and poorly finished restorations include a change in the subgingival microflora, leading to plaque accumulation, gingivitis, and recurrent caries.[212-215] The selection of proper finishing and polishing techniques is essential for achieving high-quality margins through enhanced surface and marginal polish. Numerous reports corroborate that the smoothest composite resin surface can be achieved by using aluminum oxide finishing discs.[216] Unless some means of gingival retraction is utilized, it is impossible to gain intraoral access to subgingival margins with discs. When burs and rubber rotaries are used in an attempt to render the restoration margin smooth, the result is far from ideal. Quite the reverse, extraoral finishing and polishing of Class V inlays provide unrivaled surface smoothness, which in turn promotes less plaque retention and a healthier periodontal environment.

Restorative Protocols: Adhesive Bonding, Materials, and Techniques

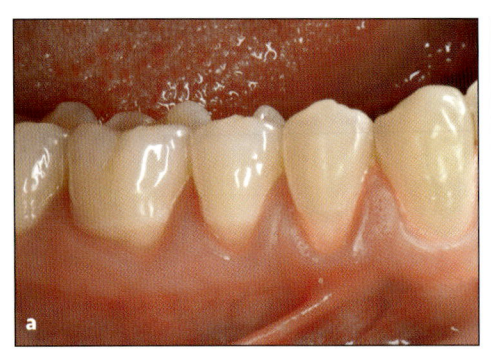

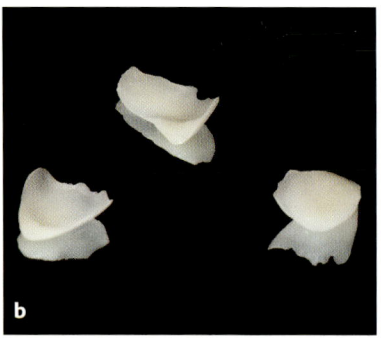

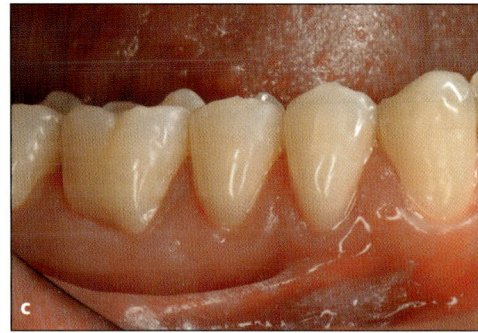

Fig 9-11 *(a)* NCCLs on mandibular teeth. *(b)* Class V composite inlays. *(c)* Completed restorations with the direct-indirect technique. Note the lack of damage to the teeth and periodontium and the sound integration between the soft tissue and restorations.

Patient comfort

Ultimately, the direct-indirect Class V technique is a remarkable improvement in patient well-being compared with the direct approach. Patients are allowed to close their mouths and rest between restorative steps because there is minimal intraoral working time. Anesthesia is rarely needed, even when packing retraction cords is required. The greatest comfort provided by the inlay technique possibly results from the absence of subgingival finishing. There is no true aggressive contact with the soft tissue other than removing minor flashes of luting resin at the gel stage with a sickle scaler and buffing the restoration surface with rubber cups. As indicated previously, scarring of gingival tissue and nicking the cementum/root surface during operative procedures are annoyances and causes of great anxiety to patients. This advantage becomes apparent immediately after completing treatment, when no damage to either tooth or periodontium results, and sound integration between soft tissue and restoration is perceived (Fig 9-11).

Step-By-Step Direct-Indirect Technique

Step 1: Composite selection

Physical properties

The important physical properties for the restorative composites used in direct-indirect Class V inlays include modulus of elasticity, handling, resistance to wear, and polishability. Although most state-of-the-art composites could be indicated for restoring NCCLs, the author prefers to use microfilled or nanofilled restoratives for direct-indirect Class V inlays because of the superior inherent properties related to their filler size and distribution. Their handling and polishability allow proper manipulation and adaptation, thus promoting exceptional surface smoothness and gloss.[217–219] Of equal clinical relevance is wear rate; however, wear by itself should not dictate restorative composite resin selection for NCCLs because the clinical assessment of wear is not easily accomplished. Submicron-filled composites have been reported to exhibit both high gloss and low wear rates,[220] which provides a strong indication for their clinical application in NCCLs.

Shade and optical properties

The selection of composite resins is dependent on the type of NCCL, which can be categorized into coronal cavitation, radicular cavitation, and coronal and radicular cavitation (Fig 9-12). In cases of no or minor root exposure with coronal cavitation, tooth-colored composites are indicated. The cervical third of the natural dentition presents higher opacity and accentuated chroma because the dentin is at its thickest and the enamel is at its thinnest, making the inner dentin color show through the thin outer enamel. This requires the use of composite resins that optically emulate natural dentin and enamel to achieve a seamless restoration.

This can be achieved with two techniques: *(1)* using artificial dentin and enamel composites as separate layers, and *(2)* using a single layer of a composite shade of an interme-

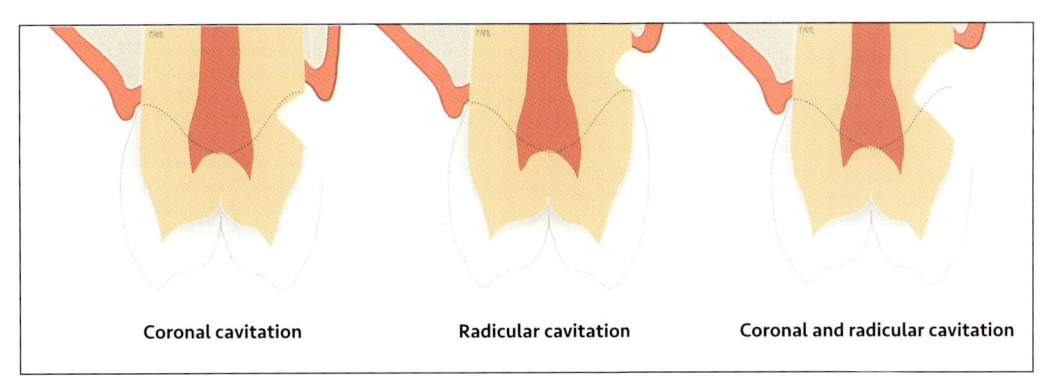

Fig 9-12 Categories of NCCL cavitation.

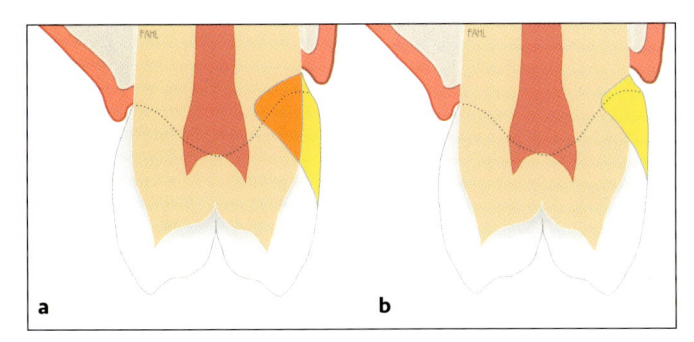

Fig 9-13 Layering of an NCCL employs one of two techniques: *(a)* Using artificial dentin and enamel composites as separate layers. *(b)* Using a single layer of a composite shade of an intermediate opacity between that of enamel and dentin.

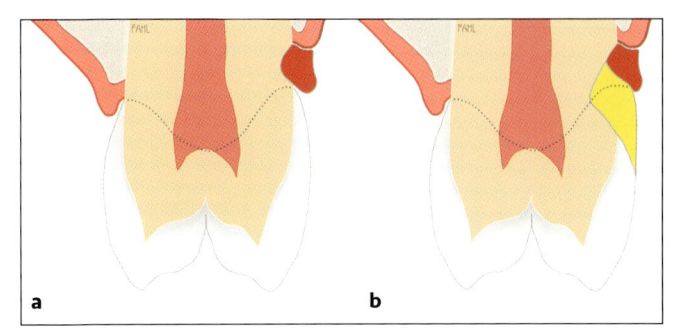

Fig 9-14 *(a)* Gingiva-colored composite is indicated if the lesion extends to the dentinoenamel junction with no coronal cavitation. *(b)* VITA-based enamel and pink composites are indicated in lesions that are longer and deeper.

diate opacity between that of enamel and dentin (Fig 9-13). The first technique requires selecting a higher chroma dentin shade than that intended. The veneering enamel composite can be selected according to either a polychromatic[221] or natural layering[222] approach. The polychromatic method uses a VITA-based[223] veneering enamel composite of the intended hue and chroma and a dentin of the same hue but with a higher chroma. The natural layering technique employs a VITA or non-VITA dentin composite of the desired hue with a higher-than-intended final chroma and a non-VITA enamel shade that modulates the dentin color to the desired chroma and value, while maintaining the same hue of the underlying dentin composite. Both techniques are equally effective, and the decision to use one over the other depends on the operator's preference and mastery of the selected technique. The author favors the use of VITA enamel shades over non-VITA shades because they provide more predictability in attaining the final hue, chroma, and value of the cervical tooth color. Cavities deeper than 2.5 mm may be restored with the dual-layer (ie, dentin and enamel) approach. In the majority of cases, however, a higher-opacity VITA enamel suffices to provide the proper opacity/value while imparting a natural depth and blending effect with the surrounding tooth structure and adjacent dentition.

In cases of short and shallow root lesions that extend up to the dentinoenamel junction with no coronal cavitation and when grafting procedures are waived as a primary option, gingiva-colored composites may be a better choice (Fig 9-14a). In longer and deeper lesions affecting both the root and crown, a combination of VITA-based enamel and pink composite is indicated to reestablish a more natural and esthetic transition between the color of the soft and hard tissues alone or in combination with tooth-colored composites (Fig 9-14b). This approach minimizes the appearance of a long clinical crown that arises if only tooth-colored composites are used, which invariably creates an unesthetic result, especially if the restorations are displayed during the smile (Figs 9-15 and 9-16).

Step 2: Cavity preparation

The type of cavity preparation is dependent on the lesion type and varies from none, in cases of biocorrosive/abrasive lesions, to beveling of the enamel for wedge-shaped lesions

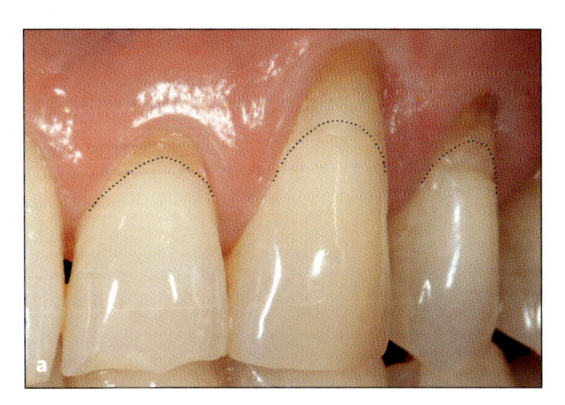

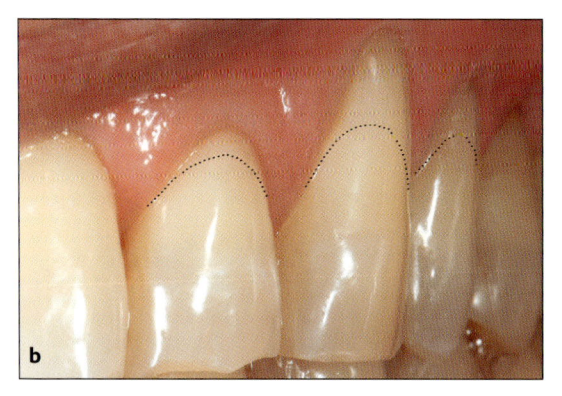

Fig 9-15 *(a and b)* Using tooth-colored composites alone to restore NCCLs with large root involvement invariably results in the appearance of unesthetic long clinical crowns.

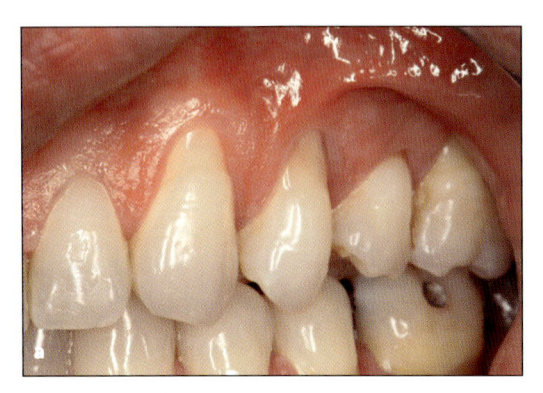

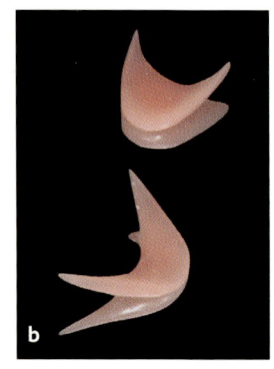

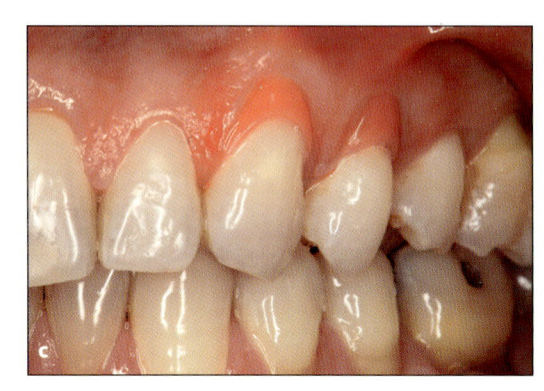

Fig 9-16 *(a to c)* In cases when grafting procedures are waived as a primary option, gingiva-colored composites may be a better option for treating root lesions that extend up to the dentinoenamel junction with no coronal cavitation.

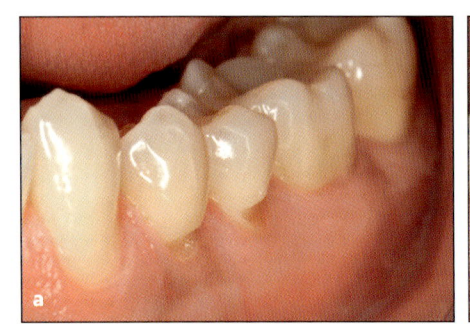

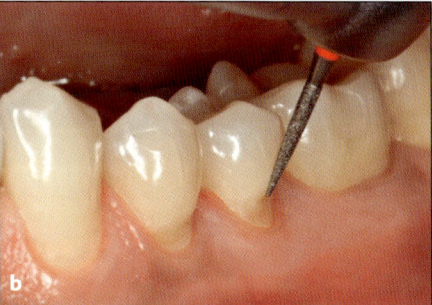

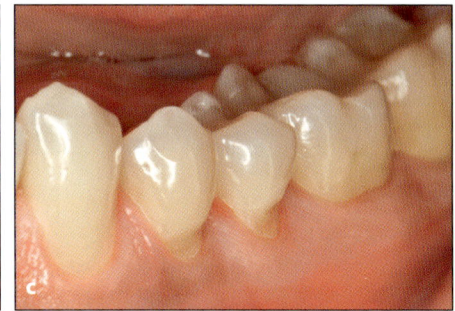

Fig 9-17 *(a to c)* Beveling of the enamel should be performed where wedge-shaped lesions with sharp enamel occlusal cavosurface margins exist to provide a seamless tooth-composite transition.

with sharp enamel occlusal cavosurface margins (Fig 9-17). In the former situation, Class V restorations may seem more like a thin contact lens veneer that may extend onto the middle and occlusal thirds, and in the latter, it assumes the actual shape of a Class V inlay.

Step 3: Composite application

If the cervical margin is equigingival or slightly subgingival, packing retraction cords is unnecessary. However, packing a nonimpregnated cord of adequate thickness may reveal margins that are deeper subgingivally and consequently assist in imprinting the margins on the composite (Fig 9-18). For lesions shallower than 2.5 mm, the selected single composite shade is made into a small ball that is rolled between the fingers and then pressed onto the cervical lesion, covering the cavity and also extending beyond its borders over the beveled enamel, interproximally, and most importantly, over the free gingival margin (Fig 9-19). An accurate imprint of the gingival margin into the compressed composite increment is achieved by tender finger pressure. Because all gross

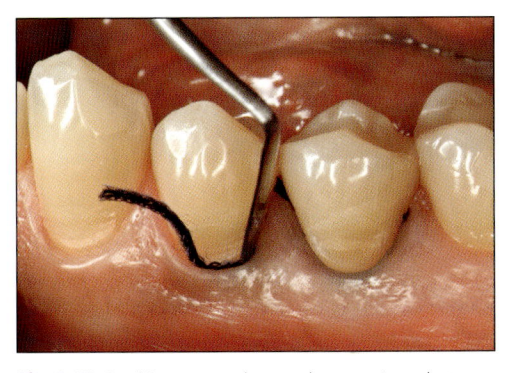

Fig 9-18 Packing a cord reveals margins that are deeper subgingivally and assists in imprinting the margins on the composite inlay.

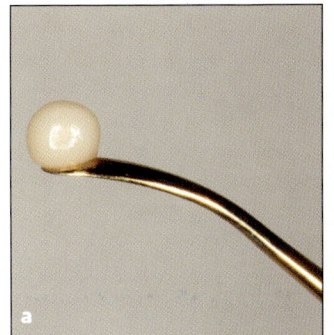

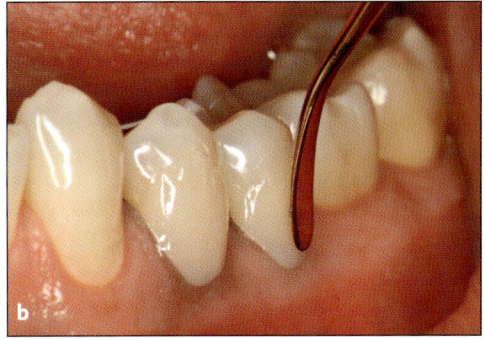

Fig 9-19 *(a and b)* A small ball of composite is rolled between the fingers and pressed onto the cervical lesion, covering the free gingival margin.

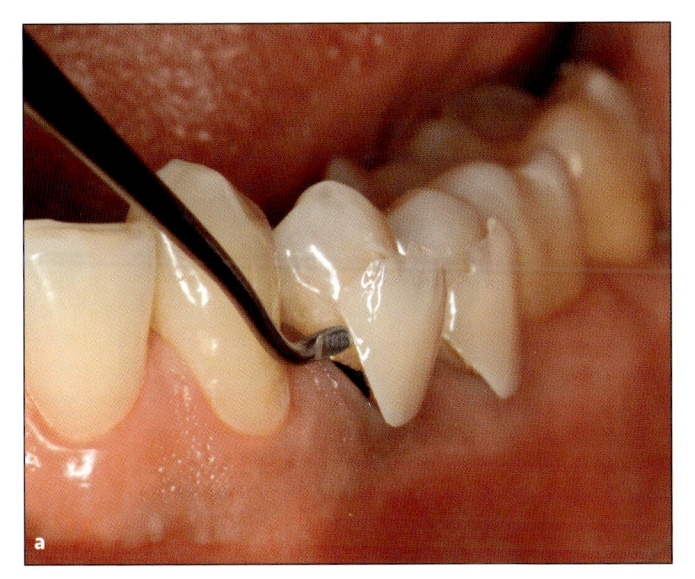

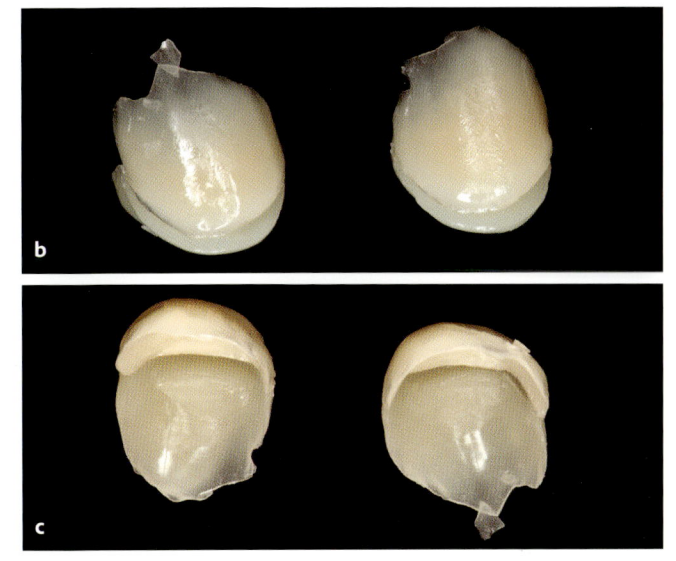

Fig 9-20 *(a to c)* After light curing, the restoration is detached from the lesion with a curette.

excess is removed through extraoral finishing and polishing, the use of instruments for further contour refinement is often unnecessary.

Step 4: Light activation and restoration removal

The restoration is thoroughly light cured by providing proper light intensity and cure time, according to the type of curing unit employed (ie, halogen, LED, plasma arc). Using a curette, the restoration is detached (Fig 9-20) and further light cured extraorally from its outer and inner aspects to ensure thorough polymerization (Fig 9-21). A thick Class V inlay restored through the bulk fill technique would normally require an extended light cure for maximum polymerization, and this prolonged curing time may have harmful consequences to the pulp.[224,225] Performing the final light curing extraorally for the direct-indirect Class V restoration allows for extended light exposure as needed without concern for potential pulp damage arising from increased temperature.

Although its clinical benefits are still in question, heat tempering has been shown to improve the physical properties of light-activated composite resins and may be used in addition to supplemental extraoral light curing to enhance their clinical performance. In this case, the composite inlays must be submitted to a heat-generating appliance such as a light and heat oven.

Step 5: Extraoral finishing and polishing

The imprinted cervical margin is clearly apparent on the cured inlay, and a pencil is used to outline its fine edges, facilitating visualization during the finishing step (Fig 9-22). Aluminum oxide discs of varying grits are used sequentially to remove the gross excess and to finish and polish the margins to ideal con-

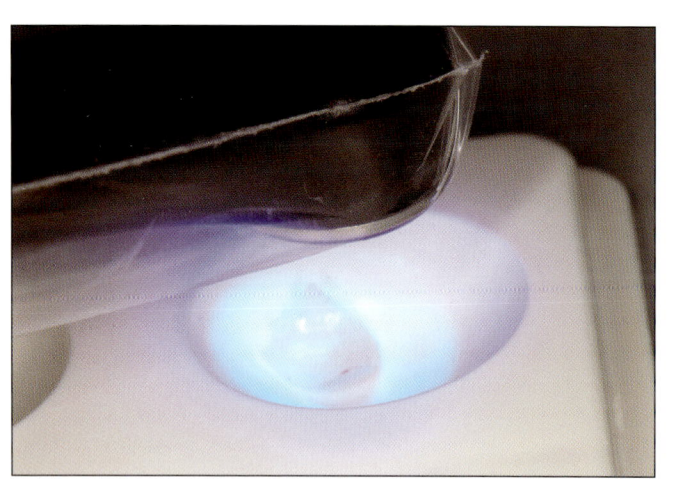

9 Restorative Protocols: Adhesive Bonding, Materials, and Techniques

Fig 9-21 The Class V inlay receives supplemental extraoral light polymerization to guarantee maximum monomer conversion.

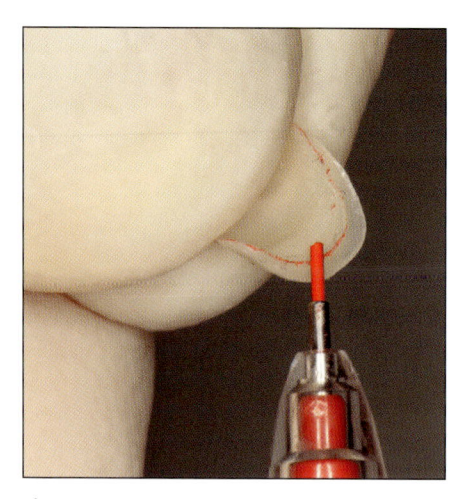

Fig 9-22 The imprinted cervical margin of the cured inlay is outlined with a pencil to facilitate visualization during the finishing step.

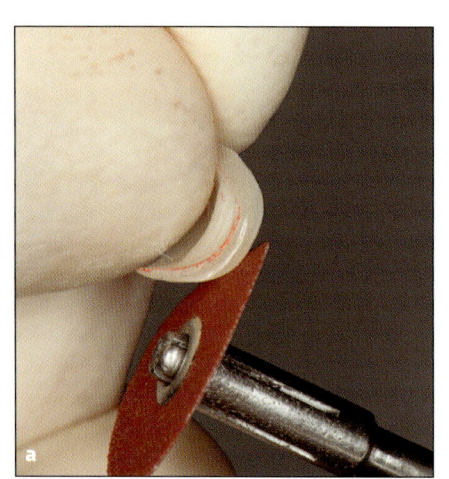

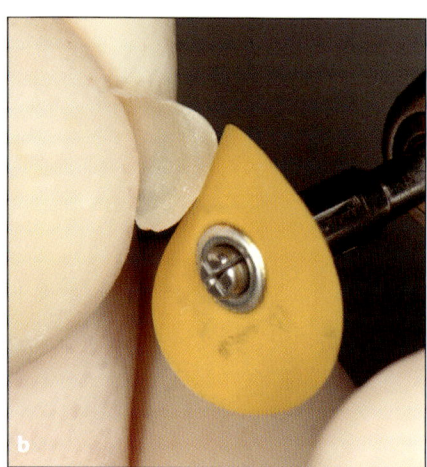

Fig 9-23 *(a and b)* Aluminum oxide discs of varying grits are used sequentially to remove the gross excess and to finish and polish the margins to ideal contour, smoothness, and gloss.

tour, smoothness, and gloss (Fig 9-23). As a result, the minute inlays exhibit superior contour, marginal finish, and polish.

Step 6: Precementation surface treatment of restoration

The inner surface of the restoration is airborne-particle abraded with 27- or 50-μm aluminum oxide particles or alternatively with a 30-μm silicate ceramic (Fig 9-24). Although composite resin compositions vary considerably and may require different protocols for adhesive cementation, mechanical roughening is reported to produce effective bond strengths on microfills, hybrids, and nanofills.[226,227] After air abrasion, the intaglio of the restoration is rinsed and dried and attached to a sticky handle for ease of handling (Fig 9-25). It is then cleaned with 35% to 40% phosphoric acid for 10 seconds, rinsed, and dried (Fig 9-26).

Silanation has been demonstrated to enhance bond strengths of laboratory-processed composites[228] and may be incorporated as an additional step for the direct-indirect Class V technique. This step is optional, as the advantages of silanation in Class V inlays have not yet been reported despite the proven benefits.

Next, a hydrophobic adhesive is applied and air thinned (Fig 9-27). The inlay is set aside under a light-protective shield until cementation (Fig 9-28). Extra care must be tak-

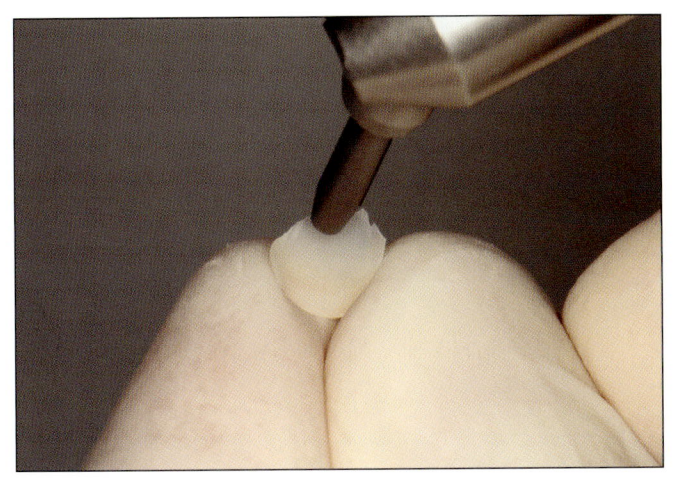

Fig 9-24 The inner surface of the restoration is airborne-particle abraded with 27- or 50-μm aluminum oxide particles or alternatively with a 30-μm silicate ceramic to enhance bond strength.

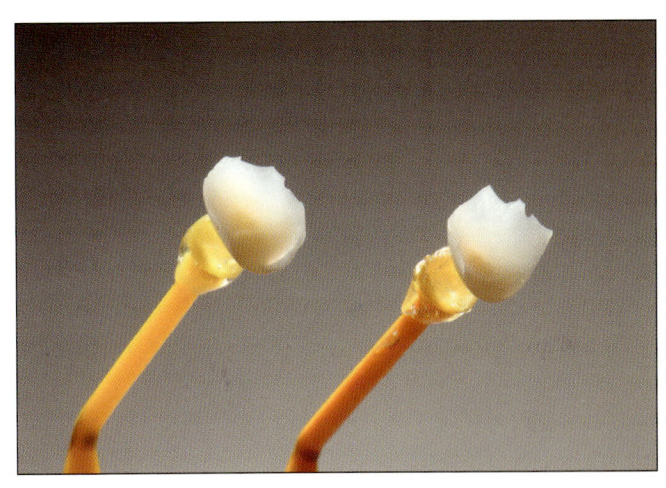

Fig 9-25 The restoration is attached to a sticky handle for ease of handling.

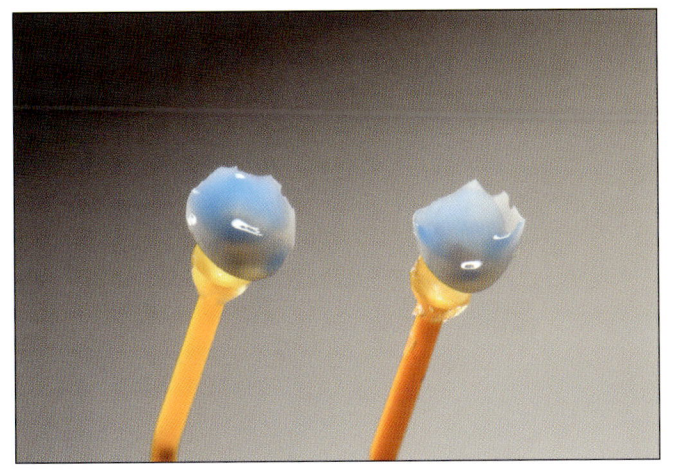

Fig 9-26 The particle-abraded surface is cleaned with 35% to 40% phosphoric acid.

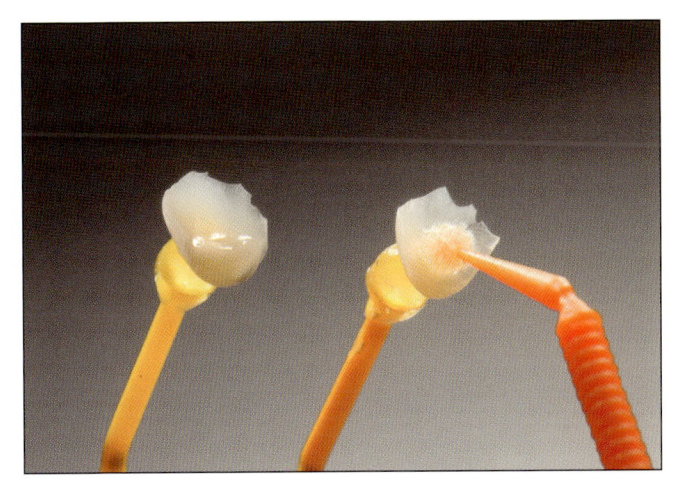

Fig 9-27 A hydrophobic adhesive is applied and air-thinned.

en to organize the restorations in the sequence according to which they will be cemented, if more than one inlay is at hand, as they are usually of similar size, and the operator may end up switching them.

Step 7: Precementation surface treatment of NCCL

Following the packing of nonimpregnated retraction cord, the dentin and enamel surfaces of the cavity are airborne-particle abraded with 27- or 50-μm aluminum oxide (Fig 9-29). This step enhances bond strengths by roughening and increasing tag penetration into dentin, in addition to removing the aprismatic layer of uninstrumented enamel beyond the bevel line, thus enhancing bonding in that area.[229,230] Air abrasion of enamel and dentin generates similar bond strengths for both etch-and-rinse and self-etch adhesives, although the tag formation seems to be more evident for self-etch adhesives.[230] There is insufficient evidence to support one adhesive or bonding protocol over another when comparing the effectiveness of self-etch versus etch-and-rinse adhesives for treating NCCLs.[212] Clinical judgment at the time of the procedure should determine adhesive selection. For instance, if gingival inflammation is present, using a three-step total-etch adhesive that requires phosphoric acid application may be contraindicated, because the acid will likely promote bleeding. Con-

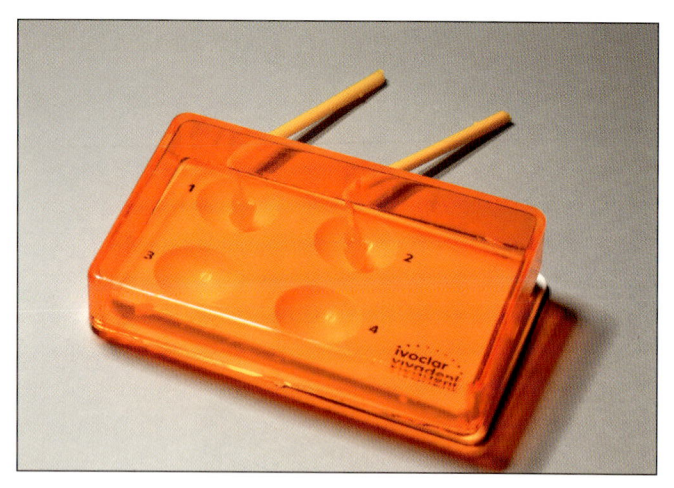

9 Restorative Protocols: Adhesive Bonding, Materials, and Techniques

Fig 9-28 The inlay is set aside under a light-protective shield until cementation.

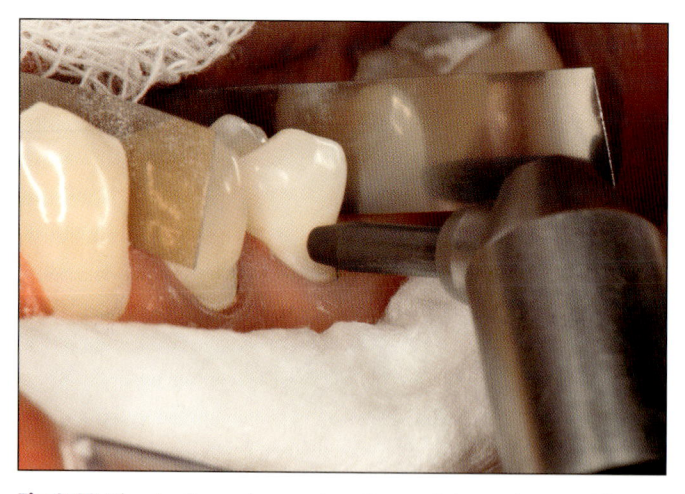

Fig 9-29 The dentin and enamel surfaces of the cavity are airborne-particle abraded with 27- or 50-μm aluminum oxide.

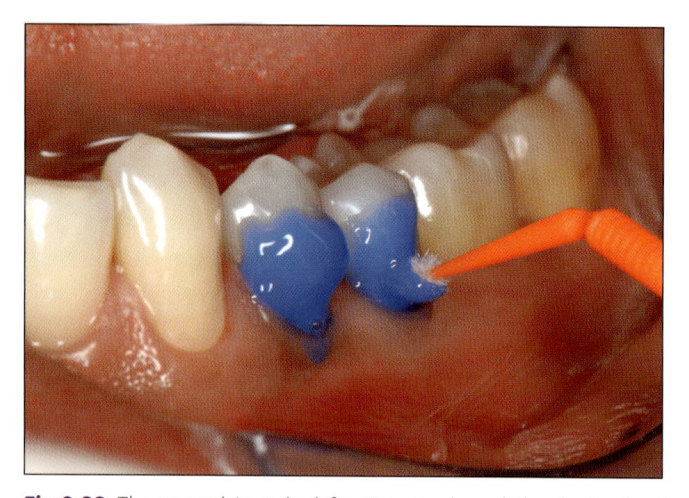

Fig 9-30 The enamel is etched for 15 seconds and the dentin for 5 to 10 seconds to comply with an etch-and-rinse three-step adhesive protocol.

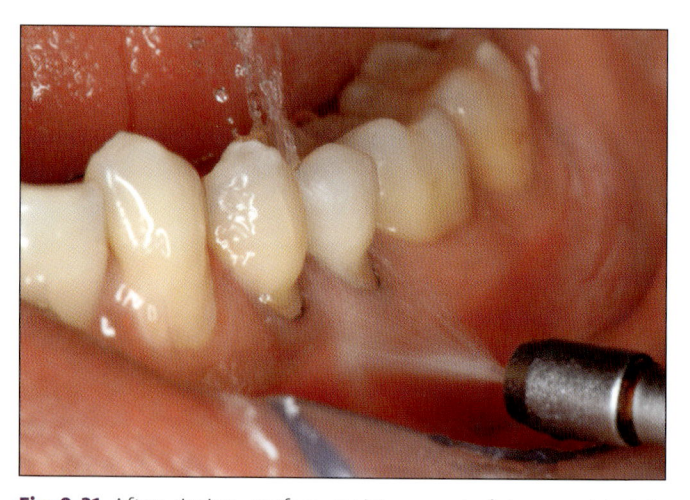

Fig 9-31 After rinsing, surface moisture control is completed by aspirating excess water.

versely, self-etching adhesives tend to be milder on the soft tissue and do not provoke bleeding upon contact with the gingiva, even if moderately inflamed. Three-step total-etch adhesives are considered the gold standard and therefore may be considered a primary choice over other adhesives for the direct-indirect Class V technique.[231]

The enamel is etched for 15 seconds and the dentin for 5 to 10 seconds to comply with an etch-and-rinse three-step adhesive protocol (Fig 9-30). After rinsing, surface moisture control is completed by aspirating excess water (Fig 9-31). Three-step total-etch adhesives with a high filler load are preferable for this technique based on the benefits they present.[232] A primer is applied and agitated onto the dentin surface for at least 20 seconds (Fig 9-32). Excess primer is aspirated, and the remnant solvent is further volatilized by a gentle spray of air (Fig 9-33). A thin coat of hydrophobic adhesive is applied, and the excess is aspirated before light activation (Fig 9-34). The high filler content of the adhesive creates a slight-

ly thicker layer that enhances bond strength and reduces microleakage, promoting longer life expectancy of the Class V restoration.[233,234] Although the adhesive is cured prior to cementation, the composite inlay will fit accurately, because airborne-particle abrasion provides room to accommodate adhesive thickness.

Step 8: Cementation of the Class V inlay

A light-cured luting cement or flowable restorative composite resin can be used for cementing the Class V inlay. Translucent resins of any shade usually provide good color blending and produce natural-looking results. The intaglio of the inlay is covered with the selected luting resin, and it is carried onto the prehybridized lesion with tweezers or a sticky handle (Fig 9-35). Once positioned, the inlay is gently pressed to ooze the excess luting resin. If the oozing of excessive luting resin prevents proper visualization of the margins, it can be carefully removed with a brush. A small-tipped light is used

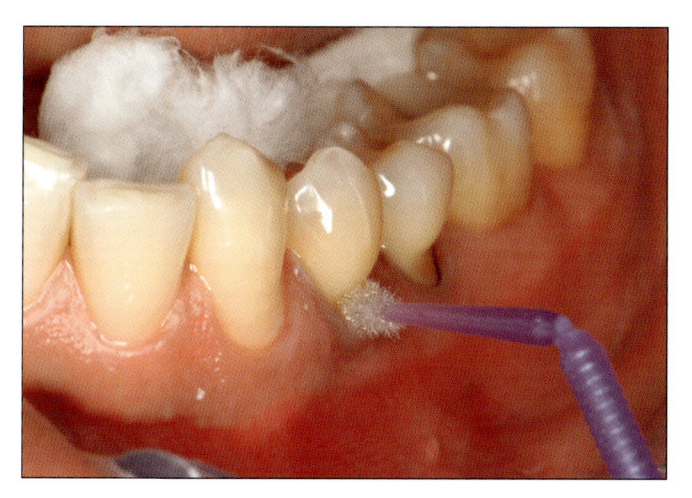

Newton Fahl's Direct-Indirect Class V Technique with Composite Resins

Fig 9-32 A primer is applied and agitated onto the dentin surface.

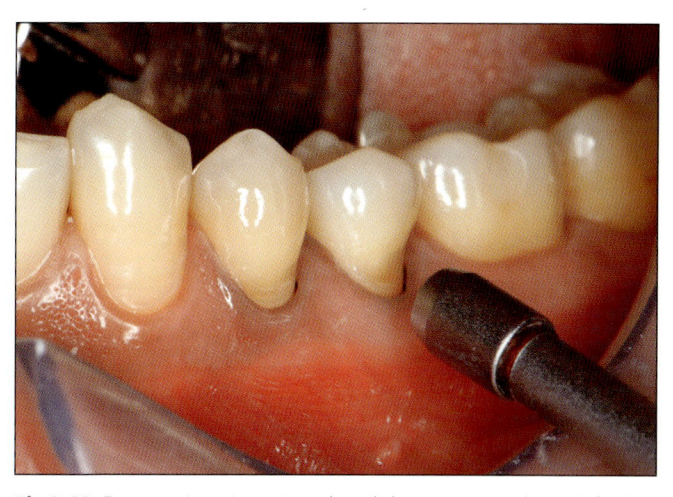

Fig 9-33 Excess primer is aspirated, and the remnant solvent is further volatilized by gentle air spray.

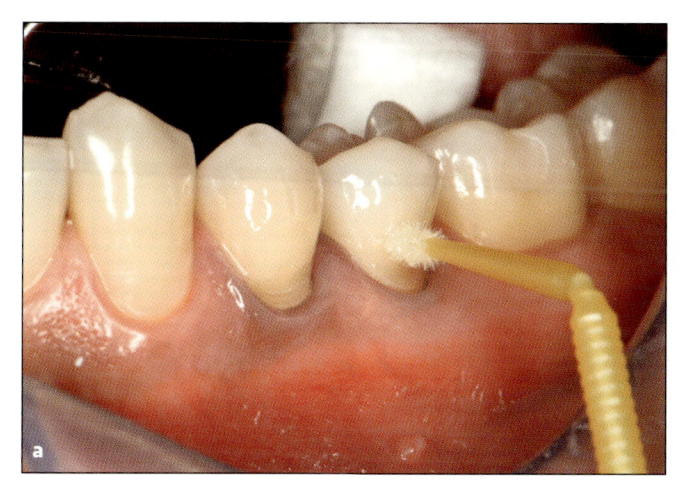

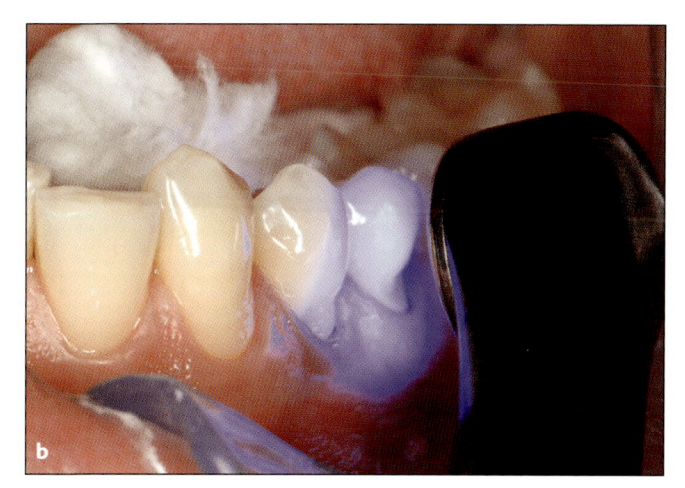

Fig 9-34 A thin coat of hydrophobic adhesive is applied *(a)*; after the excess is aspirated, the adhesive is light activated *(b)*.

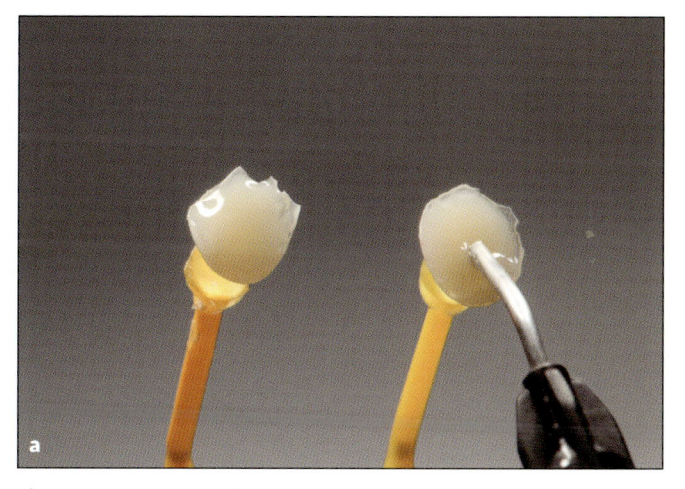

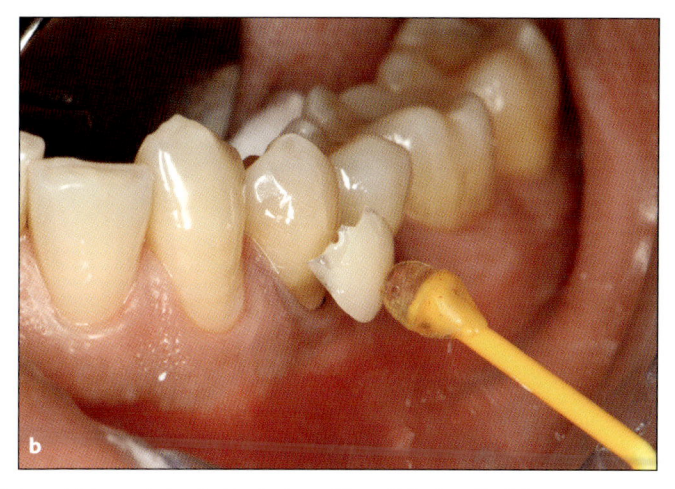

Fig 9-35 The intaglio of the inlay is covered with the selected luting resin *(a)*, and it is carried onto the lesion with a sticky handle *(b)*.

to push the inlay into position away from the cervical margin, and it is spot light cured for 1 to 3 seconds, depending on the light intensity of the curing unit (Fig 9-36). The luting resin, which has reached a gel stage, is removed with a sickle, and the interproximal areas are checked with dental floss to ensure complete removal of luting resin (Fig 9-37). An air-inhibiting gel is applied over the spot-cured inlay, and final light curing is performed for the length of time necessary according to the curing unit used (Fig 9-38).

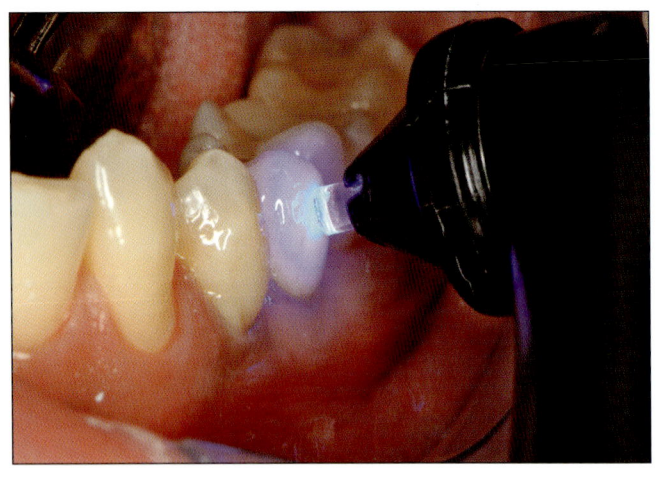

9 | Restorative Protocols: Adhesive Bonding, Materials, and Techniques

Fig 9-36 A small-tipped light guide is used to push the inlay into position away from the cervical margin, and it is spot light cured for 1 to 3 seconds.

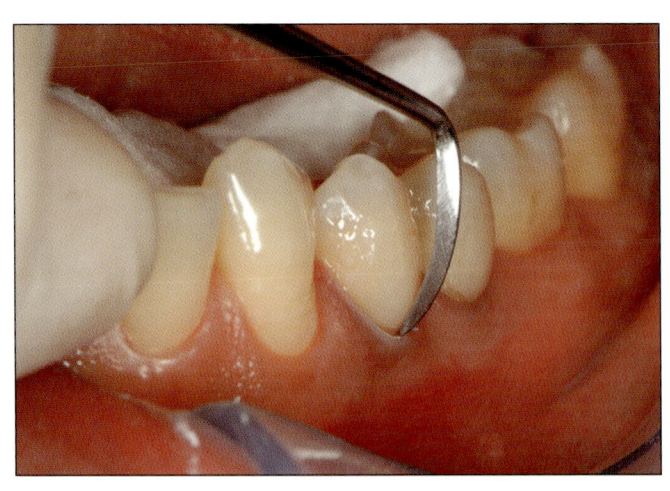

Fig 9-37 The partially cured luting resin is flaked off with a sickle, and the interproximal areas are checked with dental floss.

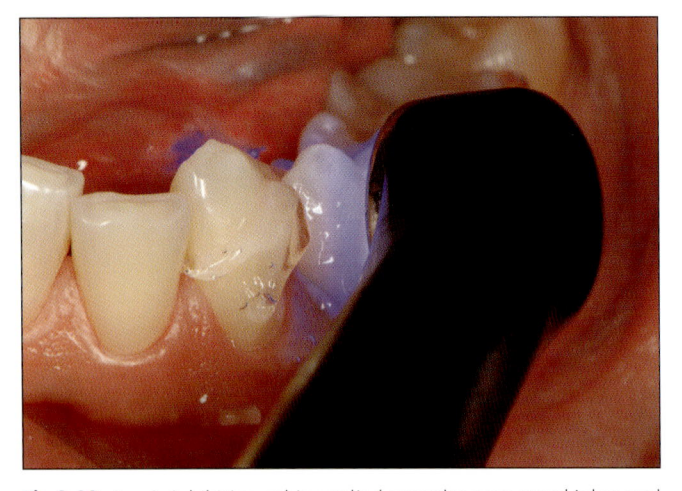

Fig 9-38 An air-inhibiting gel is applied over the spot-cured inlay, and final light curing is achieved.

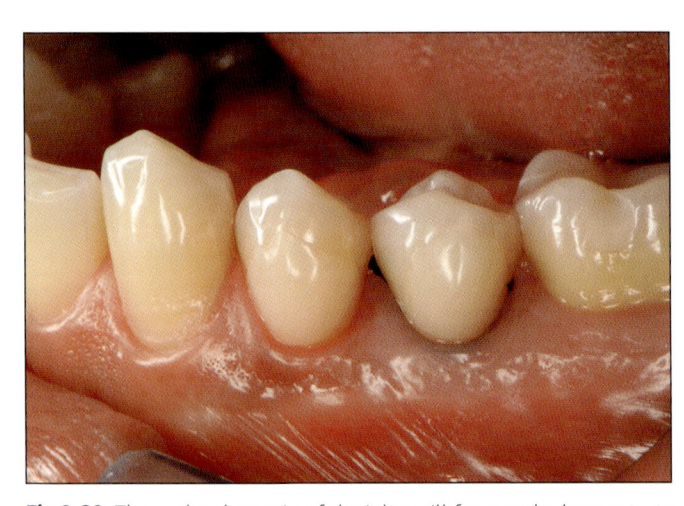

Fig 9-39 The occlusal margin of the inlay will frequently demonstrate a rougher and thicker edge, requiring additional intraoral refining.

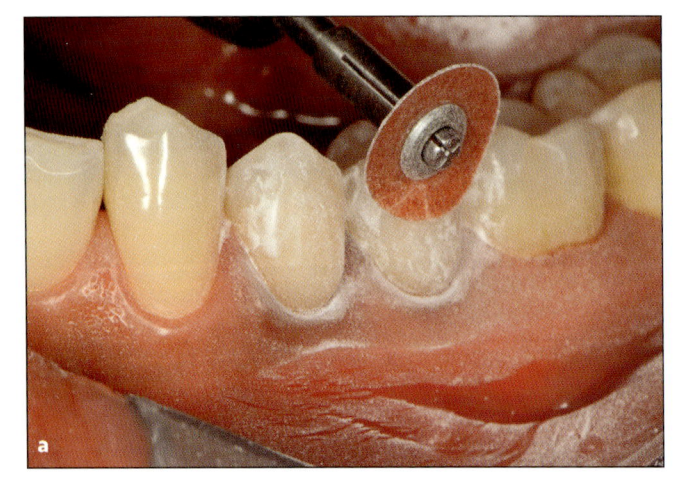

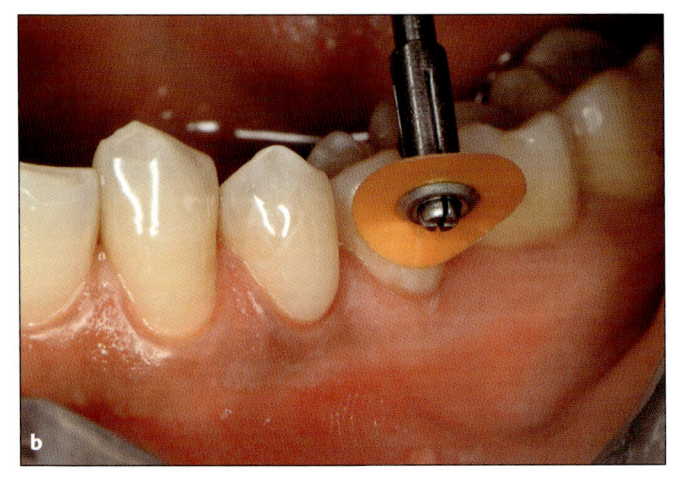

Fig 9-40 *(a and b)* Finishing discs of varying grits are used sequentially for finessing and polishing the rough margins.

Step 9: Final finishing and polishing

The occlusal margin of the inlay will frequently demonstrate a thicker edge, requiring additional intraoral refining (Fig 9-39). Finishing discs of varying grits are used sequentially to finesse any roughness and execute minor contour changes (Fig 9-40). Because the gingival margins of the inlay have been previously finished and polished, rotary instruments should be avoided to prevent unnecessary scratching of the smooth and glossy surface. For final surface polish

154

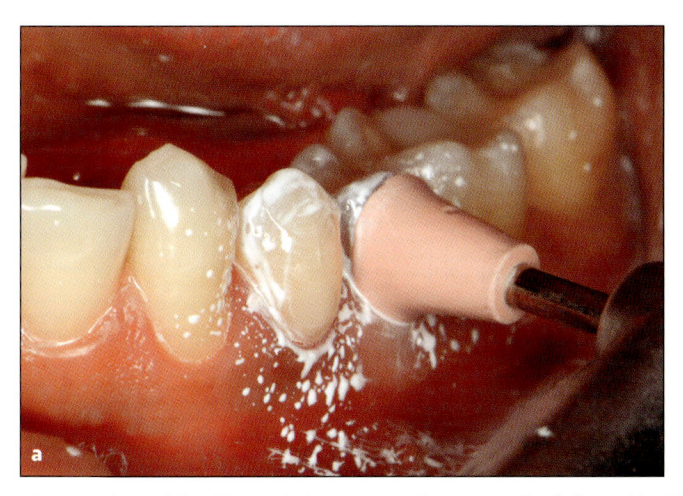

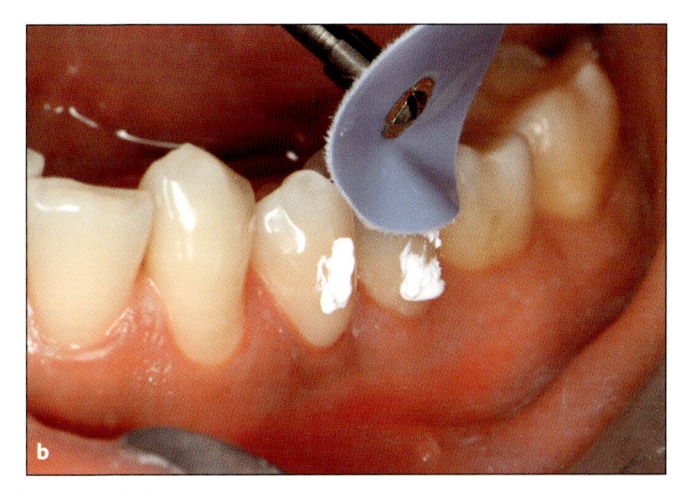

Newton Fahl's Direct-Indirect Class V Technique with Composite Resins

Fig 9-41 *(a and b)* Rubber polishers are used sequentially, followed by felt discs and polishing pastes.

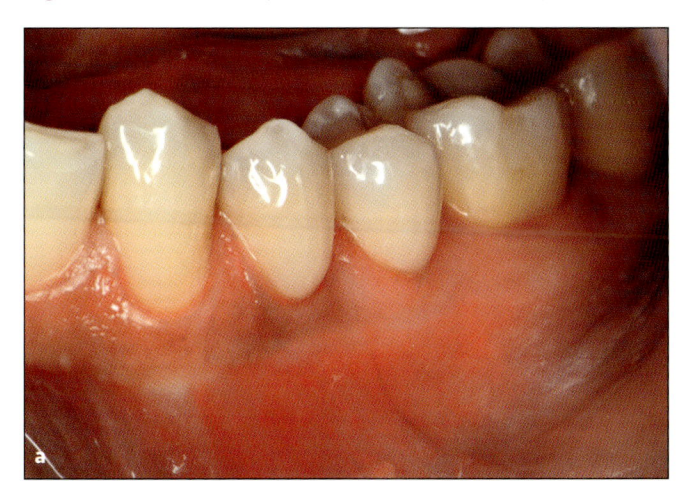

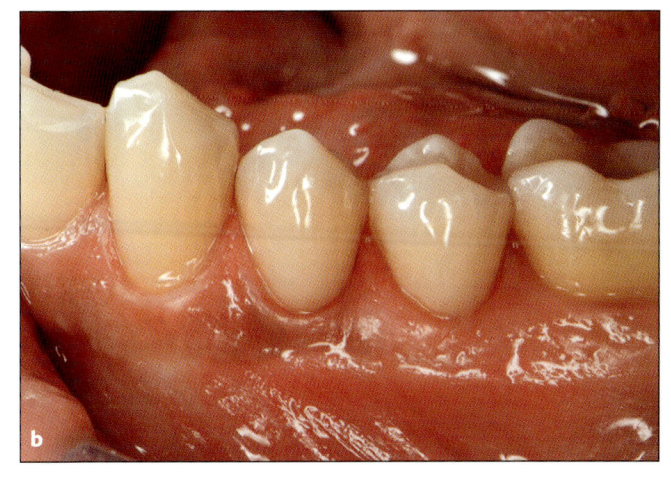

Fig 9-42 *(a and b)* The immediate postoperative evaluation of a direct-indirect Class V restoration depicts an extraordinary integration of form and color, in addition to no visible signs of soft tissue scarring.

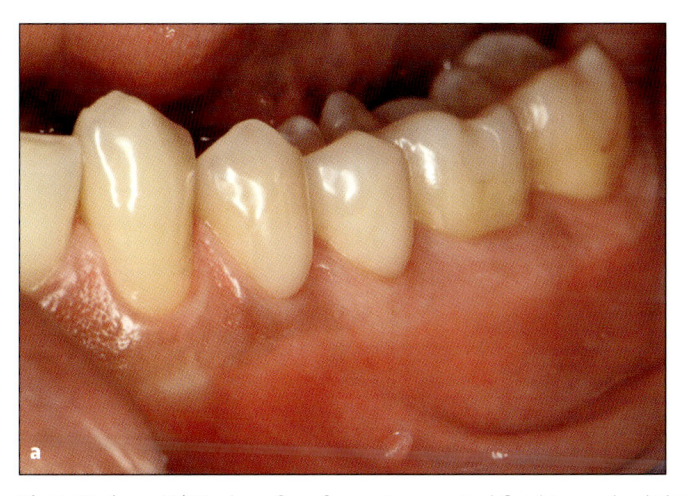

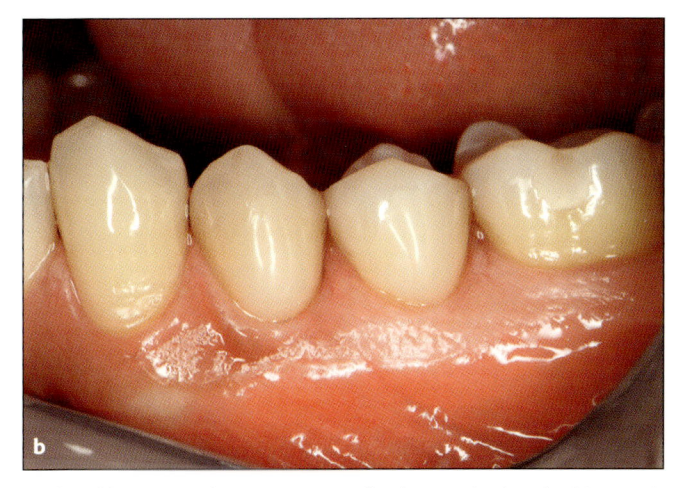

Fig 9-43 *(a and b)* The benefits of superior marginal finishing and polishing rendered by extraoral maneuvers are clearly perceived at the 24-month recall appointment.

and gloss of the inlay, rubber polishing points and cups are used sequentially, followed by felt discs and polishing pastes (Fig 9-41). The immediate postoperative evaluation of a direct-indirect Class V restoration depicts an extraordinary integration of form and color, in addition to no visible sign of soft tissue scarring (Fig 9-42). The benefits of superior marginal finishing and polishing rendered by extraoral maneuvers are clearly corroborated by the long-term clinical appraisal, which depicts a healthy periodontium (Fig 9-43).

155

9 Restorative Protocols: Adhesive Bonding, Materials, and Techniques

Other Considerations for the Direct-Indirect Technique

While the traditional direct approach is an excellent option for restoring NCCLs, the direct-indirect Class V composite inlay eliminates some of its disadvantages and offers precise extraoral margin finishing and polishing, good composite handling, periodontal health, and low polymerization shrinkage stress. However, like any new technique, it will require a paradigm shift and involves a learning curve before the clinician can become proficient. A great change in mentality begins with working with minuscule inlays intra- and extraorally. Working with high-magnification loupes or microscopes is therefore essential for precise handling of the inlays. Once a comfort zone is reached, the clinician will become more confident and be extremely pleased with the results.

Indirect Technique

The notable optical and mechanical properties of strengthened glass-ceramics as well as their good survival rates[167,235] have allowed their use in areas subjected to high mechanical stress and esthetic demands. Consequently, it can be assumed that this indirect restorative material, which is widely used for veneers and crowns, can be predictably applied in NCCL restorations. However, it is important that clinicians consider the financial feasibility of this procedure because it involves more costs than composite direct restorations.

Step-By-Step Indirect Technique

The following case illustrates the indirect technique for placing ceramic restorations in NCCLs.

A 35-year-old man presented with claims of CDH and poor esthetics (Fig 9-44a). Clinical and radiographic examination revealed good oral hygiene, no gingival inflammation or bleeding during probing, and a lack of periodontal disease. However, buccal NCCLs of different dimensions and gingival recessions were found on the maxillary right canine, premolar, and first molar (Fig 9-44b). After control of the oral acidic environment and occlusal adjustments, the NCCLs were evaluated according to the amount of structure loss. The restorative treatment plan included using a nanofilled composite resin core to build up the dentin on the premolar (Fig 9-44c) and Class V lithium disilicate–reinforced glass-ceramic partial laminate veneers to replace the remaining lost structures. The direct composite buildup procedure was performed according to the direct technique previously described.

The teeth with NCCL involvement were prepared for ceramic laminate veneers by producing a 0.5-mm bevel in the occlusal margin of enamel with fine-grit diamond burs (Fig 9-44d). Prior to impression-making, gingival displacement was performed using retraction cords size #00 and #000. The cords were removed, and a polyvinyl siloxane material was used to make impressions of the teeth using a double impression technique (Figs 9-44e and 9-44f). After polymerization, the impression tray was removed and disinfected, and full-arch type IV stone casts were poured. The shade of teeth was identified as A2 using the VITA Classical shade guide.

Class V lithium disilicate–reinforced glass-ceramic approximately 0.4 to 0.5 mm in thickness was processed using a conventional pressing technique associated with extrinsic characterization with ceramic stains (Figs 9-44g and 9-44h). The adaptation of the ceramic laminate veneers to the tooth structures and their relationship with periodontal tissues were checked (Fig 9-44i), and the shade of the ceramic restorations was verified against the tooth structure. The same shade value, A2, was selected for the resin cement on the basis of try-in pastes from the resin cement set used to simulate the final shade of the ceramic laminate veneers after luting (Fig 9-44j).

Surface treatment of the laminate veneers was performed by etching the internal surfaces with 10% hydrofluoric acid for 20 seconds (Fig 9-44k). After they were rinsed with water and air dried, 37% phosphoric acid was actively applied for 60 seconds to remove any compounds precipitated after the previous etching (Fig 9-44l). Finally, a silane coupling agent was actively applied for 20 seconds and left to react for 1 minute (Fig 9-44m).

Selective etching of the enamel was then performed with 37% phosphoric acid for 30 seconds (Fig 9-44n), followed by active application of a one-step self-etching

Indirect Technique

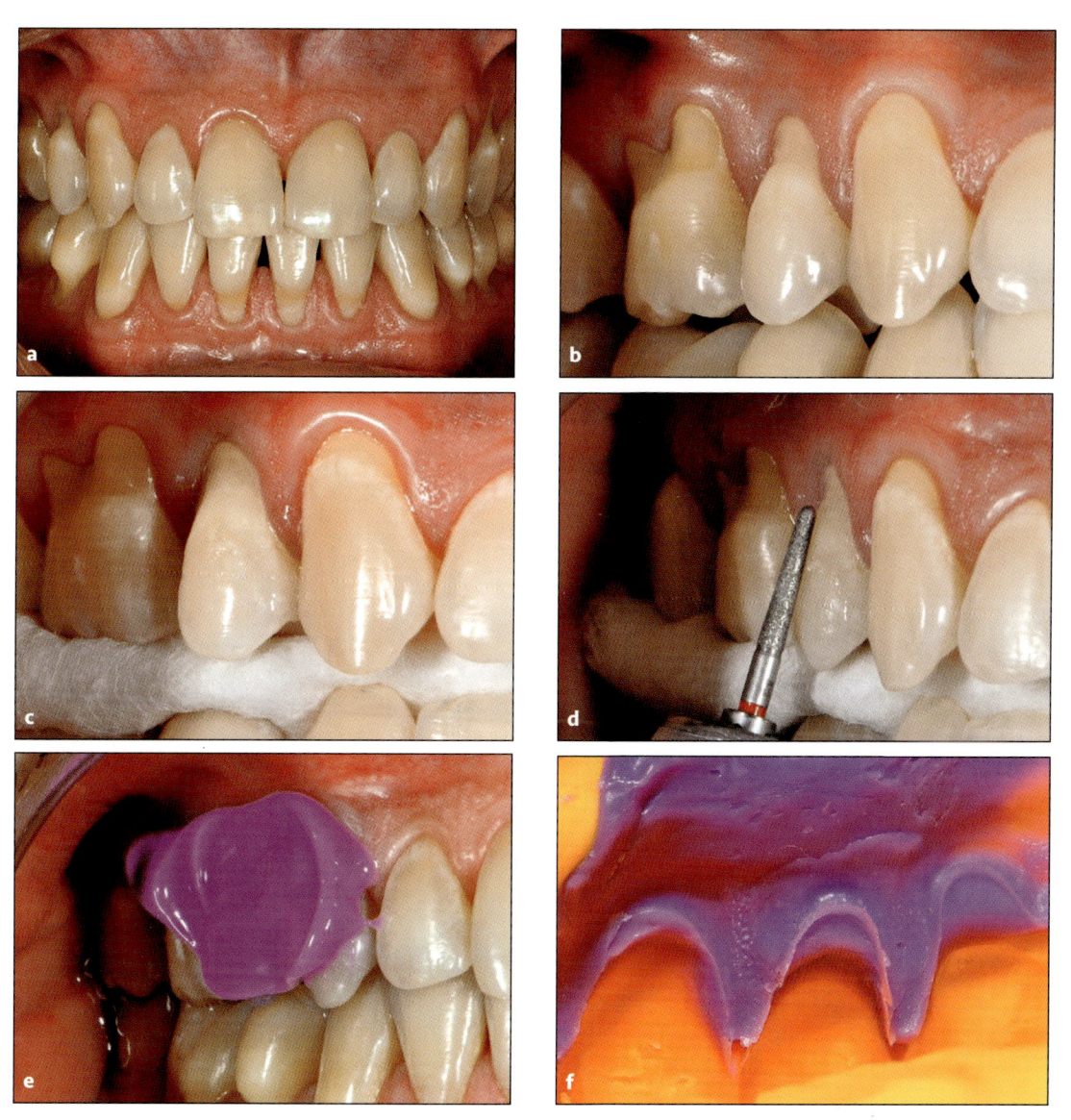

Fig 9-44 *(a)* A 35-year-old man sought treatment for CDH and was concerned about his dental esthetics. *(b)* Intraoral examination revealed good oral hygiene and no gingival inflammation or bleeding during probing, but several buccal NCCLs of different dimensions were found on the maxillary right canine, premolar, and first molar. (Note that the patient has only one premolar.) *(c)* A composite resin core was built up in the premolar to replace lost dentin. *(d)* Ultrafine-grit diamond burs were used to place a 0.5-mm bevel at the enamel margins of the NCCLs. *(e and f)* After the placement and removal of retraction cords to displace the gingiva, a polyvinyl siloxane material was used to make impressions of the teeth using a double-step impression technique. →

adhesive system (Fig 9-44o) and photoactivation for 20 seconds (Fig 9-44p). Light-curing resin cement was then used for luting the ceramic laminate veneers. After positioning the veneers on the NCCLs, excess resin cement was removed with disposable applicators, and photoactivation was performed for 60 seconds with an LED light-curing unit. Cervical finishing was carried out using ultrafine-grit diamond burs (#2135FF) and silicone rubber points with diamond paste to improve adaptation and esthetics. Figure 9-44q shows the completed ceramic veneers.

Table 9-2 presents some dental materials recommended for NCCL restoration.

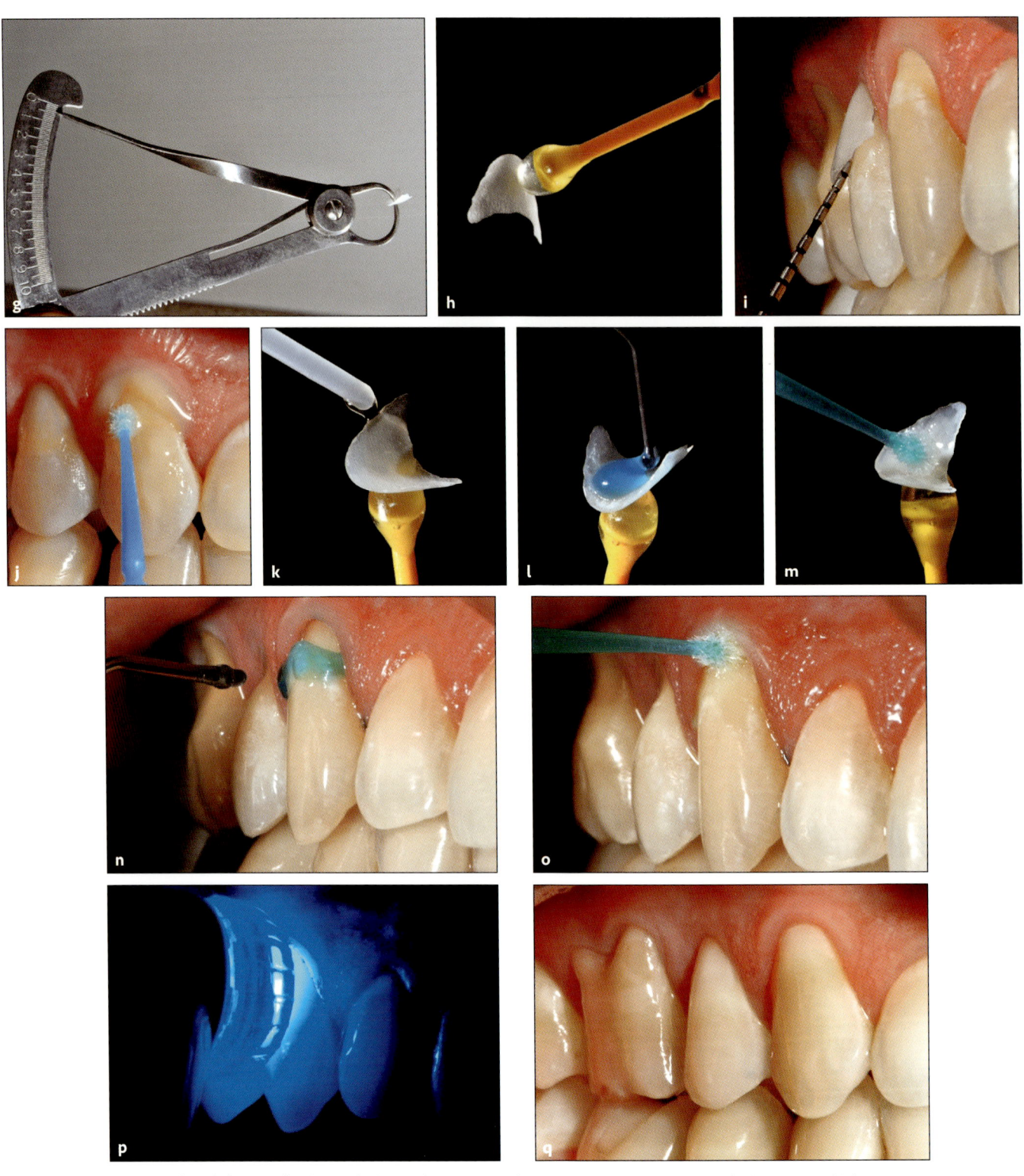

9 Restorative Protocols: Adhesive Bonding, Materials, and Techniques

Fig 9-44 *(cont)* *(g and h)* Lithium disilicate glass-ceramic laminate veneers approximately 0.5 mm in thickness were fabricated using a pressing technique associated with extrinsic characterization with stains. *(i)* Adaptation of the ceramic laminate veneers was checked. *(j)* The shade of the ceramic was checked against the tooth substrate, and the same resin cement shade was selected using try-in pastes from the resin cement set. *(k)* Surface treatment of the ceramic laminate veneers was performed with 10% hydrofluoric acid for 20 seconds. *(l)* After rinsing with water spray and air drying, 37% phosphoric acid was applied for 60 seconds to remove compounds precipitated after the previous etching. *(m)* The internal surfaces were treated with a silane coupling agent applied actively for 20 seconds and left to react for 1 minute. *(n)* Selective etching of enamel was performed with 37% phosphoric acid for 15 seconds. *(o and p)* A one-step self-etching adhesive system was applied and light cured. *(q)* After positioning the laminate veneers on the NCCLs, excess resin cement was removed, and photoactivation was performed for 60 seconds with an LED light-curing unit. The final aspect of the lithium disilicate glass-ceramic laminate veneers shows the esthetic result.

Table 9-2 Dental materials recommended for NCCL restoration

Material	Classification	Manufacturer
Gingival cord		
Ultrapak (sizes #000 and #00)	100% cotton	Ultradent
Adhesive system		
Adper Scotchbond Multi-Purpose Plus	Etch-and-rinse three-step system	3M ESPE
Adper Single Bond Plus	Etch-and-rinse two-step system	3M ESPE
Scotchbond Universal	Universal adhesive	3M ESPE
Peak Universal Bond and Peak SE Primer	Universal adhesive	Ultradent
AdheSE	Self-etching two-step system	Ivoclar Vivadent
Adhese Universal	Universal adhesive	Ivoclar Vivadent
ExciTE F	Etch-and-rinse two-step system	Ivoclar Vivadent
GO!	Self-etching single-step system	SDI
Futurabond M+	Self-etching single-step system	Voco
Futurabond NR	Self-etching single-step system	Voco
One Up Bond F Plus	Self-etching two-step system	Tokuyama
Bond Force	Self-etching single-step system	Tokuyama
Palfique Bond	Self-etching single-step system	Tokuyama
iBOND Self Etch	Self-etching single-step system	Heraeus Kulzer
Clearfil SE Bond	Self-etching two-step system	Kuraray
Clearfil Universal Bond	Universal adhesive	Kuraray
Xeno III	Self-etching two-step system	Dentsply
Xeno IV	Self-etching single-step system	Dentsply
OptiBond XTR	Self-etching two-step system	Kerr
OptiBond FL	Self-etching two-step system	Kerr
OptiBond All-in-One	Self-etching single-step system	Kerr
BeautiBond	Self-etching single-step system	Shofu
One Coat 7 Universal	Universal adhesive	Coltene
Prime & Bond Elect	Universal adhesive	Dentsply
All-Bond 2	Self-etching two-step system	Bisco
All-Bond Universal	Universal adhesive	Bisco
Composite resin		
Filtek Supreme	Nanofilled	3M ESPE
Vit-I-escence Syringes/Amelogen Plus	Microhybrid	Ultradent
IPS Empress Direct	Nanohybrid	Ivoclar Vivadent
Tetric EvoCeram	Nanohybrid	Ivoclar Vivadent
Brilliant NG	Nanohybrid	Coltene
Aura	Nanohybrid (dentin) and microfilled (enamel)	SDI
GradioSO	Nanohybrid	Voco
Amaris and Amaris Gingiva	Nanohybrid	Voco
Estelite Sigma Quick/Palfique LXS	Supra nanohybrid	Tokuyama
Estelite Omega	Supra nanohybrid	Tokuyama
Venus Diamond/Charisma Diamond	Nanohybrid	Heraeus Kulzer
Aelite	Nanohybrid	Bisco
Admira Fusion	Nanohybrid	Bisco
Beautifil II/Beautifil Gingiva	Nanohybrid	Shofu
Harmonize	Nanohybrid	Kerr
TPH Spectra LV	Nanohybrid	Dentsply

Conclusion

Let's review what we have covered in this chapter:
- Adhesive bonding requires field isolation, selection of an appropriate adhesive system, multiple coats of adhesive application, a high work time before air drying, and careful light curing.
- Composite resins are composed of an organic matrix, reinforcing fillers, a silane coupling agent, and chemical agents that promote polymerization.
- Composites are classified according to their consistency (ie, flowable vs packable) and the characteristics of their reinforcing fillers (ie, conventional/macrofilled, microfilled, nanofilled).
- Composites are an excellent choice for the restoration of NCCLs because of their similar biomechanical properties to tooth structure.
- Ceramics can also be used for restoration of NCCLs, particularly those associated with gingival recession that require soft tissue grafting.
- Polymerization success for composite resins or cements depends on the efficiency of the light-curing unit and depth of cure.
- The direct technique for adhesive Class V restorations is a simple, affordable, and universally used protocol for reproducing esthetics and function of natural tooth structure.
- The direct-indirect Class V inlay eliminates some of the disadvantages of the direct technique and offers precise extraoral margin finishing and polishing, good composite handling, periodontal health, and low polymerization shrinkage stress.
- The indirect technique can be used to restore NCCLs with ceramics, which have superior strength and smoothness compared with composite resins.
- Future controlled clinical trials are indicated to compare direct and indirect techniques.

References

1. Buonocore MG. A simple method of increasing the adhesion of acrylic filling materials to enamel surfaces. J Dent Res 1955;34:849–853.
2. Asmussen E, Peutzfeldt A. Influence of selected components on crosslink density in polymer structures. Eur J Oral Sci 2001;109:282–285.
3. Pashley DH, Tay FR, Carvalho RM, et al. From dry bonding to water-wet bonding to ethanol-wet bonding. A review of the interactions between dentin matrix and solvated resins using a macromodel of the hybrid layer. Am J Dent 2007;20:7–20.
4. Nishiyama N, Tay FR, Fujita K, et al. Hydrolysis of functional monomers in a single-bottle self-etching primer—correlation of 13C NMR and TEM findings. J Dent Res 2006;85:422–426.
5. Nishiyama N, Suzuki K, Yoshida H, Teshima H, Nemoto K. Hydrolytic stability of methacrylamide in acidic aqueous solution. Biomaterials 2004;25:965–969.
6. Collares FM, Ogliari FA, Zanchi CH, Petzhold CL, Piva E, Samuel SM. Influence of 2-hydroxyethyl methacrylate concentration on polymer network of adhesive resin. J Adhes Dent 2011;13:125–129.
7. Abedin F, Ye Q, Parthasarathy R, Misra A, Spencer P. Polymerization behavior of hydrophilic-rich phase of dentin adhesive. J Dent Res 2015;94:500–507.
8. Takahashi M, Nakajima M, Hosaka K, Ikeda M, Foxton RM, Tagami J. Long-term evaluation of water sorption and ultimate tensile strength of HEMA-containing/-free one-step self-etch adhesives. J Dent 2011;39:506–512.
9. Van Landuyt KL, Snauwaert J, De Munck J, et al. Systematic review of the chemical composition of contemporary dental adhesives. Biomaterials 2007;28:3757–3785.
10. Feitosa VP, Sauro S, Ogliari FA, et al. Impact of hydrophilicity and length of spacer chains on the bonding of functional monomers. Dent Mater 2014;30:e317–e323.
11. Van Landuyt KL, Yoshida Y, Hirata I, et al. Influence of the chemical structure of functional monomers on their adhesive performance. J Dent Res 2008;87:757–761.
12. Feitosa VP, Ogliari FA, Van Meerbeek B, et al. Can the hydrophilicity of functional monomers affect chemical interaction? J Dent Res 2014;93:201–206.
13. Reis A, Loguercio AD, Azevedo CL, de Carvalho RM, da Julio Singer M, Grande RH. Moisture spectrum of demineralized dentin for adhesive systems with different solvent bases. J Adhes Dent 2003;5:183–192.
14. Lima Gda S, Ogliari FA, da Silva EO, et al. Influence of water concentration in an experimental self-etching primer on the bond strength to dentin. J Adhes Dent 2008;10:167–172.
15. Emamieh S, Sadr A, Ghasemi A, Torabzadeh H, Akhavanzanjani V, Tagami J. Effects of solvent drying time and water storage on ultimate tensile strength of adhesives. J Investig Clin Dent 2014;5:51–57.
16. Ikemura K, Endo T. A review of the development of radical photopolymerization initiators used for designing light-curing dental adhesives and resin composites. Dent Mater J 2010;29:481–501.
17. Loguercio AD, Stanislawczuk R, Mittelstadt FG, Meier MM, Reis A. Effects of diphenyliodonium salt addition on the adhesive and mechanical properties of an experimental adhesive. J Dent 2013;41:653–658.
18. Munchow EA, Valente LL, Peralta SL, et al. 1,3-Diethyl-2-thiobarbituric acid as an alternative coinitiator for acidic photopolymerizable dental materials. J Biomed Mater Res B Appl Biomater 2013;101:1217–1221.
19. Belli R, Kreppel S, Petschelt A, Hornberger H, Boccaccini AR, Lohbauer U. Strengthening of dental adhesives via particle reinforcement. J Mech Behav Biomed Mater 2014;37:100–108.
20. Pongprueksa P, Kuphasuk W, Senawongse P. The elastic moduli across various types of resin/dentin interfaces. Dent Mater 2008;24:1102–1106.
21. Andre CB, Gomes BP, Duque TM, et al. Dentine bond strength and antimicrobial activity evaluation of adhesive systems. J Dent 2015;43:466–475.
22. Brambilla E, Ionescu A, Fadini L, et al. Influence of MDPB-containing primer on *Streptococcus mutans* biofilm formation in simulated Class I restorations. J Adhes Dent 2013;15:431–438.
23. Uysal T, Amasyali M, Ozcan S, Koyuturk AE, Sagdic D. Effect of antibacterial monomer-containing adhesive on enamel demineralization around orthodontic brackets: An in-vivo study. Am J Orthod Dentofacial Orthop 2011;139:650–656.
24. Sabatini C, Scheffel DL, Scheffel RH, et al. Inhibition of endogenous human dentin MMPs by Gluma. Dent Mater 2014;30:752–758.
25. Hebling J, Pashley DH, Tjaderhane L, Tay FR. Chlorhexidine arrests subclinical degradation of dentin hybrid layers in vivo. J Dent Res 2005;84:741–746.
26. Nakabayashi N, Ashizawa M, Nakamura M. Identification of a resin-dentin hybrid layer in vital human dentin created in vivo: Durable bonding to vital dentin. Quintessence Int 1992;23:135–141.
27. Van Meerbeek B, De Munck J, Yoshida Y, et al. Buonocore memorial lecture. Adhesion to enamel and dentin: Current status and future challenges. Oper Dent 2003;28:215–235.
28. Sano H. Microtensile testing, nanoleakage, and biodegradation of resin-dentin bonds. J Dent Res 2006;85:11–14.

References

29. Breschi L, Mazzoni A, Ruggeri A, Cadenaro M, Di Lenarda R, De Stefano Dorigo E. Dental adhesion review: Aging and stability of the bonded interface. Dent Mater 2008;24:90–101.
30. Peumans M, De Munck J, Mine A, Van Meerbeek B. Clinical effectiveness of contemporary adhesives for the restoration of non-carious cervical lesions. A systematic review. Dent Mater 2014;30:1089–1103.
31. Heintze SD, Ruffieux C, Rousson V. Clinical performance of cervical restorations—A meta-analysis. Dent Mater 2010;26:993–1000.
32. Daudt E, Lopes GC, Vieira LC. Does operatory field isolation influence the performance of direct adhesive restorations? J Adhes Dent 2013;15:27–32.
33. Loguercio AD, Luque-Martinez I, Lisboa AH, et al. Influence of isolation method of the operative field on gingival damage, patients' preference, and restoration retention in noncarious cervical lesions. Oper Dent 2015;40:581–593.
34. van Dijken JW. Durability of three simplified adhesive systems in Class V non-carious cervical dentin lesions. Am J Dent 2004;17:27–32.
35. Schroeder M, Reis A, Luque-Martinez I, Loguercio AD, Masterson D, Maia LC. Effect of enamel bevel on retention of cervical composite resin restorations: A systematic review and meta-analysis. J Dent 2015;43:777–788.
36. Da Costa TR, Loguercio AD, Reis A. Effect of enamel bevel on the clinical performance of resin composite restorations placed in non-carious cervical lesions. J Esthet Restor Dent 2013;25:346–356.
37. Perdigao J, Carmo AR, Anauate-Netto C, et al. Clinical performance of a self-etching adhesive at 18 months. Am J Dent 2005;18:135–140.
38. Perdigao J, Carmo AR, Geraldeli S. Eighteen-month clinical evaluation of two dentin adhesives applied on dry vs moist dentin. J Adhes Dent 2005;7:253–258.
39. Zander-Grande C, Ferreira SQ, da Costa TR, Loguercio AD, Reis A. Application of etch-and-rinse adhesives on dry and rewet dentin under rubbing action: A 24-month clinical evaluation. J Am Dent Assoc 2011;142:828–835.
40. Loguercio AD, Raffo J, Bassani F, et al. 24-month clinical evaluation in non-carious cervical lesions of a two-step etch-and-rinse adhesive applied using a rubbing motion. Clin Oral Investig 2011;15:589–596.
41. Can Say E, Yurdaguven H, Ozel E, Soyman M. A randomized five-year clinical study of a two-step self-etch adhesive with or without selective enamel etching. Dent Mater J 2014;33:757–763.
42. Peumans M, De Munck J, Van Landuyt K, Van Meerbeek B. Thirteen-year randomized controlled clinical trial of a two-step self-etch adhesive in non-carious cervical lesions. Dent Mater 2015;31:308–314.
43. Luque-Martinez I, Munoz MA, Mena-Serrano A, Hass V, Reis A, Loguercio AD. Effect of EDTA conditioning on cervical restorations bonded with a self-etch adhesive: A randomized double-blind clinical trial. J Dent 2015;43:1175–1183.
44. Loguercio AD, de Paula EA, Hass V, Luque-Martinez I, Reis A, Perdigao J. A new universal simplified adhesive: 36-month randomized double-blind clinical trial. J Dent 2015;43:1083–1092.
45. Dutra-Correa M, Saraceni CH, Ciaramicoli MT, Kiyan VH, Queiroz CS. Effect of chlorhexidine on the 18-month clinical performance of two adhesives. J Adhes Dent 2013;15:287–292.
46. Sartori N, Stolf SC, Silva SB, Lopes GC, Carrilho M. Influence of chlorhexidine digluconate on the clinical performance of adhesive restorations: A 3-year follow-up. J Dent 2013;41:1188–1195.
47. Araujo MS, Souza LC, Apolonio FM, et al. Two-year clinical evaluation of chlorhexidine incorporation in two-step self-etch adhesive. J Dent 2015;43:140–148.
48. Reis A, Leite TM, Matte K, et al. Improving clinical retention of one-step self-etching adhesive systems with an additional hydrophobic adhesive layer. J Am Dent Assoc 2009;140:877–885.
49. Perdigao J, Dutra-Correa M, Saraceni CH, Ciaramicoli MT, Kiyan VH, Queiroz CS. Randomized clinical trial of four adhesion strategies: 18-month results. Oper Dent 2012;37:3–11.
50. Loguercio AD, Reis A. Application of a dental adhesive using the self-etch and etch-and-rinse approaches: An 18-month clinical evaluation. J Am Dent Assoc 2008;139:53–61.
51. Zander-Grande C, Amaral RC, Loguercio AD, Barroso LP, Reis A. Clinical performance of one-step self-etch adhesives applied actively in cervical lesions: 24-month clinical trial. Oper Dent 2014;39:228–238.
52. Hill EE, Rubel BS. Do dental educators need to improve their approach to teaching rubber dam use? J Dent Educ 2008;72:1177–1181.
53. Gilbert GH, Litaker MS, Pihlstrom DJ, Amundson CW, Gordan VV, Group DC. Rubber dam use during routine operative dentistry procedures: Findings from the Dental PBRN. Oper Dent 2010;35:491–499.
54. Eliguzeloglu E, Omurlu H, Eskitascioglu G, Belli S. Effect of surface treatments and different adhesives on the hybrid layer thickness of non-carious cervical lesions. Oper Dent 2008;33:338–345.
55. van Dijken JW. Clinical evaluation of three adhesive systems in class V non-carious lesions. Dent Mater 2000;16:285–291.
56. Camargo MA, Roda MI, Marques MM, de Cara AA. Micro-tensile bond strength to bovine sclerotic dentine: Influence of surface treatment. J Dent 2008;36:922–927.
57. Lopes GC, Vieira LC, Monteiro S Jr, Caldeira de Andrada MA, Baratieri CM. Dentin bonding: Effect of degree of mineralization and acid etching time. Oper Dent 2003;28:429–439.
58. Hashimoto M. A review—Micromorphological evidence of degradation in resin-dentin bonds and potential preventional solutions. J Biomed Mater Res B Appl Biomater 2010;92:268–280.
59. Hashimoto M, Ohno H, Kaga M, et al. Over-etching effects on microtensile bond strength and failure patterns for two dentin bonding systems. J Dent 2002;30:99–105.
60. Stanislawczuk R, Reis A, Loguercio AD. A 2 year in vitro evaluation of a chlorhexidine-containing acid on the durability of resin-dentin interfaces. J Dent 2011;39:40–47.
61. Stanislawczuk R, Amaral RC, Zander-Grande C, Gagler D, Reis A, Loguercio AD. Chlorhexidine-containing acid conditioner preserves the longevity of resin-dentin bonds. Oper Dent 2009;34:481–490.
62. Sabatini C, Patel SK. Matrix metalloproteinase inhibitory properties of benzalkonium chloride stabilizes adhesive interfaces. Eur J Oral Sci 2013;121:610–616.
63. Tjaderhane L, Nascimento FD, Breschi L, et al. Strategies to prevent hydrolytic degradation of the hybrid layer—A review. Dent Mater 2013;29:999–1011.
64. Sabatini C, Pashley DH. Mechanisms regulating the degradation of dentin matrices by endogenous dentin proteases and their role in dental adhesion. A review. Am J Dent 2014;27:203–214.
65. Frankenberger R, Lohbauer U, Roggendorf MJ, Naumann M, Taschner M. Selective enamel etching reconsidered: Better than etch-and-rinse and self-etch? J Adhes Dent 2008;10:339–344.
66. Erickson RL, Barkmeier WW, Latta MA. The role of etching in bonding to enamel: A comparison of self-etching and etch-and-rinse adhesive systems. Dent Mater 2009;25:1459–1467.
67. Osorio R, Erhardt MC, Pimenta LA, Osorio E, Toledano M. EDTA treatment improves resin-dentin bonds' resistance to degradation. J Dent Res 2005;84:736–740.
68. Sauro S, Toledano M, Aguilera FS, et al. Resin-dentin bonds to EDTA-treated vs. acid-etched dentin using ethanol wet-bonding. Part II: Effects of mechanical cycling load on microtensile bond strengths. Dent Mater 2011;27:563–572.
69. Luque-Martinez IV, Mena-Serrano A, Munoz MA, Hass V, Reis A, Loguercio AD. Effect of bur roughness on bond to sclerotic dentin with self-etch adhesive systems. Oper Dent 2013;38:39–47.
70. Bogra P, Kaswan S. Etching with EDTA—An in vitro study. J Indian Soc Pedod Prev Dent 2003;21:79–83.
71. Perdigao J, Kose C, Mena-Serrano AP, et al. A new universal simplified adhesive: 18-month clinical evaluation. Oper Dent 2014;39:113–127.
72. Munoz MA, Luque-Martinez I, Malaquias P, et al. In vitro longevity of bonding properties of universal adhesives to dentin. Oper Dent 2015;40:282–292.
73. Chee B, Rickman LJ, Satterthwaite JD. Adhesives for the restoration of non-carious cervical lesions: A systematic review. J Dent 2012;40:443–452.
74. King NM, Tay FR, Pashley DH, et al. Conversion of one-step to two-step self-etch adhesives for improved efficacy and extended application. Am J Dent 2005;18:126–134.
75. de Andrade e Silva SM, Carrilho MR, Marquezini Junior L, et al. Effect of an additional hydrophilic versus hydrophobic coat on the quality of dentinal sealing provided by two-step etch-and-rinse adhesives. J Appl Oral Sci 2009;17:184–189.

76. Cadenaro M, Antoniolli F, Sauro S, et al. Degree of conversion and permeability of dental adhesives. Eur J Oral Sci 2005;113:525–530.
77. Breschi L, Cadenaro M, Antoniolli F, et al. Polymerization kinetics of dental adhesives cured with LED: Correlation between extent of conversion and permeability. Dent Mater 2007;23:1066–1072.
78. Reis A, Albuquerque M, Pegoraro M, et al. Can the durability of one-step self-etch adhesives be improved by double application or by an extra layer of hydrophobic resin? J Dent 2008;36:309–315.
79. Hashimoto M, De Munck J, Ito S, et al. In vitro effect of nanoleakage expression on resin-dentin bond strengths analyzed by microtensile bond test, SEM/EDX and TEM. Biomaterials 2004;25:5565–5574.
80. Ito S, Tay FR, Hashimoto M, et al. Effects of multiple coatings of two all-in-one adhesives on dentin bonding. J Adhes Dent 2005;7:133–141.
81. Reis A, de Carvalho Cardoso P, Vieira LC, Baratieri LN, Grande RH, Loguercio AD. Effect of prolonged application times on the durability of resin-dentin bonds. Dent Mater 2008;24:639–644.
82. Cardoso Pde C, Loguercio AD, Vieira LC, Baratieri LN, Reis A. Effect of prolonged application times on resin-dentin bond strengths. J Adhes Dent 2005;7:143–149.
83. Toledano M, Proenca JP, Erhardt MC, et al. Increases in dentin-bond strength if doubling application time of an acetone-containing one-step adhesive. Oper Dent 2007;32:133–137.
84. Erhardt MC, Osorio R, Pisani-Proenca J, et al. Effect of double layering and prolonged application time on MTBS of water/ethanol-based self-etch adhesives to dentin. Oper Dent 2009;34:571–577.
85. Miyazaki M, Onose H, Iida N, Kazama H. Determination of residual double bonds in resin-dentin interface by Raman spectroscopy. Dent Mater 2003;19:245–251.
86. Wang Y, Spencer P. Hybridization efficiency of the adhesive/dentin interface with wet bonding. J Dent Res 2003;82:141–145.
87. Hashimoto M, Ohno H, Kaga M, Sano H, Endo K, Oguchi H. The extent to which resin can infiltrate dentin by acetone-based adhesives. J Dent Res 2002;81:74–78.
88. Reis A, Pellizzaro A, Dal-Bianco K, Gones OM, Patzlaff R, Loguercio AD. Impact of adhesive application to wet and dry dentin on long-term resin-dentin bond strengths. Oper Dent 2007;32:380–387.
89. Jacobsen T, Soderholm KJ. Effect of primer solvent, primer agitation, and dentin dryness on shear bond strength to dentin. Am J Dent 1998;11:225–228.
90. Dal-Bianco K, Pellizzaro A, Patzlaft R, de Oliveira Bauer JR, Loguercio AD, Reis A. Effects of moisture degree and rubbing action on the immediate resin-dentin bond strength. Dent Mater 2006;22:1150–1156.
91. Loguercio AD, Munoz MA, Luque-Martinez I, Hass V, Reis A, Perdigao J. Does active application of universal adhesives to enamel in self-etch mode improve their performance? J Dent 2015;43:1060–1070.
92. Reis A, Carrilho M, Breschi L, Loguercio AD. Overview of clinical alternatives to minimize the degradation of the resin-dentin bonds. Oper Dent 2013;38:E1–E25.
93. Cuadros-Sanchez J, Szesz A, Hass V, Patzlaff RT, Reis A, Loguercio AD. Effects of sonic application of adhesive systems on bonding fiber posts to root canals. J Endod 2014;40:1201–1205.
94. Mena-Serrano A, Garcia EJ, Loguercio AD, Reis A. Effect of sonic application mode on the resin-dentin bond strength and nanoleakage of simplified self-etch adhesive. Clin Oral Investig 2014;18:729–736.
95. Loguercio AD, Loeblein F, Cherobin T, Ogliari F, Piva E, Reis A. Effect of solvent removal on adhesive properties of simplified etch-and-rinse systems and on bond strengths to dry and wet dentin. J Adhes Dent 2009;11:213–219.
96. Hass V, Folkuenig MS, Reis A, Loguercio AD. Influence of adhesive properties on resin-dentin bond strength of one-step self-etching adhesives. J Adhes Dent 2011;13:417–424.
97. Reis A, Grandi V, Carlotto L, et al. Effect of smear layer thickness and acidity of self-etching solutions on early and long-term bond strength to dentin. J Dent 2005;33:549–559.
98. Takahashi A, Sato Y, Uno S, Pereira PN, Sano H. Effects of mechanical properties of adhesive resins on bond strength to dentin. Dent Mater 2002;18:263–268.
99. Takai T, Hosaka K, Kambara K, et al. Effect of air-drying dentin surfaces on dentin bond strength of a solvent-free one-step adhesive. Dent Mater J 2012;31:558–563.
100. Spreafico D, Semeraro S, Mezzanzanica D, et al. The effect of the air-blowing step on the technique sensitivity of four different adhesive systems. J Dent 2006;34:237–244.
101. Hiraishi N, Breschi L, Prati C, Ferrari M, Tagami J, King NM. Technique sensitivity associated with air-drying of HEMA-free, single-bottle, one-step self-etch adhesives. Dent Mater 2007;23:498–505.
102. Luque-Martinez IV, Perdigao J, Munoz MA, Sezinando A, Reis A, Loguercio AD. Effects of solvent evaporation time on immediate adhesive properties of universal adhesives to dentin. Dent Mater 2014;30:1126–1135.
103. el-Din AK, Abd el-Mohsen MM. Effect of changing application times on adhesive systems bond strengths. Am J Dent 2002;15:321–324.
104. Magne P, Mahallati R, Bazos P, So WS. Direct dentin bonding technique sensitivity when using air/suction drying steps. J Esthet Restor Dent 2008;20:130–138.
105. Aziz TM, Anwar MN, El-Askary FS. Push-out bond strength of fiber posts to root canal dentin using a one-step self-etching adhesive: the effect of solvent removal and light-curing methods. J Adhes Dent 2014;16:79–86.
106. Hinoura K, Miyazaki M, Onose H. Effect of irradiation time to light-cured resin composite on dentin bond strength. Am J Dent 1991;4:273–276.
107. Reis A, Ferreira SQ, Costa TR, Klein-Junior CA, Meier MM, Loguercio AD. Effects of increased exposure times of simplified etch-and-rinse adhesives on the degradation of resin-dentin bonds and quality of the polymer network. Eur J Oral Sci 2010;118:502–509.
108. Yamamoto A, Tsubota K, Takamizawa T, et al. Influence of light intensity on dentin bond strength of self-etch systems. J Oral Sci 2006;48:21–26.
109. Hass V, Luque-Martinez I, Sabino NB, Loguercio AD, Reis A. Prolonged exposure times of one-step self-etch adhesives on adhesive properties and durability of dentine bonds. J Dent 2012;40:1090–1102.
110. Peutzfeldt A. Resin composites in dentistry: The monomer systems. Eur J Oral Sci 1997;105:97–116.
111. Bouillaguet S, Caillot G, Forchelet J, Cattani-Lorente M, Wataha JC, Krejci I. Thermal risks from LED- and high-intensity QTH-curing units during polymerization of dental resins. J Biomed Mater Res B Appl Biomater 2005;72:260–267.
112. Bagis B, Bagis Y, Ertas E, Ustaomer S. Comparison of the heat generation of light curing units. J Contemp Dent Pract 2008;9:65–72.
113. Sakaguchi RL, Powers JM. Craig's Restorative Dental Materials, ed 13. St Louis: Mosby, 2011.
114. Sideridou I, Tserki V, Papanastasiou G. Effect of chemical structure on degree of conversion in light-cured dimethacrylate-based dental resins. Biomaterials 2002;23:1819–1829.
115. Ferracane JL. Resin composite: State of the art. Dent Mater 2011;27:29–38.
116. Charton C, Falk V, Marchal P, Pla F, Colon P. Influence of Tg, viscosity and chemical structure of monomers on shrinkage stress in light-cured dimethacrylate-based dental resins. Dent Mater 2007;23:1447–1459.
117. Braga RR, Ballester RY, Ferracane JL. Factors involved in the development of polymerization shrinkage stress in resin-composites: A systematic review. Dent Mater 2005;21:962–970.
118. Ilie N, Hickel R. Investigations on mechanical behaviour of dental composites. Clin Oral Investig 2009;13:427–438.
119. Asmussen E, Peutzfeldt A. Influence of UEDMA, BisGMA and TEGDMA on selected mechanical properties of experimental resin composites. Dent Mater 1998;14:51–56.
120. Floyd CJ, Dickens SH. Network structure of Bis-GMA- and UDMA-based resin systems. Dent Mater 2006;22:1143–1149.
121. Atai M, Watts DC. A new kinetic model for the photopolymerization shrinkage-strain of dental composites and resin-monomers. Dent Mater 2006;22:785–791.
122. Dewaele M, Truffier-Boutry D, Devaux J, Leloup G. Volume contraction in photocured dental resins: The shrinkage-conversion relationship revisited. Dent Mater 2006;22:359–365.
123. Kramer N, Lohbauer U, Garcia-Godoy F, Frankenberger R. Light curing of resin-based composites in the LED era. Am J Dent 2008;21:135–142.
124. Turssi CP, Ferracane JL, Vogel K. Filler features and their effects on wear and degree of conversion of particulate dental resin composites. Biomaterials 2005;26:4932–4937.
125. Emami N, Sjodahl M, Soderholm KJ. How filler properties, filler fraction, sample thickness and light source affect light attenuation in particulate filled resin composites. Dent Mater 2005;21:721–730.

References

126. Wilson KS, Antonucci JM. Interphase structure-property relationships in thermoset dimethacrylate nanocomposites. Dent Mater 2006;22:995–1001.
127. Watts DC. Reaction kinetics and mechanics in photo-polymerised networks. Dent Mater 2005;21:27–35.
128. Stojanac IL, Premovic MT, Ramic BD, Drobac MR, Stojsin IM, Petrovic LM. Noncarious cervical lesions restored with three different tooth-colored materials: Two-year results. Oper Dent 2013;38:12–20.
129. Perdigão J, Dutra-Correa M, Saraceni SHC, Ciaramicoli MT, Kiyan VH. Randomized clinical trial of two resin-modified glass ionomer materials: 1-year results. Oper Dent 2012;37:591–601.
130. Santiago SL, Passos VF, Vieira AHM, Navarro MF, Lauris JR, Franco EB. Two-year clinical evaluation of resinous restorative systems in non-carious cervical lesions. Braz Dent J 2010;21:229–234.
131. Onal B, Pamir T. The two-year clinical performance of esthetic restorative materials in noncarious cervical lesions. J Am Dent Assoc 2005;136:1547–1555.
132. Namgung C, Rho YJ, Jin BH, Lim BS, Cho BH. A retrospective clinical study of cervical restorations: Longevity and failure-prognostic variables. Oper Dent 2013;38:376–385.
133. Peumans M, De Munck J, Van Landuyt K, Van Meerbeek B. Thirteen-year randomized controlled clinical trial of a two-step self-etch adhesive in non-carious cervical lesions. Dent Mater 2013;31:308–314.
134. Çelik Ç, Ozgunaltay O, Attar N. Clinical evaluation of flowable resins in non-carious cervical lesions: Two-year results. Oper Dent 2007;32:313–321.
135. Baroudi K, Rodrigues JC. Flowable resin composites: A systematic review and clinical considerations. J Clin Diagn Res 2015;9:ZE18–ZE24.
136. Labella R, Lambrechts P, Van Meerbek B, Vanherle G. Polymerizations shrinkage and elasticity of flowable composites and filled adhesives. Dent Mater 1999;15:128–137.
137. Qin W, Song Z, Ye YY, Lin ZM. Two-year clinical evaluation of composite resins in non-carious cervical lesions. Clin Oral Investig 2013;17:799–804.
138. Leprince JG, Palin WM, Vanacker J, Sabbagh J, Devaux J, Leloup G. Physico-mechanical characteristics of commercially available bulk-fill composites. J Dent 2014;42:993–1000.
139. Furness A, Tadros MY, Looney SW, Rueggeberg FA. Effect of bulk/incremental fill on internal gap formation of bulk-fill composites. J Dent 2014;42:439–449.
140. Lohbauer U, Frankenberger R, Kramer N, Petschelt A. Strength and fatigue performance versus filler fractions of different types of direct dental restoratives. J Biomed Mater Res B Appl Biomater 2006;76:114–120.
141. Peumans M, De Munck J, Van Landuyt KL, et al. Restoring cervical lesions with flexible composites. Dent Mater 2007;23:749–754.
142. Borges AL, Borges AB, Xavier TA, Bottino MC, Platt JA. Impact of quantity of resin, C-factor, and geometry on resin composite polymerization shrinkage stress in Class V restorations. Oper Dent 2014;39:144–151.
143. Wilson AD, Kent BE. The glass-ionomer cement, a new translucent dental filling material. J Appl Chem Biotechnol 1971;21:313.
144. Baig MS, Fleming GJP. Conventional glass-ionomer materials: A review of the developments in glass powder, polyacid liquid and the strategies of reinforcement. J Dent 2015;43:897–912.
145. Fagundes TC, Barata TJE, Bresciani E, et al. Seven-year clinical performance of resin composite versus resin-modified glass ionomer restorations in noncarious cervical lesions. Oper Dent 2014;39:578–587.
146. Ichim I, Li Q, Loughran J, Swain MV, Kieser J. Restorations of non-carious cervical lesions—Part I. Modelling of restorative fracture. Dent Mater 2007;23:1553–1561.
147. Anusavice KJ, Shen C, Rawls HR. Phillips' Science of Dental Materials, ed 12. Philadelphia: Elsevier, 2012.
148. Antonson SA, Anusavice KJ. Contrast ratio of veneering and core ceramics as a function of thickness. Int J Prosthodont 2001;14:316–320.
149. da Silva EM, de Sa Rodrigues CU, Dias DA, et al. Effect of toothbrushing-mouthrinse-cycling on surface roughness and topography of nano-filled, microfilled, and microhybrid resin composites. Oper Dent 2014;39:521–529.
150. de Paula AB, de Fucio SB, Alonso RC, Ambrosano GM, Puppin-Rontani RM. Influence of chemical degradation on the surface properties of nano restorative materials. Oper Dent 2014;39:E109–E117.
151. Vieira AC, Oliveira MC, Lima EM, Rambob I, Leite M. Evaluation of the surface roughness in dental ceramics submitted to different finishing and polishing methods. J Ind Prosthodont Soc 2013;13:290–295.
152. Deliberador TM, Martins TM, Furlaneto FA, Klingenfuss M, Bosco AF. Use of the connective tissue graft for the coverage of composite resin-restored root surfaces in maxillary central incisors. Quintessence Int 2012;43:597–602.
153. Santamaria MP, Ambrosano GM, Casati MZ, et al. Connective tissue graft and resin glass ionomer for the treatment of gingival recession associated with noncarious cervical lesions: A case series. Int J Periodontics Restorative Dent 2011;31:e57–63.
154. Santamaria MP, Ambrosano GM, Casati MZ, et al. Connective tissue graft plus resin-modified glass ionomer restoration for the treatment of gingival recession associated with non-carious cervical lesion: A randomized-controlled clinical trial. J Clin Periodontol 2009;36:791–798.
155. Pereira AG, Teixeira DN, Soares MP, Gonzaga RC, Fernandes-Neto AJ, Soares PV. Periodontal and restorative treatment of gingival recession associated with non-carious cervical lesions: Case study. J Int Acad Periodontol 2016;18:16–22.
156. Carty WM, Senapati U. Porcelain—Raw materials, processing, phase evolution and machanical behavior. J Am Ceram Soc 1998;81:3–20.
157. McLean JW, Hughes TH. The reinforcement of dental porcelain with ceramic oxides. Br Dent J 1965;119:251–267.
158. Gomes EA, Assunção WG, Rocha EP, Santos PH. Cerâmicas odontológicas: O estado atual. Cerâmica 2008;54:319–325.
159. Callister WD Jr, Rethwisch DG. Structures and properties of ceramics. In: Materials Science and Engineering: An Introduction, ed 8. Hoboken, NJ: Wiley, 1999.
160. Cesar PF, Soki FN, Yoshimura HN, Gonzaga CC, Styopkin V. Influence of leucite content on slow crack growth of dental porcelains. Dent Mater 2008;24:1114–1122.
161. Gonzaga CC, Cesar PF, Miranda WG Jr, Yoshimura HN. Slow crack growth and reliability of dental ceramics. Dent Mater 2011;27:394–406.
162. Denry IL, Mackert JR Jr, Holloway JA, Rosenstiel SF. Effect of cubic leucite stabilization on the flexural strength of feldspathic dental porcelain. J Dent Res 1996;75:1928–1935.
163. Pieger S, Salman A, Bidra AS. Clinical outcomes of lithium disilicate single crowns and partial fixed dental prostheses: A systematic review. J Prosthet Dent 2014;112:22–30.
164. Albakry M, Guazzato M, Swain MV. Biaxial flexural strength, elastic moduli, and x-ray diffraction characterization of three pressable all-ceramic materials. J Prosthet Dent 2003;89:374–380.
165. Gehrt M, Wolfart S, Rafai N, Reich S, Edelhoff D. Clinical results of lithium-disilicate crowns after up to 9 years of service. Clin Oral Investig 2013;17:275–284.
166. Machado AC, Soares CJ, Reis BR, Bicalho AA, Raposo LHA, Soares PV. Management of cervical lesions with different restorative techniques: Influence of load type and mechanical fatigue on the biomechanical behavior of affected teeth. Oper Dent [in press].
167. Soares PV, Spini PH, Carvalho VF, et al. Esthetic rehabilitation with laminated ceramic veneers reinforced by lithium disilicate. Quintessence Int 2014;45:129–133.
168. Wegehaupt FJ, Taubock TT, Attin T, Belibasakis GN. Influence of light-curing mode on the cytotoxicity of resin-based surface sealants. BMC Oral Health 2014;14:48.
169. Bicalho AA, Pereira RD, Zanatta RF, et al. Incremental filling technique and composite material—Part I: Cuspal deformation, bond strength, and physical properties. Oper Dent 2014;39:E71–E82.
170. Bicalho AA, Valdivia AD, Barreto BC, et al. Incremental filling technique and composite material—Part II: Shrinkage and shrinkage stresses. Oper Dent 2014;39:E83–E92.
171. Bortolotto T, Guillarme D, Gutemberg D, Veuthey JL, Krejci I. Composite resin vs resin cement for luting of indirect restorations: Comparison of solubility and shrinkage behavior. Dent Mater J 2013;32:834–838.
172. May LG, Kelly JR. Influence of resin cement polymerization shrinkage on stresses in porcelain crowns. Dent Mater 2013;29:1073–1079.
173. Stahl F, Ashworth SH, Jandt KD, Mills RW. Light-emitting diode (LED) polymerisation of dental composites: Flexural properties and polymerisation potential. Biomaterials 2000;21:1379–1385.
174. Mills RW, Uhl A, Blackwell GB, Jandt KD. High power light emitting diode (LED) arrays versus halogen light polymerization of oral biomaterials: Barcol hardness, compressive strength and radiometric properties. Biomaterials 2002;23:2955–2963.

175. Jandt KD, Mills RW. A brief history of LED photopolymerization. Dent Mater 2013;29:605–617.
176. Rueggeberg FA. State-of-the-art. Dental photocuring—A review. Dent Mater 2011;27:39–52.
177. Runnacles P, Correr GM, Baratto Filho F, Gonzaga CC, Furuse AY. Degree of conversion of a resin cement light-cured through ceramic veneers of different thicknesses and types. Braz Dent J 2014;25:38–42.
178. Christensen RP, Palmer TM, Ploeger BJ, Yost MP. Resin polymerization problems—Are they caused by resin curing lights, resin formulations, or both? Compend Contin Educ Dent Suppl 1999:S42–S54.
179. Flury S, Lussi A, Hickel R, Ilie N. Light curing through glass ceramics: Effect of curing mode on micromechanical properties of dual-curing resin cements. Clin Oral Investig 2014;18:809–818.
180. Kopperud HM, Johnsen GF, Lamolle S, et al. Effect of short LED lamp exposure on wear resistance, residual monomer and degree of conversion for Filtek Z250 and Tetric EvoCeram composites. Dent Mater 2013;29:824–834.
181. Rencz A, Hickel R, Ilie N. Curing efficiency of modern LED units. Clin Oral Investig 2012;16:173–179.
182. Ergun G, Egilmez F, Yilmaz S. Effect of reduced exposure times on the cytotoxicity of resin luting cements cured by high-power LED. J Appl Oral Sci 2011;19:286–292.
183. Ozturk E, Chiang YC, Cosgun E, et al. Effect of resin shades on opacity of ceramic veneers and polymerization efficiency through ceramics. J Dent 2013;41(suppl 5):e8–e14.
184. Diamantopoulou S, Papazoglou E, Margaritis V, Kakaboura A. Change of optical properties of contemporary polychromatic resin composites after light curing and finishing. Int J Esthet Dent 2014;9:224–237.
185. Ozturk E, Bolay S, Hickel R, Ilie N. Effects of ceramic shade and thickness on the micro-mechanical properties of a light-cured resin cement in different shades. Acta Odontol Scand 2015;73:503–507.
186. Aguiar FH, Lazzari CR, Lima DA, Ambrosano GM, Lovadino JR. Effect of light curing tip distance and resin shade on microhardness of a hybrid resin composite. Braz Oral Res 2005;19:302–306.
187. Aguirar FH, e Oliveria TR, Lima DA, Ambrosano G, Lovadino JR. Microhardness of different thicknesses of resin composite polymerized by conventional photocuring at different distances. Gen Dent 2008;56:144–148.
188. Ichim I, Schmidlin PR, Kieser JA, Swain MV. Mechanical evaluation of cervical glass-ionomer restorations: 3D finite element study. J Dent 2007;35:28–35.
189. Kim SY, Lee KW, Seong SR, et al. Two-year clinical effectiveness of adhesives and retention form on resin composite restorations of non-carious cervical lesions. Oper Dent 2009;34:507–515.
190. Perez CR. Alternative technique for class V resin composite restorations with minimum finishing/polishing procedures. Oper Dent 2010;35:375–379.
191. Miller N, Penaud J, Ambrosini P, Bisson-Boutelliez C, Briançon S. Analysis of etiologic factors and periodontal conditions involved with 309 abfractions. J Clin Periodontol 2003;30:828–832.
192. Osborne-Smith KL, Burke FJ, Wilson NH. The aetiology of the non-carious cervical lesion. Int Dent J 1999;49:139–143.
193. Wood I, Jawad Z, Paisley C, Brunton P. Non-carious cervical tooth surface loss: A literature review. J Dent 2008;36:759–766.
194. Litonjua LA, Andreana S, Cohen RE. Toothbrush abrasions and noncarious cervical lesions: Evolving concepts. Compend Contin Educ Dent 2005;26:767–768,770–774,776.
195. Bassiouny MA. Effects of common beverages on the development of cervical erosion lesions. Gen Dent 2009;57:212–223.
196. Grippo JO, Simring M, Coleman TA. Abfraction, abrasion, biocorrosion, and the enigma of noncarious cervical lesions: A 20-year perspective. J Esthet Restor Dent 2012;24:10–23.
197. Grippo JO. Abfractions: A new classification of hard tissue lesions of teeth. J Esthet Dent 1991;3:14–19.
198. Grippo JO, Chaiyabutr Y, Kois JC. Effects of cyclic fatigue stress-biocorrosion on noncarious cervical lesions. J Esthet Restor Dent 2013;25:265–272.
199. Levitch LC, Bader JD, Shugars DA, Heymann HO. Non-carious cervical lesions. J Dent 1994;22:195–207.
200. Lussi AR, Schaffner M, Hotz P, Suter P. Epidemiology and risk factors of wedge-shaped defects in a Swiss population. Schweiz Monatsschr Zahnmed 1993;103:276–280.
201. Al-Dlaigan YH, Shaw L, Smith A. Dental erosion in a group of British 14-year-old, school children. Part I: Prevalence and influence of differing socioeconomic backgrounds. Br Dent J 2001;190:145–149.
202. Smith WA, Marchan S, Rafeek RN. The prevalence and severity of non-carious cervical lesions in a group of patients attending a university hospital in Trinidad. J Oral Rehabil 2008;35:128–134.
203. Borcic J, Anic I, Urek MM, Ferreri S. The prevalence of non-carious cervical lesions in permanent dentition. J Oral Rehabil 2004;31:117–123.
204. Estafan A, Bartlett D, Goldstein G. A survey of management strategies for noncarious cervical lesions. Int J Prosthodont 2014;27:87–90.
205. Grippo JO. Noncarious cervical lesions: The decision to ignore or restore. J Esthet Dent 1992;4(suppl):55–64.
206. Tackas VJ. Root coverage techniques: A review. J West Soc Periodontol Periodontal Abstr 1995;43:5–14.
207. Weeks DB. Surgical coverage of exposed root surfaces: A review of available techniques and applications. Compend Contin Educ Dent 1993;14:1098,1100.
208. Zucchelli G, De Sanctis M. Treatment of multiple recession-type defects in patients with esthetic demands. J Periodontol 2000;71:1506–1514.
209. Zucchelli G, De Sanctis M. The coronally advanced flap for the treatment of multiple recession defects: A modified surgical approach for the upper anterior teeth. J Int Acad Periodontol 2007;9:96–103.
210. Bherwani C, Kulloli A, Kathariya R, et al. Zucchelli's technique or tunnel technique with subepithelial connective tissue graft for treatment of multiple gingival recessions. J Int Acad Periodontol 2014;16:34–42.
211. Haller B, Klaiber B, Secknus A. Marginal seal of cervical composite inlays in vitro. Dtsch Zahnarztl Z 1990;45:296–299.
212. Folwaczny M, Loher C, Mehl A, Kunzelmann KH, Hinkel R. Tooth-colored filling materials for the restoration of cervical lesions: A 24-month follow-up study. Oper Dent 2000;25:251–258.
213. Smales RJ, Ng KK. Longevity of a resin-modified glass ionomer cement and a polyacid-modified resin composite restoring non-carious cervical lesions in a general dental practice. Aust Dent J 2004;49:196–200.
214. Burgess JO, Gallo JR, Ripps AH, Walker RS, Ireland EJ. Clinical evaluation of four Class 5 restorative materials: 3-year recall. Am J Dent 2004;17:147–150.
215. Folwaczny M, Loher C, Mehl A, Kunzelmann KH, Hickel R. Class V lesions restored with four different tooth-colored materials—3-year results. Clin Oral Investig 2001;5:31–39.
216. Sidhu SK. A comparative analysis of techniques of restoring cervical lesions. Quintessence Int 1993;24:553–559.
217. Fahl N Jr. The direct/indirect composite resin veneers: A case report. Pract Periodontics Aesthet Dent 1996;8:627–638.
218. Diestchi D, Spreafico R. Adhesive Metal-Free Restorations: Current Concepts for the Esthetic Treatment of Posterior Teeth. Chicago: Quintessence, 1997.
219. Ferracane JL, Condon JR. Post-cure heat treatments for composites: Properties and fractography. Dent Mater 1992;8:290–295.
220. Wassell RW, McCabe JF, Walls AW. Wear rates of regular and tempered composites. J Dent 1997;25:49–52.
221. Ferracane JL, Mitchem JC, Condon JR, Todd R. Wear and marginal breakdown of composites with various degrees of cure. J Dent Res 1997;76:1508–1516.
222. Alomari QD, Barrieshi-Nusair K, Ali M. Effect of C-factor and LED curing mode on microleakage of Class V resin composite restorations. Eur J Dent 2011;5:400–408.
223. Borges AL, Borges AB, Xavier TA, Bottino MC, Platt JA. Impact of quantity of resin, C-factor, and geometry on resin composite polymerization shrinkage stress in Class V restorations. Oper Dent 2014;39:144–151.
224. Linden JJ, Swift EJ Jr. Microleakage of two new dentin adhesives. Am J Dent 1994;7:31–34.
225. Aranha AC, Pimento LA. Effect of two different restorative techniques using resin based composites on microleakage. Am J Dent 2004;17:99–103.
226. Owens BM, Johnson WW. Effect of insertion technique and adhesive system on microleakage of Class V resin composite restorations. J Adhes Dent 2005;7:303–308.

227. Winkler MM, Katona TR, Paydar NH. Finite element stress analysis of three filling techniques for class V light-cured composite restorations. J Dent Res 1996;75:1477–1483.
228. Sensi LG, Marson FC, Baratieri LN, Monteiro Junior S. Effect of placement techniques on the marginal adaptation of Class V composite restorations. J Contemp Dent Pract 2005;6(4):17–25.
229. da Silva MA, de Oliveira GJ, Tonholo J, Júnior JG, Santos Lde M, Dos Reis JI. Effect of the insertion and polymerization technique in composite resin restorations: Analysis of marginal gap by atomic force microscopy. Microsc Microanal 2010;16:779–784.
230. Freeman R, Klaiber B, Secknus A. Effect of air abrasion and thermocycling on resin adaptation and shear bond strength to dentin for an etch-and-rinse and self-etch resin adhesive. Dent Mater J 2012;31:180–188.
231. Paolantonio M, D'ercole S, Perinetti G, et al. Clinical and microbiological effects of different restorative materials on the periodontal tissues adjacent to subgingival class V restorations. J Clin Periodontol 2004;31:200–207.
232. Quirynen M, Bollen CM. The influence of surface roughness and surface-free energy on supra- and subgingival plaque formation in man. A review of the literature. J Clin Periodontol 1995;22:1–14.
233. Carlén A, Nikdel K, Wennerberg A, et al. Surface characteristics and in vitro biofilm formation on glass ionomer and composite resin. Biomaterials 2001;22:481–487.
234. Flausino JS, Soares PBF, Carvalho VF, et al. Biofilm formation on different materials for tooth restoration: Analysis of surface characteristics. J Mater Sci 2014;49:6820–6829.
235. Soares CJ, Soares PV, De Freitas Santos-Filho PC, Castro CG, Magalhaes D, Versluis A. The influence of cavity design and glass fiber posts on biomechanical behavior of endodontically treated premolars. J Endod 2008;34:1015–1019.

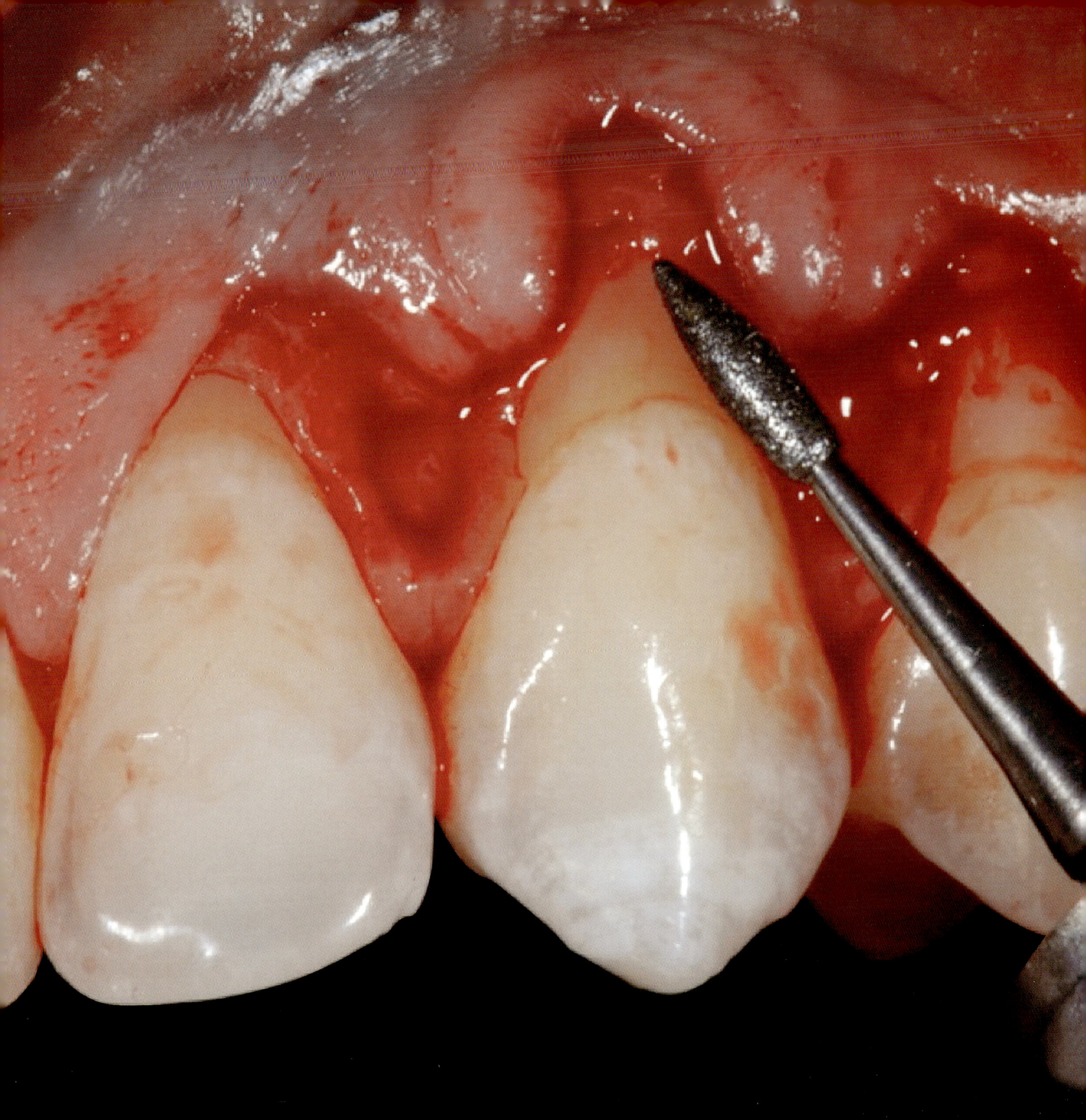

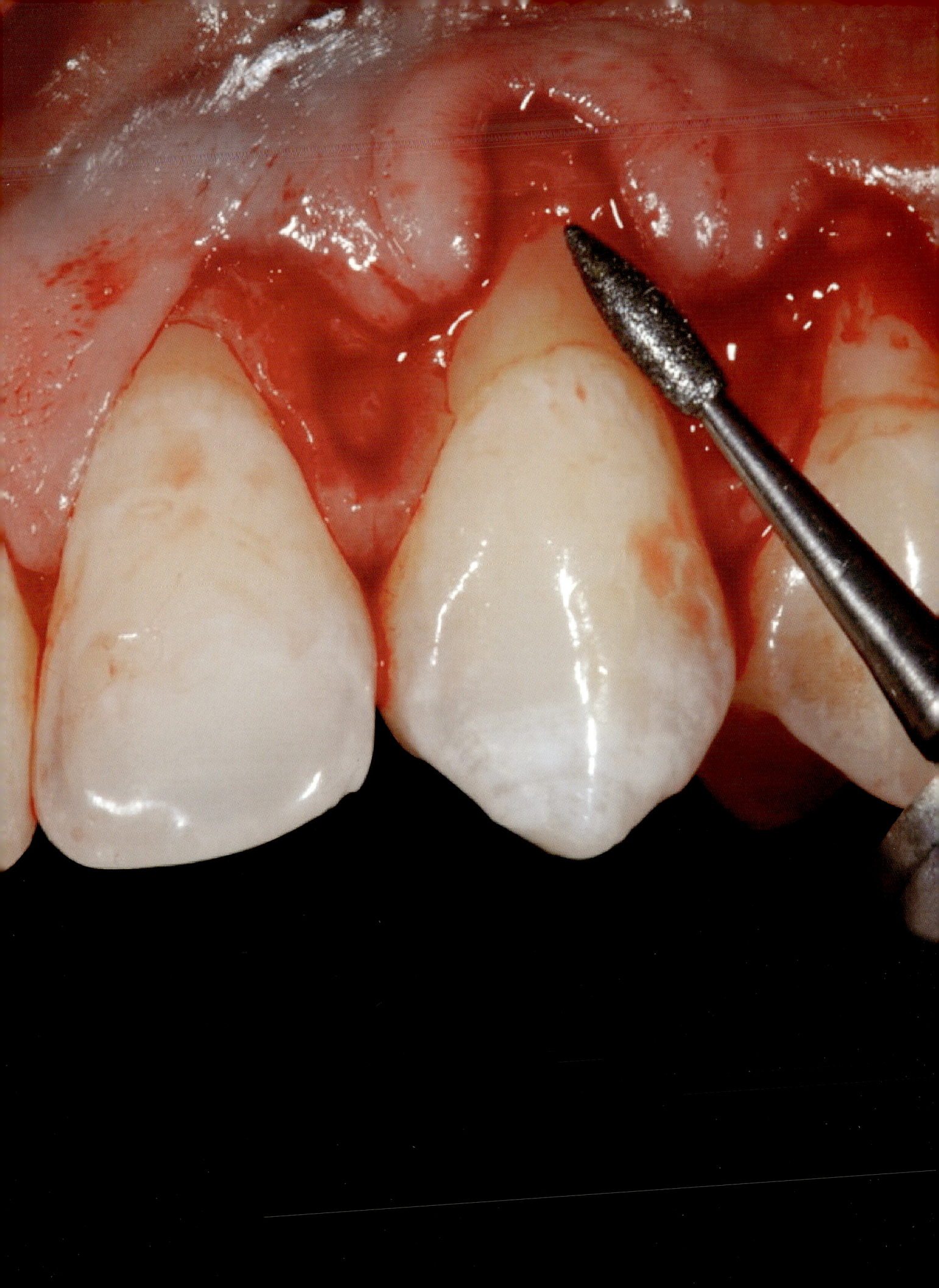

10

Surgical Protocols: Periodontal Therapy and Root Coverage

In addition to creating esthetic and functional problems, gingival recessions may render teeth more susceptible to root caries, abrasion, and/or biocorrosion and may also cause cervical dentin hypersensitivity (CDH).[1-3] Several root coverage procedures have therefore been developed to surgically treat these recession defects.[1,4-7] This chapter describes the different approaches and illustrates how they can be used to manage patients with noncarious cervical lesions (NCCLs) and/or CDH. When NCCLs are found with gingival recessions involving the cementoenamel junction (CEJ), the authors advocate combined restorative-surgical therapy in which the cervical area is first restored using composites before root coverage surgery is performed with connective tissue grafting.[8,9]

Recession Defects and Root Coverage

The Miller classification is a useful recession defect classification based on the height of the interproximal bone adjacent to the defect region and the relationship of the gingival margin to the mucogingival junction (MGJ).[10] The Miller classification has four categories:

- *Class I:* Marginal tissue recession not extending to the MGJ and no loss of interdental bone or soft tissue
- *Class II:* Recession extending to or beyond the MGJ and no loss of interdental bone or soft tissue
- *Class III:* Recession extending to or beyond the MGJ with loss of interdental bone or soft tissue apical to the CEJ but coronal to the most apical level of the recession defect
- *Class IV:* Recession extending to or beyond the MGJ with loss of interdental bone or soft tissue apical to the CEJ and reaching the most apical level of the recession defect.

According to this classification, up to 100% root coverage can be anticipated in Class I and Class II defects, while less than 100% coverage is expected in Class III defects (but to the height of the adjacent interproximal bone peaks), and no root coverage can be anticipated in Class IV defects. However, the presence of NCCLs can make identification of the CEJ more difficult and can limit expectations for root coverage.[11]

Several surgical techniques have been used in the treatment of single and multiple recession defects. These approaches use different flap designs with or without a connective tissue graft (CTG) or substitute (such as resorbable collagen matrix or processed human skin) and with or without biologic modifiers (such as enamel matrix derivative [EMD] or platelet-rich plasma).[1,4,5,12–14] Regardless of the surgical approach, successful root coverage is defined as complete coverage with probing depths no deeper than 3 mm, no detected inflammation, and a tissue color and volume matching that of adjacent nontreated regions.[15]

Among the various surgical approaches used to treat recession defects, the subepithelial connective tissue graft (SCTG) in combination with flap advancement has demonstrated excellent predictability and is considered the gold standard for treating gingival recession.[1,4,5,12,13] It is presumed that success with this technique is due to full coverage of the graft by overlying tissue.[16–18] Therefore, several technical variants have been proposed to cover the graft.[16,19] Among these, the coronally positioned flap and the laterally positioned flaps are the most widely used.[1,4,5,12,13] The SCTG is particularly well indicated in defects associated with very thin/delicate gingival margins, a lack of keratinized tissue (Class II defects), NCCLs, and defects associated with prosthetic crowns.[6,7] The authors propose that the addition of a CTG apical to the flap can have a positive impact not only on esthetic contour appearance but also on long-term margin stability.[20] Da Silva et al[21] have shown that the SCTG associated with a coronally advanced flap (CAF) improves the percentage of root coverage compared with the CAF alone but is much more effective in improving gingival dimensions. Furthermore, the SCTG can be used in different clinical scenarios with different flap designs.[22] Several authors support the concept that the SCTG renders long-term stability and a higher percentage of complete root coverage while improving gingival dimensions.[1,4,5,12,20]

The morbidity associated with CTG harvesting is frequently indicated as the greatest drawback of the procedure.[1,5] Use of an autogenous graft, processed human cadaver skin (acellular dermal matrix [ADM]), or a porcine resorbable collagen matrix (PRCM) has been used with varying outcomes.[1,5] Joly et al[23] showed that the clinical performance of the SCTG was better than ADM in the root coverage of isolated gingival recessions. The authors do not recommend ADM as a graft material for the clinical protocol presented in this chapter due to necrosis concerns. Conversely, PRCM has been associated with good clinical outcomes similar to those observed with the SCTG.[5,24–26] Furthermore, other studies have shown combined therapies (eg, CAF with collagen) to be superior in terms of enhanced root coverage and/or gingival dimensions.[25,27] The conclusions reported by Schlee et al[28] indicate that the resorbable collagen matrix can be considered as a viable alternative to the SCTG in specific situations when the SCTG is not the primary choice for grafting material.

EMD is a healing biologic modifier originally introduced as a protein extract capable of regenerating root cementum and consequently promoting the formation of a new periodontal ligament and alveolar bone.[29–32] It has been successfully used to produce a higher mean root coverage and percentage of sites with complete coverage.[5] Moreover, recent evidence has demonstrated that this approach yields improved long-term root coverage results.[5,33,34] In addition, EMD has been shown to have a positive effect on postoperative symptoms and soft tissue healing with reduced pain or swelling and more rapid healing.[35–38] EMD can therefore be considered a viable substitute to an SCTG. However, it is important to note that EMD results in regeneration while SCTG results in repair. Therefore, EMD is indicated to improve the healing pattern and postoperative symptoms, while an SCTG is used to enhance the tissue biotype. It is the authors' opinion that both approaches (EMD + SCTG) may in fact work synergistically and should be considered in some, if not all, clinical conditions.

Treatment Approaches

This section presents specific techniques for root coverage based on the type and severity of the defect (ie, single versus multiple, 4 mm versus 7 mm). The severity of the recession defect dictates the treatment approach (Table 10-1).

Single shallow defect: Modified envelope with SCTG

The modified envelope combined with the SCTG is used to treat the single shallow defect. Whereas the original envelope technique used a split-thickness flap elevation,[16] the modified approach uses a mucoperiosteal flap parallel to the level of the mucogingival line. An intrasulcular incision is made using a 15c blade, and blunt tunneling instruments

Treatment Approaches

Table 10-1 Randomized controlled trials correlating periodontal procedures with CDH and gingival recession

Authors (year)	Patient population	Treatment	Outcome/results	Follow-up time
Tammaro et al[39] (2000)	35 patients (29–65 yo) with root dentin sensitivity requiring nonsurgical treatment for moderate to severe periodontal disease	SRP with hand and/or ultrasonic instrumentation	Meticulous plaque control diminished root dentin sensitivity, and SRP resulted in an increase in the number of teeth responding to painful stimuli	4 weeks
Taani et al[40] (2002)	295 patients (20–60 yo) evaluated for CDH at general dental clinics (n = 144) and periodontal specialty clinics (n = 151)	Questionnaires were recorded, and intraoral examination measured oral hygiene levels (plaque, tooth wear, and gingival recession)	CDH was higher in periodontal patients than in the general dental population; this indicates that periodontal disease and its treatment may increase the occurrence of CDH	NA
Santos et al[41] (2006)	12 patients (35–75 yo) with CDH after periodontal therapy	Oxagel (group 1) and Gluma Desensitizer (group 2)	Both desensitizers were effective in reducing CDH after periodontal therapy; Gluma was more effective than evaporative and thermal stimuli	60 days
Gusmão et al[42] (2010)	200 patients (18–71 yo) with CDH before and after basic periodontal treatment	Mechanical and thermal tests for CDH before and 30 days after basic periodontal instrumentation	CDH increased and persisted 30 days after supragingival and subgingival instrumentation	30 days
Yilmaz et al[43] (2011)	48 patients with 244 teeth affected by CDH	Treatment with GaAlAs laser, placebo laser, NaF varnish, and placebo NaF varnish	GaAlAs laser irradiation was effective in the treatment of CDH and was a more comfortable and faster procedure than traditional CDH treatment	6 months
Fernandes-Dias et al[44] (2015)	40 patients presenting with Miller Class I and Class II gingival recessions	CTG with or without diode laser therapy (660 nm) applied immediately after surgery and every day for 7 days (eight applications)	Low-level therapy may increase the percentage of complete root coverage when associated with a CTG	7 days

yo, years old; SRP, scaling and root planing; NA, not available; GaAlAs, gallium aluminum arsenide; NaF, sodium fluoride.

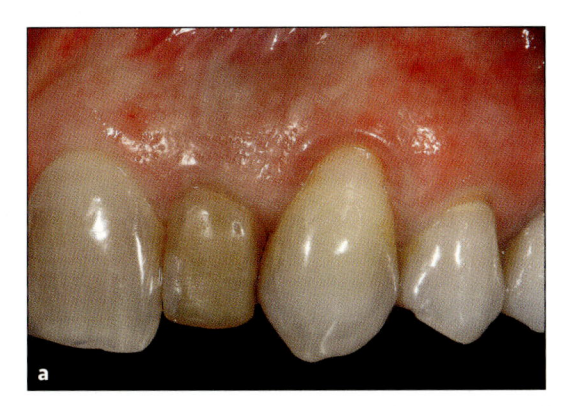

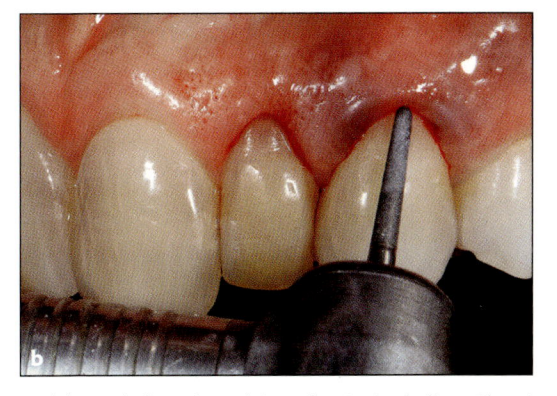

Fig 10-1 Root coverage using the modified envelope technique. *(a)* Initial clinical condition of a single shallow Class I defect on the maxillary left canine. *(b)* Old compromised composite at the cervical region is removed. →

are used to create the mucoperiosteal flap followed by apical sharp dissection using a new 15c blade.[6,7]

Papillae are not elevated in this technique. After a pouch is created, the SCTG is obtained, positioned, and stabilized with proximal isolated sutures, generally 6.0-monofilament suture material. The dimensions of the graft should be sized in accordance to the recipient site but generally approximate 5 to 6 mm in height and 1 mm in thickness. When indicated, one sling suture is used to reduce the amount of graft exposure and better stabilize the flap/graft. Some minor graft exposure is accepted and should not be a problem for its incorporation as long as it is very stable and most of it is well covered and protected by the flap[45] (Fig 10-1).

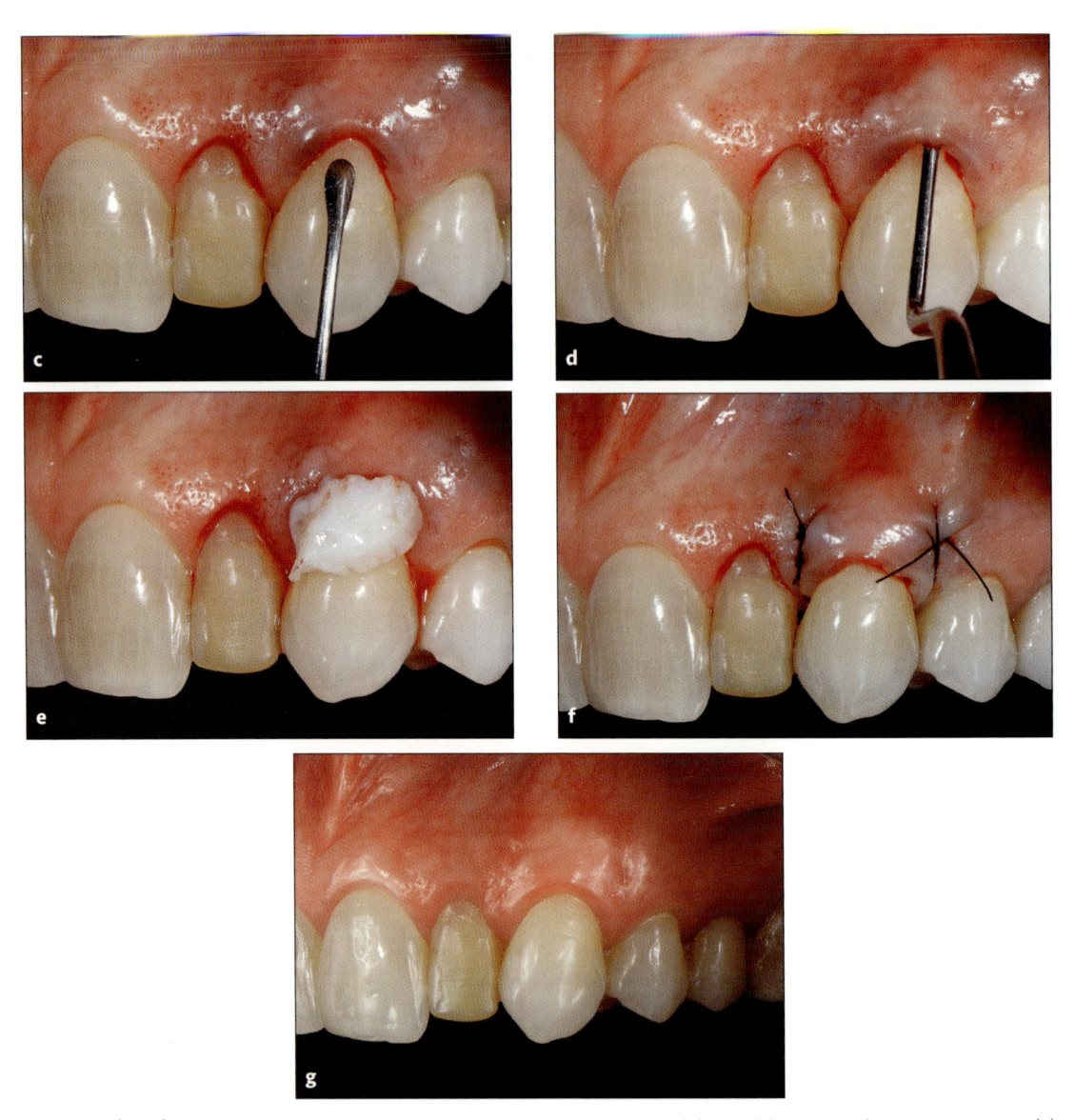

Fig 10-1 *(cont)* *(c and d)* Mucoperiosteal envelope preparation using delicate blunt tunneling instruments. *(e)* Evaluation of the SCTG dimensions. *(f)* Modified sling suture stabilizing the graft and flap in the coronal direction. Note that the graft is completely covered. *(g)* Complete root coverage at 6-month postoperative view. Observe the perfect color matching and improvement in the tissue dimensions (ie, thickness and width of keratinized tissue). (Clinical case courtesy of Robert Carvalho, Júlio César Joly, and Paulo Fernando, São Paulo, Brazil.)

Single moderate defect: Modified CAF or L-shaped CAF

In this clinical condition, two approaches are frequently used: the modified CAF or the L-shaped CAF. The modified CAF is an adaptation of the incision design suggested for the treatment of multiple adjacent defects,[46] which is described later in the chapter. With this approach, oblique paramarginal incisions are made from the CEJ of the affected tooth toward the gingival margin of the adjacent nonaffected tooth. This unique incision design creates surgical papillae (apical to the incisions) and anatomical papillae (coronal to the incisions). A mucoperiosteal flap is then reflected to the level of the mucogingival line followed by sharp dissection to release the tension of the flap during placement and suturing. The anatomical papillae are de-epithelialized with micro-

Treatment Approaches

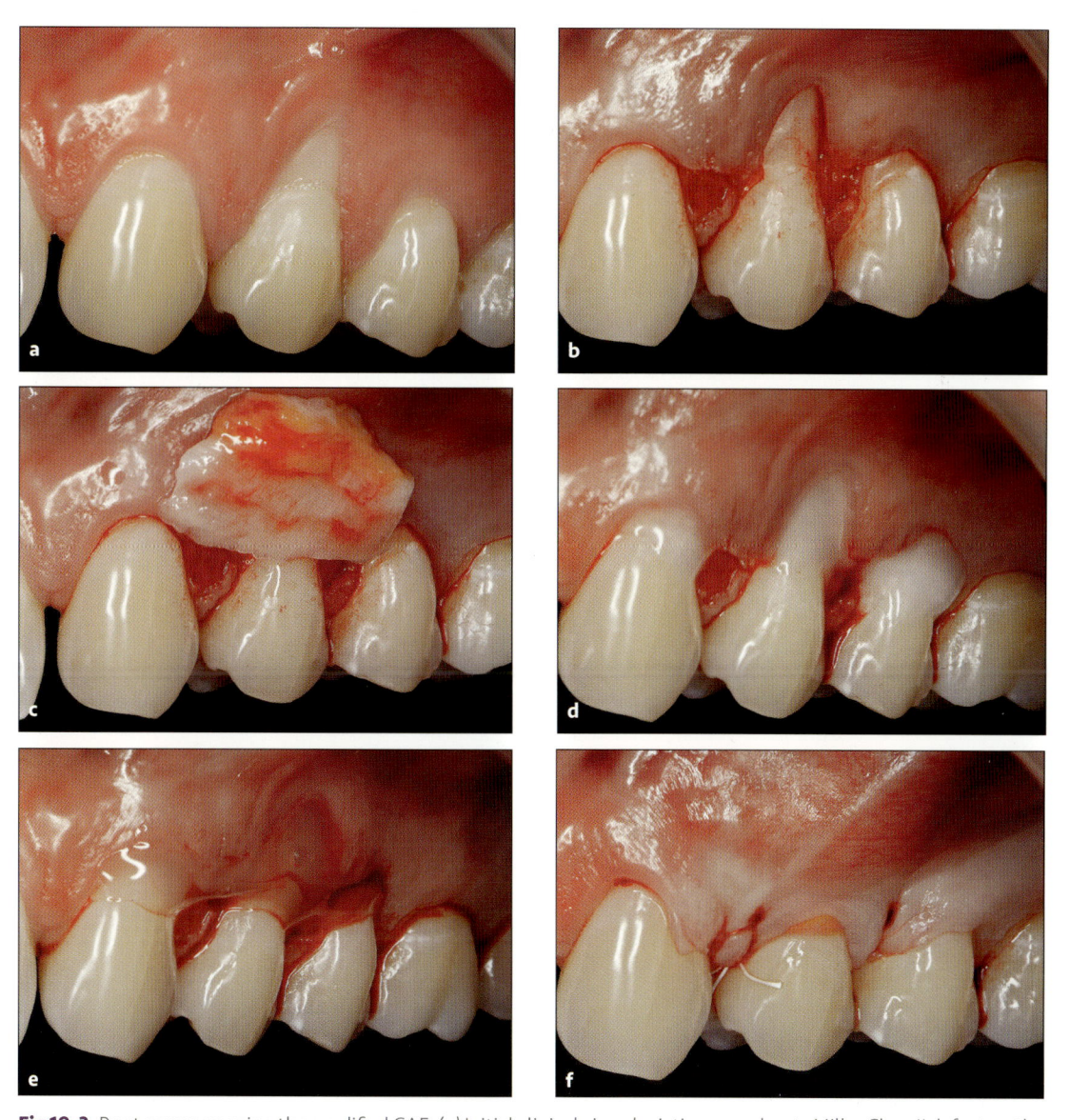

Fig 10-2 Root coverage using the modified CAF. *(a)* Initial clinical view depicting a moderate Miller Class II defect on the maxillary left first premolar. *(b)* Oblique paramarginal incisions starting close to the CEJ toward the adjacent gingival margins are continued with intrasulcular incisions, followed by mucoperiosteal flap elevation, apical sharp dissection, and papillae de-epithelialization. *(c)* SCTG in position to check its dimensions. *(d)* Chemical root decontamination using 24% ethylenediaminetetraacetic acid (EDTA) for 2 minutes. *(e)* After thorough irrigation with saline solution, EMD was applied below the flap and on the root surface. *(f)* Sling suture coronally advancing the flap and stabilizing the graft.

scissors to create a connective tissue bed for advancement of the flap (Fig 10-2).

The L-shaped CAF is based on the usage of one vertical releasing incision, generally distal to the affected tooth for esthetic reasons.[6,7] This technique is distinguished from the traditional CAF in which two vertical releasing incisions adjacent to the defect are provided.[17] Vertical incisions may jeopardize the lateral blood supply and create scarlike healing that is detrimental to the esthetics.[46–48] At the mesial aspect, if possible, the papilla is left untouched or a small paramarginal incision is rendered to aid flap placement. The L-shaped incision starts in the proximity of the distal CEJ toward the mucogingival line with a slightly curved design. This incision design creates a surgical papilla that mimics the shape of an anatomical papilla to favor interproximal flap adaptation. A mucoperiosteal flap is reflected, followed by apical

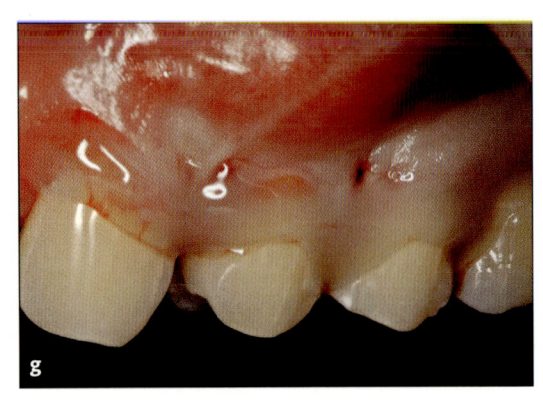

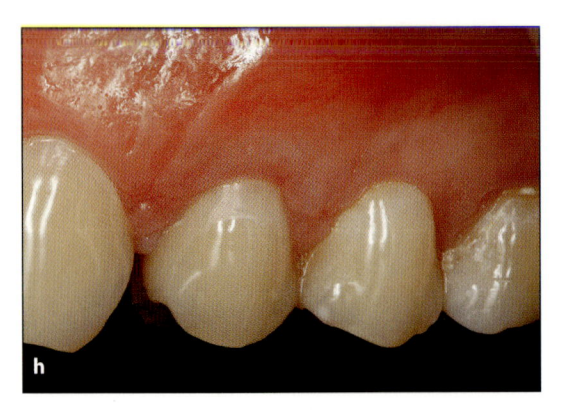

10 Surgical Protocols: Periodontal Therapy and Root Coverage

Fig 10-2 *(cont)* *(g)* EMD externally applied to improve healing. *(h)* Clinical view 6 months after surgery showing complete root coverage and soft tissue enhancement. (Clinical case courtesy of Robert Carvalho, Júlio César Joly, and Paulo Fernando, São Paulo, Brazil.)

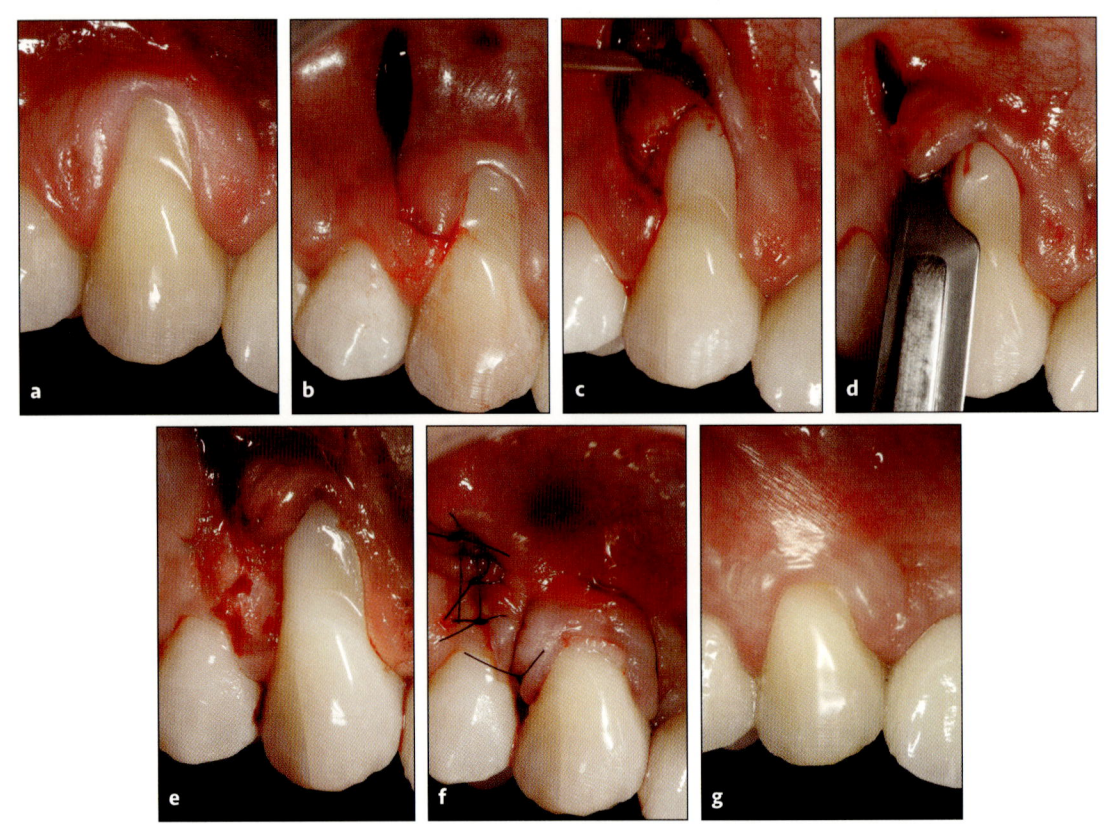

Fig 10-3 Root coverage using the L-shaped CAF. *(a)* Initial clinical view depicting a moderate Class I gingival defect on the maxillary right canine. *(b)* L-shaped incision at the distal aspect. After mucoperiosteal flap elevation *(c)* and apical sharp dissection *(d)*, the distal papilla was de-epithelialized *(e)*. *(f)* Advanced flap over the SCTG stabilized with sling and interrupted sutures. *(g)* Final view 9 months after surgery showing complete root coverage and improved soft tissue. (Clinical case courtesy of Robert Carvalho, Júlio César Joly, and Paulo Fernando, São Paulo, Brazil.)

sharp dissection. The papilla associated with the vertical incision is de-epithelialized to create a connective tissue bed for the advancement of the flap tissue. Depending on operator preference, an SCTG or a substitute could be placed. Sling sutures are used to stabilize the CAF without tension at least 1 mm coronal to the anticipated level of root coverage. Single interrupted sutures are also placed at the vertical incision in the L-shaped surgical line (Fig 10-3).

The choice of technique for moderate defects is subjective and depends on operator preference, but there is a trend to use the modified CAF when there is a smaller band of keratinized tissue and the L-shaped CAF when a wider band of keratinized tissue is present.

Treatment Approaches

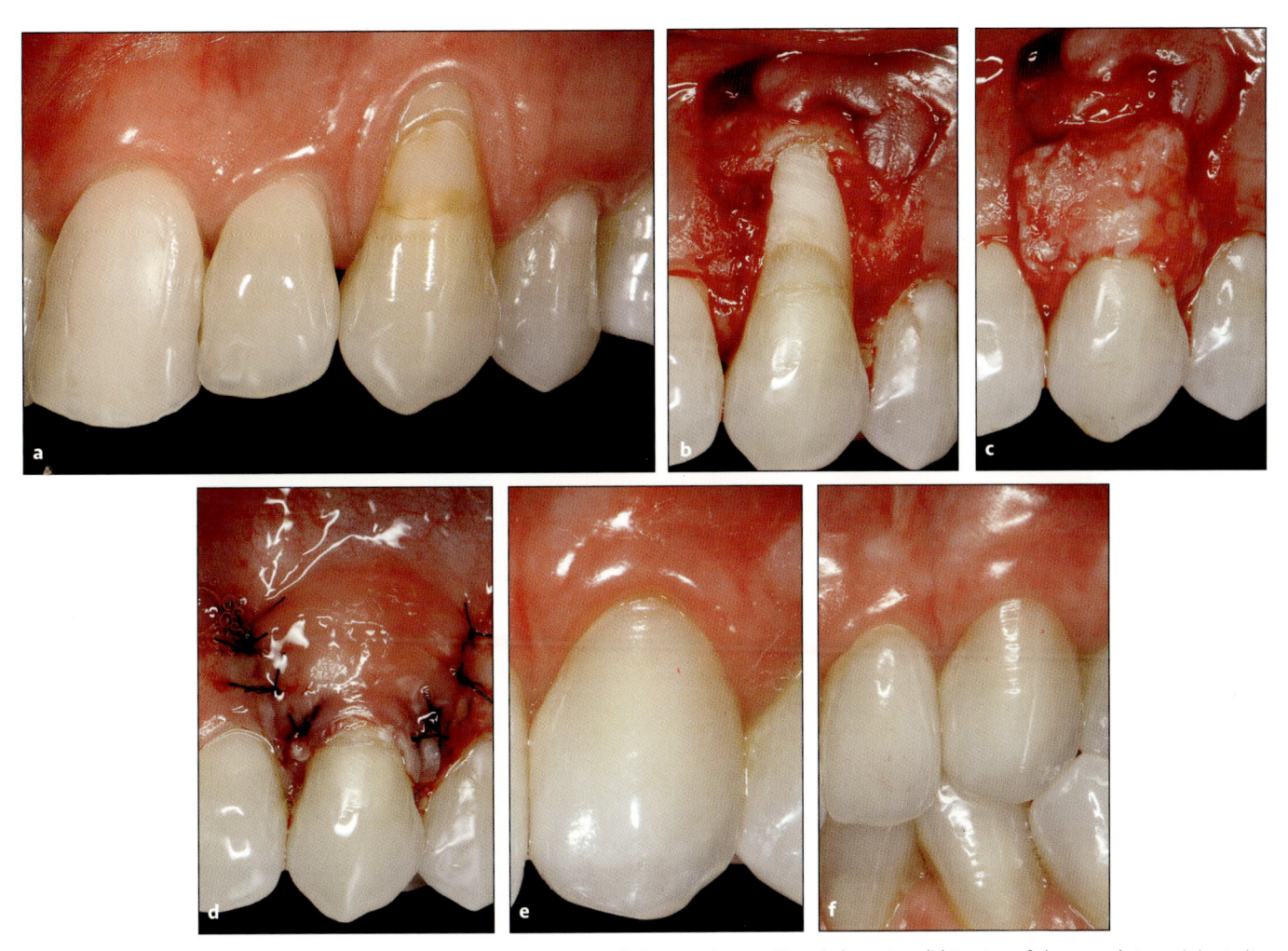

Fig 10-4 Root coverage using the traditional CAF. *(a)* A deep Class I defect on the maxillary left canine. *(b)* Design of the complete recipient site preparation, including the two vertical incisions, mucoperiosteal flap elevation and sharp dissection, papillae de-epithelialization, and removal of the old cervical restoration. *(c)* SCTG in position. *(d)* Stabilization of the advanced flap using sling and interrupted sutures. *(e)* Complete root coverage with esthetic prosthetic optimization after 6 months. *(f)* Note the stability of the outcome after 2 years. (Clinical case courtesy of Robert Carvalho, Júlio César Joly, and Paulo Fernando; prosthetic rehabilitation courtesy of prosthodontist Bruno Godoy and technician Marcos Celestrino, São Paulo, Brazil.)

Single deep defect: Traditional CAF or laterally positioned flap

Deeper defects necessarily rely on vertical incisions to facilitate advancement of the flap over the denuded root. The traditional CAF or the laterally positioned flap (LPF) may be used to address these cases.

The traditional CAF is associated with two vertical releasing incisions, similar to that described for the L-shaped incision design, mesial and distal to the affected tooth.[17,49] Following elevation of the mucoperiosteal flap, apical sharp dissection is performed and the papillae are de-epithelialized. The depth of the vestibular fornix should be carefully evaluated. In order to coronally advance the flap, there must be an acceptable distance from the gingival margin to the deepest portion of the regional vestibular fornix. A short distance may result in only partial root coverage. It is important to recognize and inform the patient that eventual multiple procedures may be required to achieve the desired amount of root coverage when this complicating factor exists (Fig 10-4).

The LPF was widely used in the past[50] but gradually lost favor as more recent approaches were developed. However, in 2004 Zucchelli et al[51] modified this technique with very specific criteria to perform the incision design. One advantage of the LPF design is that the vertical tension on the flap is minimized because flap advancement is lateral. The incision is initiated with a 3-mm-long horizontal incision of the opposite papilla (usually the mesial papilla) from where the lateral flap is rotated (usually from distal). A vertical shallow incision at the end of the horizontal incision is de-

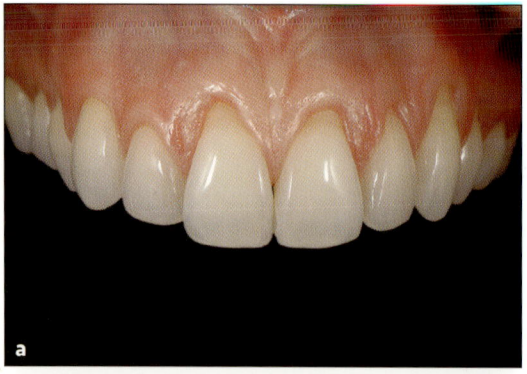

10 Surgical Protocols: Periodontal Therapy and Root Coverage

Fig 10-5 Root coverage of multiple adjacent defects using the envelope-like flap with paramarginal incisions at the base of papillae. *(a)* Initial clinical view of the recessions on the maxillary teeth. Note the NCCLs. *(b and c)* After the NCCLs were restored, oblique incisions were made starting from the maxillary right first premolar and maxillary left canine.

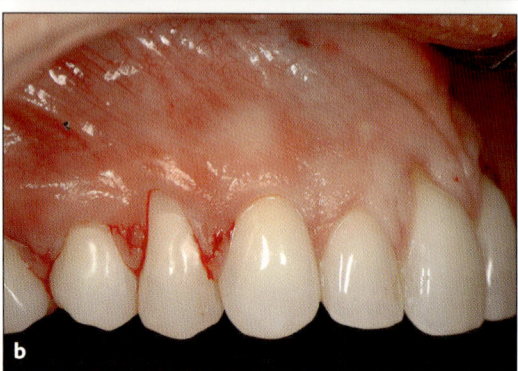

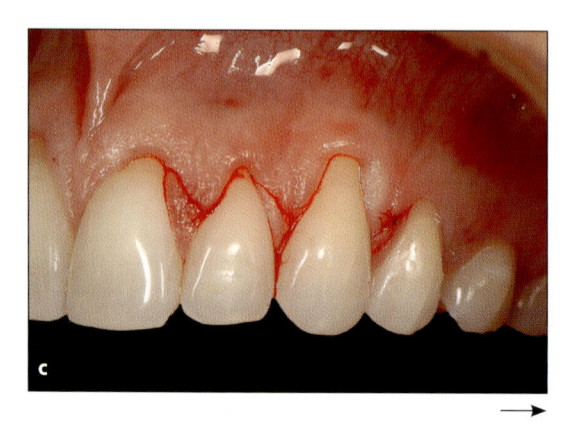

livered toward the apical direction of the gingival margin at the center of the tooth. The epithelium demarcated by both described incisions is removed, creating a connective tissue bed for the latter adaptation of the LPF. A paramarginal incision 6 mm longer than the width of the exposed root is now placed in the region of keratinized tissue that is to be laterally positioned. This incision is positioned at least 1 mm apical to the probing depth of adjacent teeth to prevent recession in the donor site. A vertical releasing incision is then prepared toward and beyond the mucogingival line, as previously described, and a cutback incision at the base of the vertical incision further facilitates the flap rotation. A mucoperiosteal flap is elevated from the gingival margin toward the vertical incision until the last 3 mm of split-thickness soft tissue remains to avoid exposure of bone following the LPF placement. Apical sharp dissection creates a tension-free advancement. To complete the flap design, the papillae are de-epithelialized to further advance the flap in the coronal direction. An SCTG can be used if the anatomy of the defect requires it, and sling sutures are used to stabilize both LPF flap designs without tension at least 1 mm coronal to the expected line of root coverage. Single interrupted sutures are also placed at the vertical incision to reduce tension.

Multiple defects: Envelope flaps with paramarginal incisions

Regardless of the severity of multiple recession defects, envelope-like flaps should be prepared with paramarginal incisions at the base of the papillae.[6,7,46] The first choice is the lateral approach suggested and described by Zucchelli and De Sanctis.[46] The incision design for this approach begins at the central affected tooth (midline). When an even number of defects is present, the incision should be initiated at the center tooth with the deeper defect. Oblique paramarginal incisions are performed starting close to the CEJ toward the most apical level at the deepest point of adjacent gingival margins mesially and distally and at each papilla adjacent to the recessions. The oblique incisions divide each papilla into a surgical papilla (apical) and an anatomical papilla (coronal). The mucoperiosteal flap is elevated to the level of the mucogingival line, followed by sharp dissection to release the tension during flap placement. The flap is coronally advanced until the surgical papillae completely cover the previously de-epithelialized anatomical papillae. Sling sutures are used to coronally advance the flap at least 1 mm more coronal than the expected line of root coverage (Fig 10-5).

A suggested modification to this technique is to perform a V-shaped incision at the base of each papilla connecting the

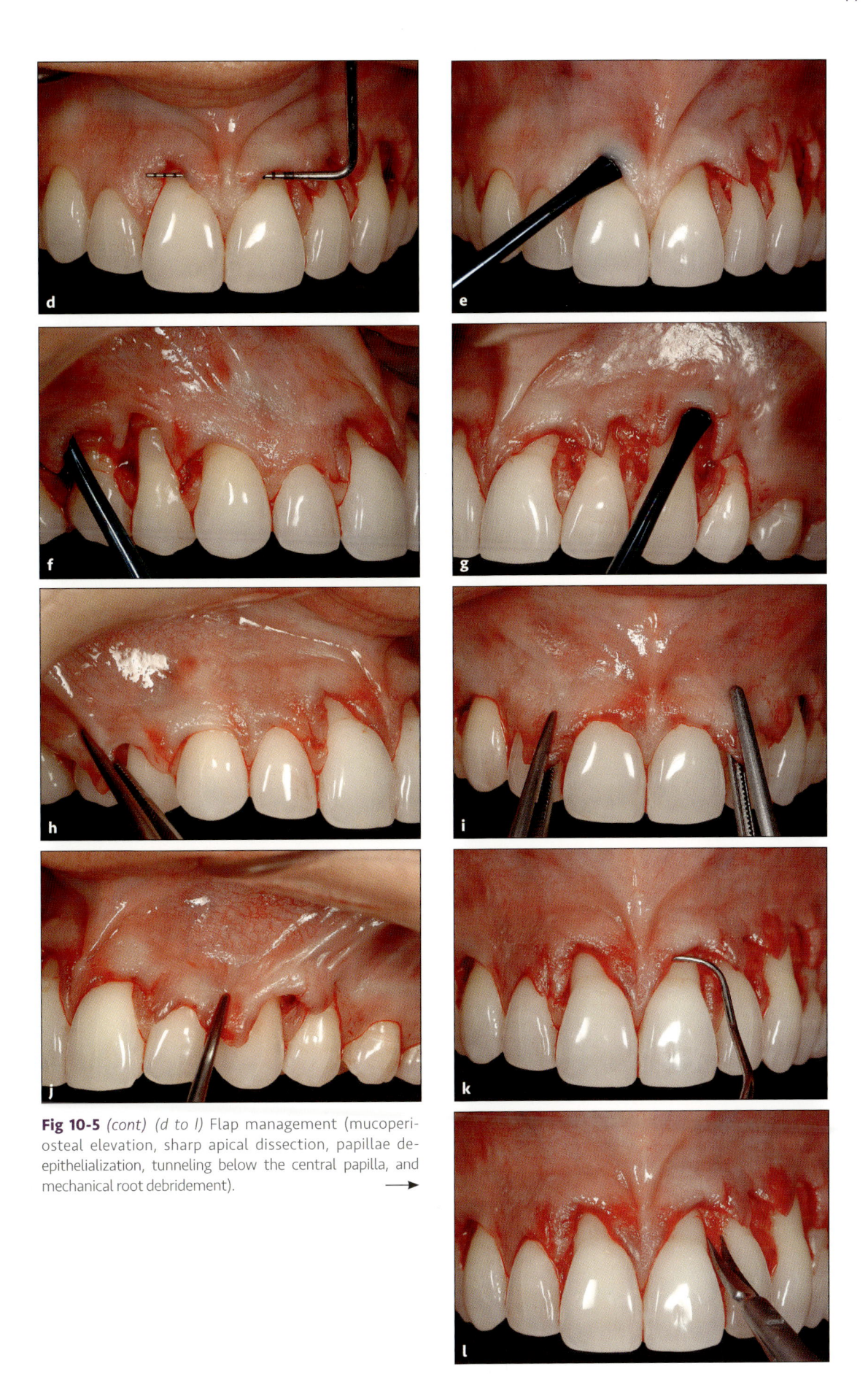

Fig 10-5 *(cont) (d to l)* Flap management (mucoperiosteal elevation, sharp apical dissection, papillae de-epithelialization, tunneling below the central papilla, and mechanical root debridement).

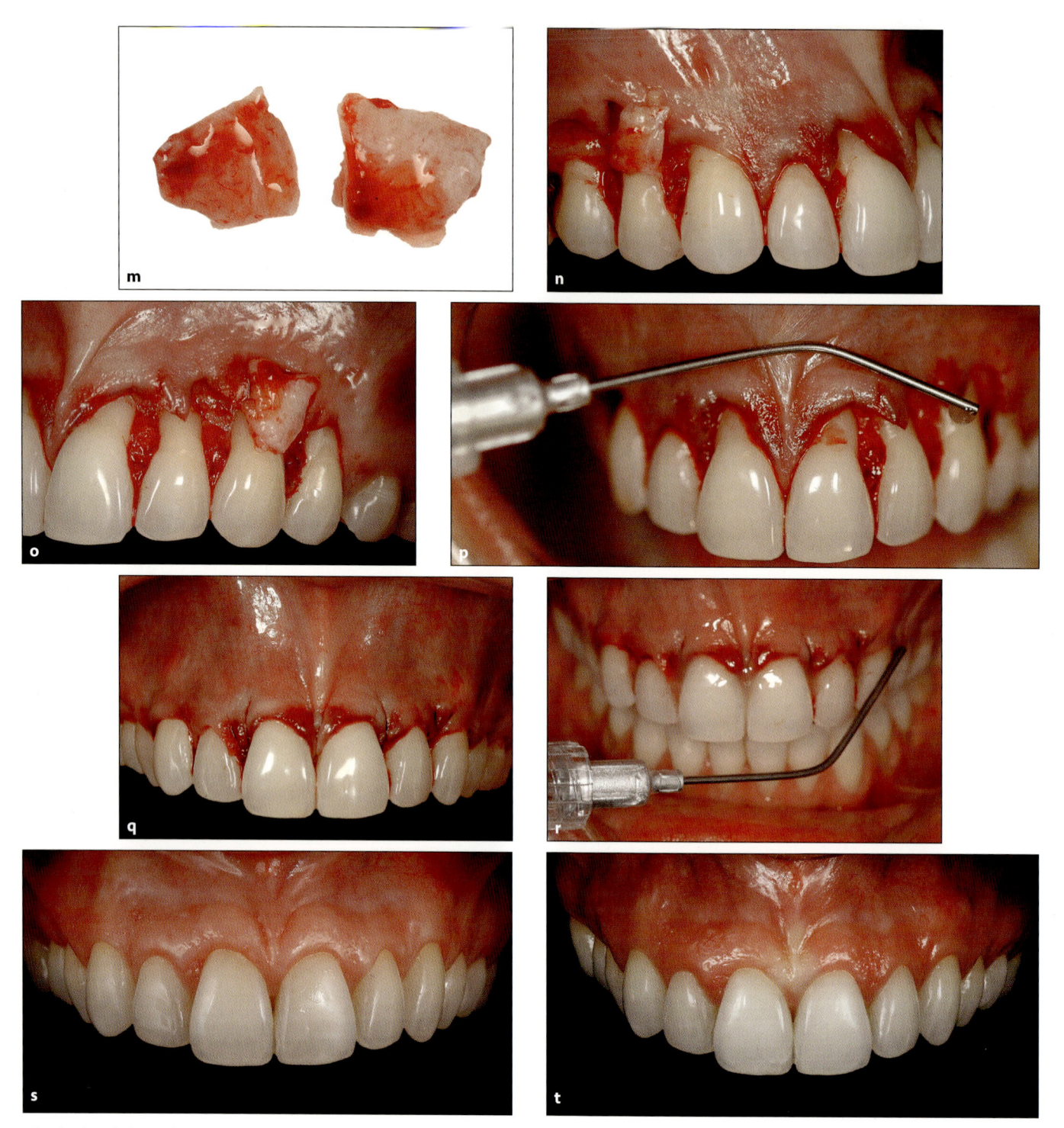

10 Surgical Protocols: Periodontal Therapy and Root Coverage

Fig 10-5 *(cont)* *(m to o)* An SCTG obtained from the palatal area was divided into two grafts that were adapted to the cervical regions of the right first premolar and left canine. *(p)* EMD was delivered on all previously prepared denuded roots. *(q)* Sling sutures stabilized the CAF. *(r)* EMD was applied over the sutures to improve soft tissue healing. *(s)* Postoperative view after 3 months. *(t)* Observe the complete root coverage and stable gingival margins at the 3-year follow-up. (Clinical case courtesy of Robert Carvalho, Júlio César Joly, and Paulo Fernando; restorations courtesy of Simone Magalhães, São Paulo, Brazil.)

CEJs of the adjacent teeth with recession defects. This allows for improved adaptation of the surgical papillae over the previously de-epithelialized anatomical papillae. For both described approaches, when the deepest defect is located at one of the extremities (not in the central area), a vertical releasing incision or an extra paramarginal incision mimicking a gingival recession defect that does not exist should be performed to facilitate the flap advancement and adaptation.

Root decontamination

For all cases of surgical root coverage, mechanical root decontamination using manual curettes or ultrasonic instrumentation is essential to ensure healthy gingival tissue.[52] It is performed immediately after flap elevation, and in the suggested clinical protocol, no chemical agents are used. However, when EMD is used, 24% ethylenediaminetetraacetic acid (EDTA) can be delivered for 2 minutes according to manufacturer instructions. The site should be thoroughly irrigated with saline solution to completely remove any EDTA residue due to its potential to retard coagulum formation.[53] EDTA is a potent chelant that is effective in the removal of the smear layer, but its clinical benefit is questionable.[5,54] Regardless, the authors recommend using this agent as part of EMD clinical application.

Case Reports of Root Coverage Associated with NCCLs or CDH

Restored NCCLs

Following restorative procedures for NCCLs (see Fig 9-44), a CTG with a CAF was used for finishing the reconstruction. After the administration of local anesthesia (2% mepivacaine with epinephrine 1:100,000), an intrasulcular incision was performed at the facial aspect from the maxillary right first molar to lateral incisor. The tissue was then divided to its mucogingival limit, which eliminated muscle tension, facilitated coronal repositioning, and provided mobility to the flap (Fig 10-6a). The buccal portions of the interdental papillae were de-epithelialized to create a connective tissue bed. Root debridement was performed using manual scraping curettes and completed using sterile saline solution irrigation (Fig 10-6b). Root surfaces were also decontaminated with 37% phosphoric acid for 60 seconds (Fig 10-6c), and tetracycline powder mixed with 0.9% saline solution was applied for 3 minutes to finish the root decontamination and its chemical preparation (Fig 10-6d).

The graft tissue was harvested from the palatal region (Fig 10-6e and 10-6f) of the right premolar and placed in position, overlaying the buccal cervical surface of the involved teeth (canine, premolar, and first molar). Sutures were placed to immobilize the graft, pull the buccal flap to the coronal position, and close the donor site (Fig 10-6g). Postoperative management included anti-inflammatory medication (ibuprofen 400 mg three times a day for 3 days) and chlorhexidine 0.12% mouthwash twice a day for 7 days until the sutures were removed and toothbrushing could be fully reestablished. After 18 months, the success of both the restorations and the root coverage procedure could be observed (Fig 10-6h). The ceramic laminate veneers showed neither stains nor marginal failure. The gingival tissue presented healthy characteristics including great volume, color, and texture without inflammation.

The biocompatibility of the ceramic materials combined with the fact that the patient was followed monthly for prophylaxis, plaque control, and oral hygiene instructions may help to explain the good gingival health observed during the follow-up period.

CDH

An otherwise healthy 21-year-old woman presented complaining of poor esthetics and increasing CDH following the formation of multiple areas of gingival recession (Fig 10-7a). The main contributing etiologic factors were thin gingival biotype and traumatic occlusion. Full-mouth radiographs, periodontal charting, study casts, and a careful medical and dental history were obtained. The treatment goals included pain relief, repositioning of the attached gingiva, and stabilization of the free gingival margins.

Before any surgery was performed, it was necessary for the patient to undergo nonsurgical periodontal therapy (scaling and oral hygiene instructions) to ensure that the dentinal tubules were free of plaque and thereby reduce the CDH. Occlusal stabilization and desensitizing treatment began shortly thereafter to enhance patient comfort while the surgical treatment was being planned. The patient's casts showed posterior occlusal interference. Once it was removed with a fine-grit diamond bur, an anterior interference appeared. Lateral excursive imbalances were also checked. Interferences were removed in this manner until occlusal balance in centric occlusion was achieved.

The patient's gingival recessions in the maxillary left quadrant were classified as Miller Class I without any interproximal loss and without reaching the mucogingival junction (Figs 10-7b and 10-7c). For this reason, the chosen surgical technique was the SCTG.

An initial sulcular incision was made with the scalpel parallel to the long axis of the teeth. The dissection was a partial-thickness flap, leaving connective tissue over existing bone and/or root surfaces (Fig 10-7d). Care was taken to extend flaps to the mucogingival junction without perforation, which could result in reduced blood supply. Figure 10-7e illustrates flap mobility, which has to be adequate for total root coverage. The convexities on the denuded roots were flattened with curettes (Fig 10-7f) and diamond burs (Fig 10-7g). Scaling of the root was performed so that no debris remained. The interproximal

10 Surgical Protocols: Periodontal Therapy and Root Coverage

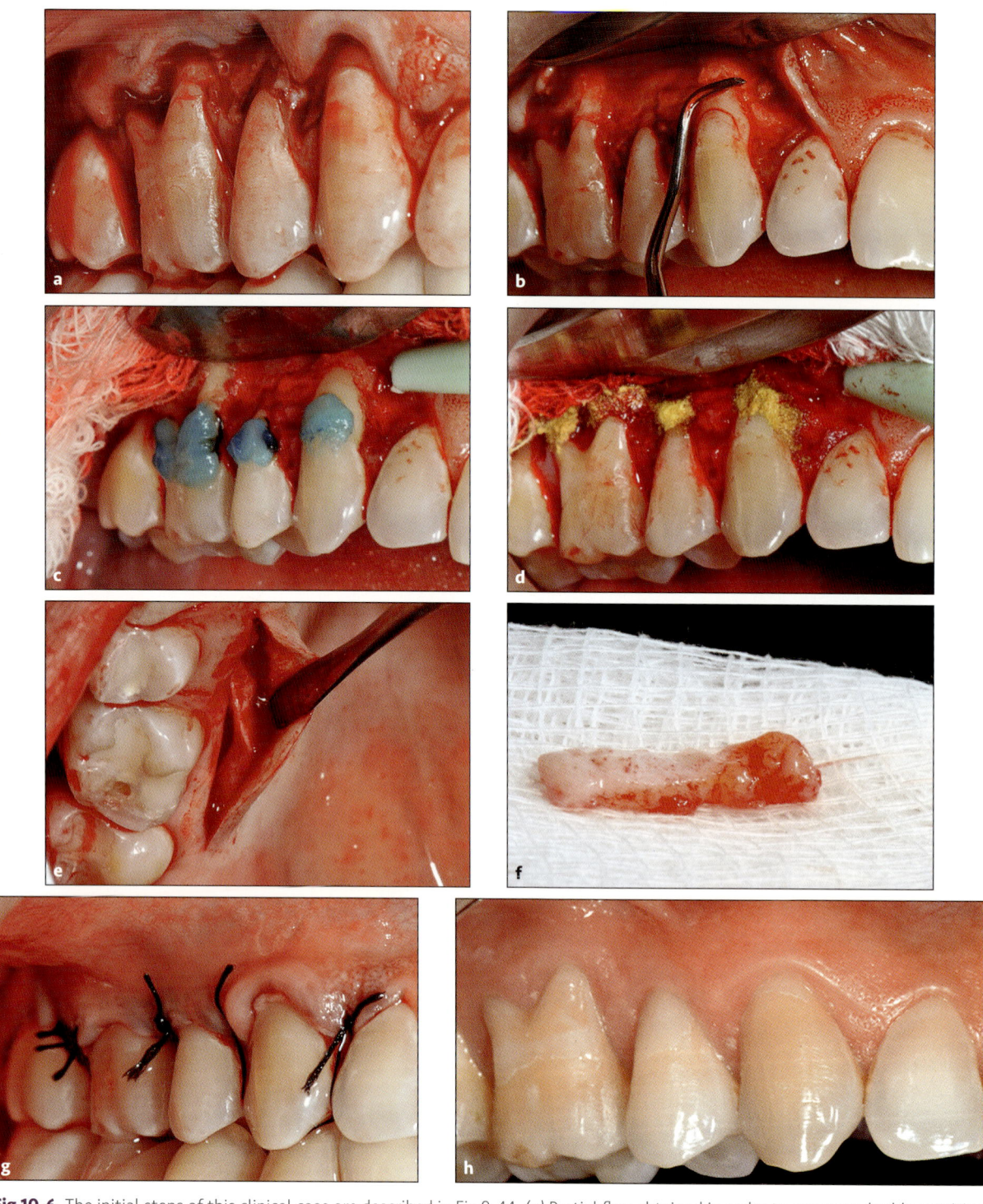

Fig 10-6 The initial steps of this clinical case are described in Fig 9-44. *(a)* Partial flap obtained in order to promote double nutrition for the graft. *(b)* For root debridement, manual scraping curettes were used with sterile saline irrigation. *(c)* Decontamination of the restorations using 37% phosphoric acid. *(d)* Chemical treatment and decontamination of root surfaces using tetracycline mixed with saline solution applied for 3 minutes and then washed with saline solution for another 3 minutes. *(e and f)* CTG harvested from palate. *(g)* Sutures were placed to immobilize the graft and pull the buccal flap to the coronal position. *(h)* The 18-month postoperative view presents healthy attached gingiva and satisfactory restorations. (Courtesy of the NCCL Research Group, Uberlândia, Brazil.)

papillae were left intact so they could be the parameter for future healing (Fig 10-7h). With these procedures concluded, the recipient site was ready to receive the graft.

The palate was chosen as the donor site. The length of the tissue was determined by the combined width of teeth to be covered (left lateral incisor to premolar). A horizontal

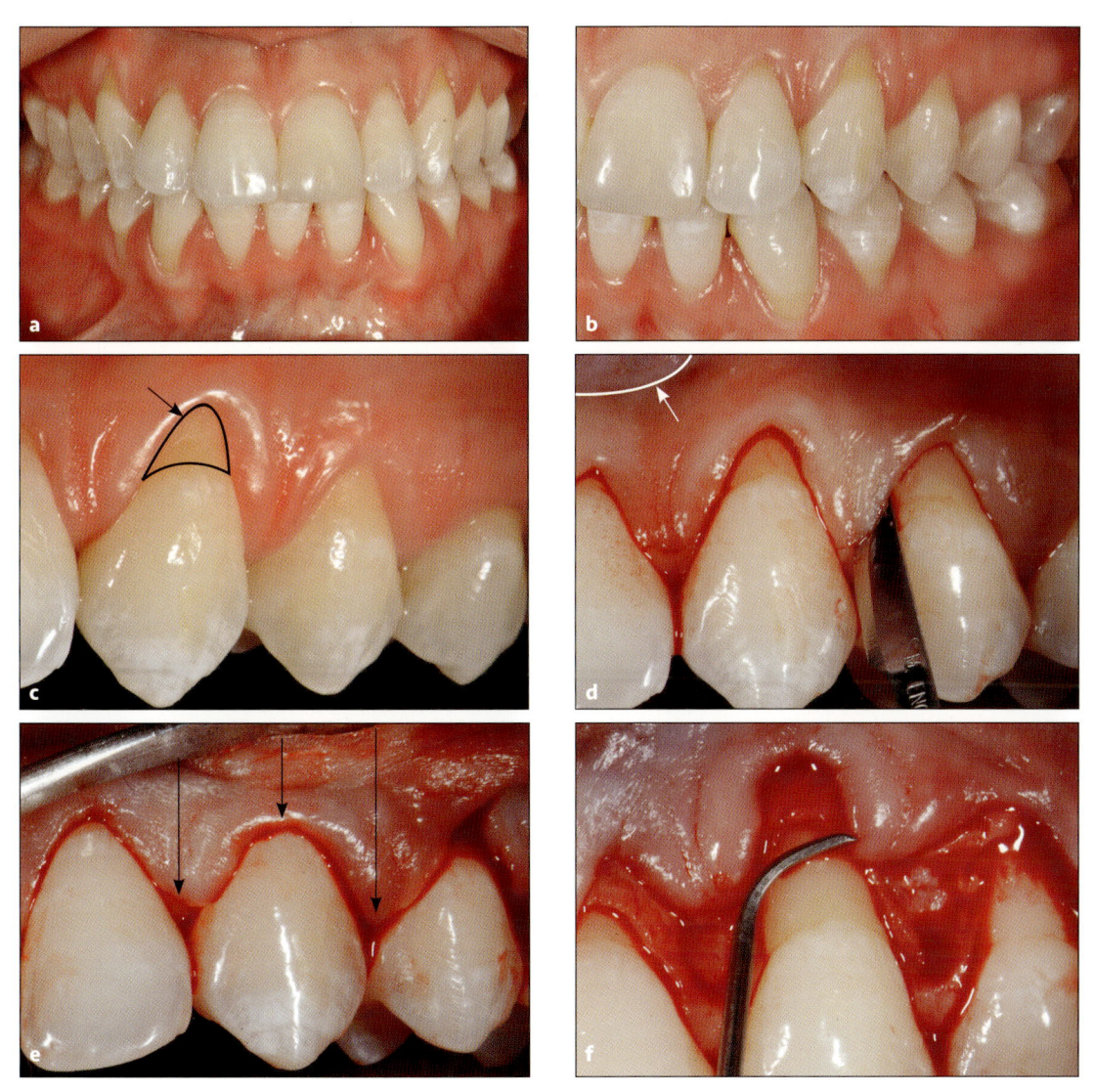

Case Reports of Root Coverage Associated with NCCLs or CDH

Fig 10-7 *(a)* Pretreatment frontal view. *(b)* Pretreatment lateral view. The lack of attached gingiva allows apical migration of the gingival margin. *(c)* Because there is no interproximal attachment loss (bone or gingiva), root coverage is predictable. Note the limited area of loss of attached gingiva on the maxillary left canine. *(d)* Initial incision. The scalpel is positioned parallel to the long axis of the tooth so that a partial flap can be promoted. For recipient placement of the flap, incisions must reach the mucogingival junction *(arrow)*. Care was taken to preserve the periosteum apical to the area of recession. *(e)* Flap mobility. The flap was reflected by a blunt instrument so that there was no danger of damaging the tissue. It was required for proper covering of the donor graft. *(f)* Root treatment with curettes. Before placing the graft, the root was decontaminated from biofilm and calculus. A thorough scaling with a curette positioned parallel to the long axis of the tooth removed existing debris.

incision was made 2 to 3 mm from the palatal free gingival margins and perpendicular to the long axis of the maxillary teeth. The donor flap was adjacent to the teeth involved so that the patient could have a more comfortable postoperative experience involving only one region of the mouth.

From the existing incision, the flap was divided with the scalpel parallel to the long axis of the respective teeth. The connective tissue's thickness was then defined and adapted so that it was favorable for graft positioning at the recipient site. Vertical incisions were made on either side of the horizontal incision, and another incision at the base of the graft was made to facilitate removal of the donor CTG. The graft was then removed (Fig 10-7i).

The graft was placed over the recipient denuded roots/periosteum and sutured in place, ensuring its immobility (Fig 10-7j) to reduce the risk of bleeding or resultant necrosis. The partial-thickness flap was positioned in a manner to cover as much of the recipient site as possible and sutured into position (Fig 10-7k).

Postoperative management included anti-inflammatory medication and 0.12% chlorhexidine mouthwash twice a day until the sutures were removed and toothbrushing could be

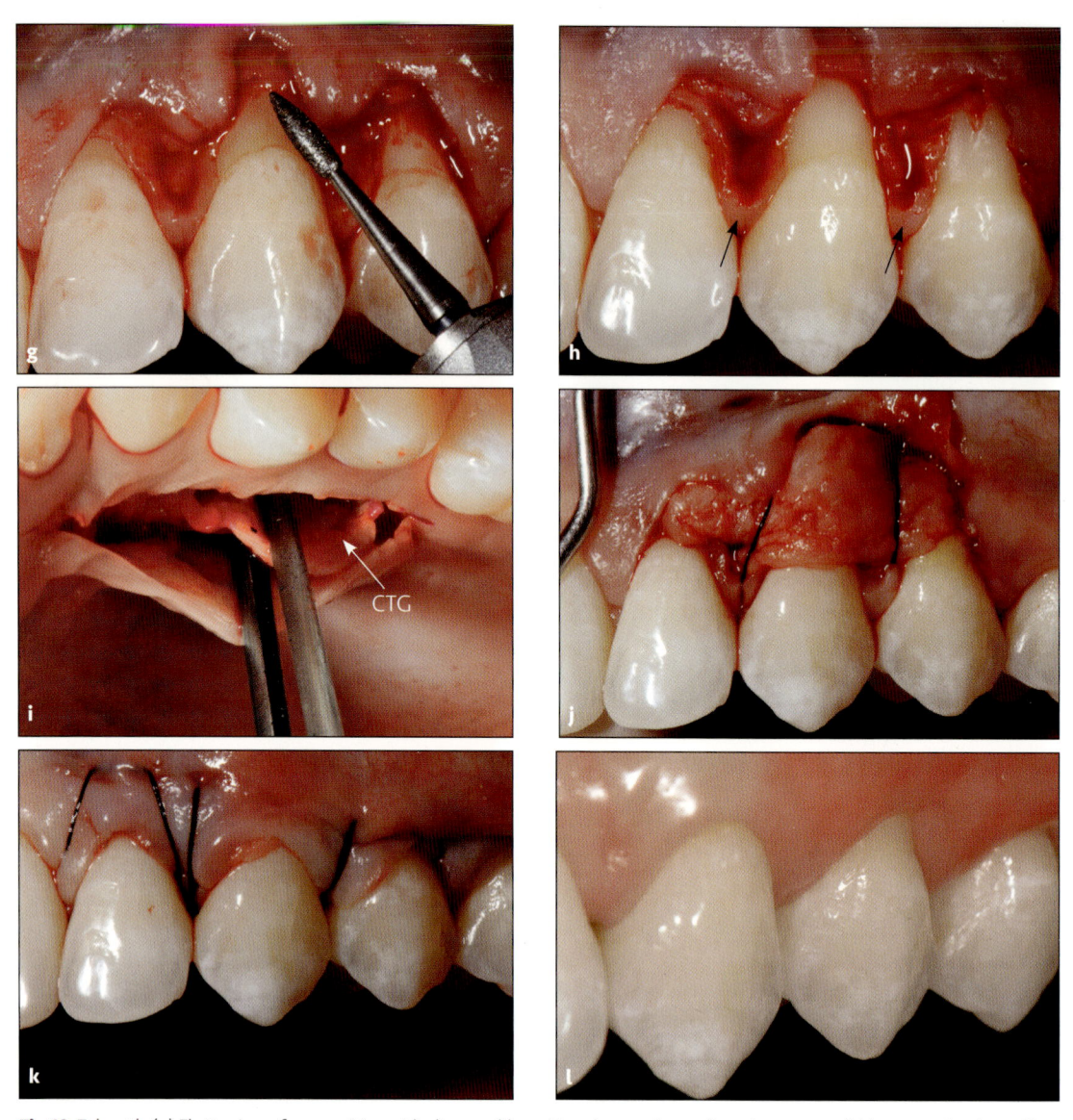

Fig 10-7 *(cont)* *(g)* Flattening of convexities with diamond burs to enhance donor flap placement. *(h)* Interproximal papillae. Preparation of the recipient site root and flap was accomplished. Note that in papillary areas, the incision was made slightly above the margin so that the existing papillae could be the parameter for future healing. *(i)* View of the palate showing the donor site. A horizontal incision was placed 2 to 3 mm apical to the free gingival margin of respective teeth. *(j)* Graft positioned and sutured. For the technique to be successful, the graft must be positioned on the root and also the underlying periosteum so that it will have double vascularization potential. Individualized suturing was provided to avoid necrosis and maximize blood flow. *(k)* Flap suturing. *(l)* Gingival aspect after 6 months. Note the full coverage of the canine.

resumed. The sutures were removed 1 week later with uneventful healing.

The outcomes of the surgery were satisfactory (Fig 10-7l). Note the full coverage of the root, healthy gingival margins, and lack of CDH at the canine. There was no periodontal probing depth greater than 3 mm, no bleeding on probing, low plaque index, and no clinical inflammation in the gingival margin region. However, the first premolar was not fully covered. The recession and CDH decreased, but the root was still exposed. A desensitizing protocol was immediately reestablished during postoperative therapy due to patient complaint of CDH (Fig 10-7m) and showed good results. A second surgery was recommended for total covering of the exposed root to eliminate CDH.

The maxillary right canine and mandibular right canine and first premolar also required periodontal surgery (Figs 10-7n and 10-7o). The same technique was used to treat these recessions. In the mandible, two surgeries were performed to obtain total root coverage of the Miller Class II recession at the canine. In the end, the CDH was eliminated and the quality of gingival tissue was restored/stabilized (Fig 10-7p).

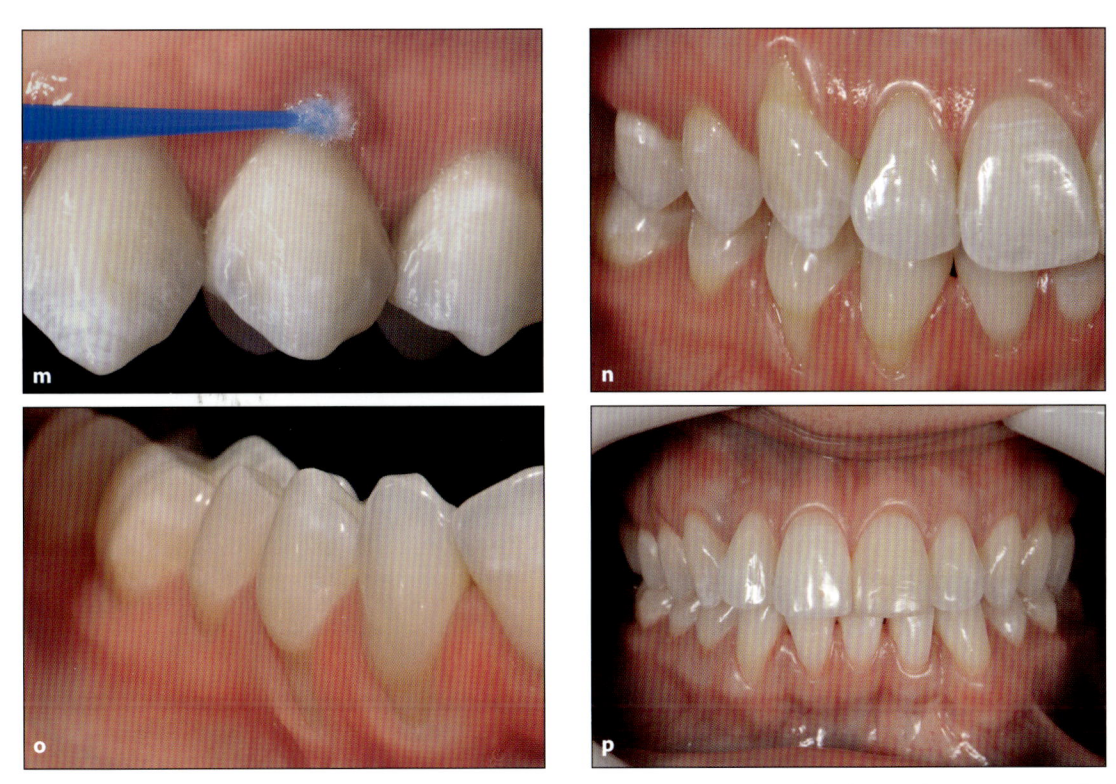

Fig 10-7 *(cont)* *(m)* Desensitizing protocol. The maxillary left first premolar still presented with CDH after surgery. *(n and o)* Multiple gingival recessions on the maxillary right canine and mandibular right canine and first premolar. *(p)* Postoperative view after 9 months. It was recommended that the patient be reevaluated every 3 months for the presence of CDH. (Clinical case courtesy of Cristianne Pacheco Ribeiro, Maria Aparecida de Oliveira Campoli, and Analice Giovani Pereira, NCCL Research Group, Uberlândia, Brazil.)

Conclusion

Let's review what we have covered in this chapter:
- The Miller classification is a useful recession defect classification based on the height of the interproximal bone and the relationship of the gingival margin to the MGJ.
- The presence of NCCLs can limit expectations for root coverage.
- The SCTG in combination with flap advancement has demonstrated excellent predictability and is considered the gold standard for treating gingival recession.
- Combined therapies (eg, CAF with collagen) have been reported to be superior to traditional root coverage.
- The severity of the recession dictates the treatment approach for gingival recession.
- For all cases of surgical root coverage, mechanical root decontamination is essential to ensure healthy gingival tissue.

References

1. Cairo F, Pagliaro U, Nieri M. Treatment of gingival recession with coronally advanced flap procedures: A systematic review. J Clin Periodontol 2008;35(8 suppl):136–162.
2. Seichter U. Root surface caries: A critical literature review. J Am Dent Assoc 1987;115:305–310.
3. Canadian Advisory Board on Dentin Hypersensitivity. Consensus-based recommendations for the diagnosis and management of dentin hypersensitivity. J Can Dent Assoc 2003;69:221–226.
4. Zucchelli G, Mounssif I. Periodontal plastic surgery. Periodontol 2000 2015;68:333–368.
5. Chambrone L, Tatakis DN. Periodontal soft tissue root coverage procedures: A systematic review from the AAP Regeneration Workshop. J Periodontol 2015;86(2 suppl):S8–S51.
6. Joly JC, Carvalho PF, da Silva RC. Reconstrução tecidual estética: Procedimentos plásticos e regenerativos periodontais e peri-implantares. São Paulo: Artes Médicas, 2009.
7. Joly JC, Carvalho PFM, Silva RC. Esthetic Perio-Implantology. São Paulo: Quintessence Editora, 2016:93–193.
8. Zucchelli G, Gori G, Mele M, et al. Non-carious cervical lesions associated with gingival recessions: A decision-making process. J Periodontol 2011;82:1713–1724.
9. Mele M, Zucchelli G, Montevecchi M, Checchi L. Bilaminar technique in the treatment of a deep cervical abrasion defect. Int J Periodontics Restorative Dent 2008;28:63–71.
10. Miller PD Jr. A classification of the marginal tissue recession. Int J Periodontics Restorative Dent 1985;5:8–13.

11. Zucchelli G, Mele M, Stefanini M, et al. Predetermination of root coverage. J Periodontol 2010;81:1019–1026.
12. Chambrone L, Pannuti CM, Tu YK, Chambrone LA. Evidence-based periodontal plastic surgery. II. An individual data meta-analysis for evaluating factors in achieving complete root coverage. J Periodontol 2012;83:477–490.
13. Wennström JL. Mucogingival therapy. Ann Periodontol 1996;1:671–701.
14. Jankovic S, Aleksic Z, Milinkovic I, Dimitrijevic B. The coronally advanced flap in combination with platelet-rich fibrin (PRF) and enamel matrix derivative in the treatment of gingival recession: A comparative study. Eur J Esthet Dent 2010;5:260–273.
15. Miller PD. Periodontal plastic surgical techniques for regeneration. In: Polson AL (ed). Periodontal Regeneration: Current Status and Directions. Chicago: Quintessence, 1994:53–70.
16. Raetzke PB. Covering localized areas of root exposure employing the "envelope" technique. J Periodontol 1985;56:397–402.
17. Langer B, Langer L. Subepithelial connective tissue graft for root coverage. J Periodontol 1985;56:715–720.
18. Bouchard P, Malet J, Borghetti A. Decision-making in aesthetics: Root coverage revisited. Periodontol 2000 2001;27:97–120.
19. Harris RJ. The connective tissue and partial thickness double pedicle graft: A predictable method of obtaining root coverage. J Periodontol 1992;63:477–486.
20. Pini-Prato GP, Cairo F, Nieri M, Franceschi D, Rotundo R, Cortellini P. Coronally advanced flap versus connective tissue graft in the treatment of multiple gingival recessions: A split-mouth study with a 5-year follow-up. J Clin Periodontol 2010;37:644–650.
21. Da Silva RC, Joly JC, de Lima AF, Takakis DN. Root coverage using the coronally positioned flap with or without a subepithelial connective tissue graft. J Periodontol 2004;75:413–419.
22. Martorelli de Lima AF, da Silva RC, Joly JC, Takakis DN. Coronally positioned flap with subepithelial connective tissue graft for root coverage: Various indications and flap designs. J Int Acad Periodontol 2006;8:53–60.
23. Joly JC, Carvalho AM, da Silva RC, Ciotti DL, Cury PR. Root coverage in isolated gingival recessions using autograft versus allograft: A pilot study. J Periodontol 2007;78:1017–1022.
24. Rotundo R, Pini-Prato G. Use of a new collagen matrix (mucograft) for the treatment of multiple gingival recessions: Case reports. Int J Periodontics Restorative Dent 2012;32:413–419.
25. Cardaropoli D, Tamagnone L, Roffredo A, Gaveglio L. Coronally advanced flap with and without a xenogenic collagen matrix in the treatment of multiple recessions: A randomized controlled clinical study. Int J Periodontics Restorative Dent 2014;34(suppl 3):S97–S102.
26. McGuire MK, Scheyer ET. Xenogeneic collagen matrix with coronally advanced flap compared to connective tissue with coronally advanced flap for the treatment of dehiscence-type recession defects. J Periodontol 2010;81:1108–1117.
27. Jepsen K, Jepsen S, Zucchelli G, et al. Treatment of gingival recession defects with a coronally advanced flap and a xenogeneic collagen matrix: A multicenter randomized clinical trial. J Clin Periodontol 2013;40:82–89.
28. Schlee M, Lex M, Rathe F, Kasaj A, Sader R. Treatment of multiple recessions by means of a collagen matrix: A case series. Int J Periodontics Restorative Dent 2014;34:817–823.
29. Heijl L, Heden G, Svärdström G, Ostgren A. Enamel matrix derivative (EMDOGAIN) in the treatment of intrabony periodontal defects. J Clin Periodontol 1997;24(9 pt 2):705–714.
30. Hammarström L, Heijl L, Gestrelius S. Periodontal regeneration in a buccal dehiscence model in monkeys after application of enamel matrix proteins. J Clin Periodontol 1997;24(9 pt 2):669–677.
31. Gestrelius S, Andersson C, Johansson AC, et al. Formulation of enamel matrix derivative for surface coating. Kinetics and cell colonization. J Clin Periodontol 1997;24(9 pt 2):678–684.
32. Gestrelius S, Lyngstadaas SP, Hammarström L. Emdogain—Periodontal regeneration based on biomimicry. Clin Oral Investig 2000;4:120–125.
33. Cortellini P, Pini Prato G. Coronally advanced flap and combination therapy for root coverage. Clinical strategies based on scientific evidence and clinical experience. Periodontol 2000 2012;59:158–184.
34. McGuire MK, Scheyer ET, Nunn M. Evaluation of human recession defects treated with coronally advanced flaps and either enamel matrix derivative or connective tissue: Comparison of clinical parameters at 10 years. J Periodontol 2012;83:1353–1362.
35. Wennström JL, Lindhe J. Some effects of enamel matrix proteins on wound healing in the dento-gingival region. J Clin Periodontol 2002;29:9–14.
36. Lyngstadaas SP, Wohlfahrt JC, Brookes SJ, Paine ML, Snead ML, Reseland JE. Enamel matrix proteins; old molecules for new applications. Orthod Craniofac Res 2009;12:243–253.
37. Tonetti MS, Fourmousis I, Suvan J, Cortellini P, Brägger U, Lang NP; European Research Group on Periodontology (ERGOPERIO). Healing, post-operative morbidity and patient perception of outcomes following regenerative therapy of deep intrabony defects. J Clin Periodontol 2004;31:1092–1098.
38. McGuire MK, Nunn M. Evaluation of human recession defects treated with coronally advanced flaps and either enamel matrix derivative or connective tissue. Part 1: Comparison of clinical parameters. J Periodontol 2003;74:1110–1125.
39. Tammaro S, Wennström JL, Bergenholtz G. Root-dentin sensitivity following non-surgical periodontal treatment. J Clin Periodontol 2000;27:690–697.
40. Taani SD, Awartani F. Clinical evaluation of cervical dentin sensitivity (CDS) in patients attending general dental clinics and periodontal specialty clinics (PSC). J Clin Periodontol 2002;29:118–122.
41. Santos RL, Gusmão ES, Jovino-Silveira RC, Tenório SB, Barbosa RPS. Clinical evaluation of obliterative desensitizers after periodontal scaling. Rev Bras Cien Saúde 2006;10:123–132.
42. Gusmão ES, Coelho RS, Farias BC, Cimões R. Dentin hypersensitivity before and after periodontal treatment. Acta Stomatol Croat 2010;44:251–261.
43. Yilmaz HG, Kurtulmus-Yilmaz S, Cengiz E. Long-term effect of diode laser irradiation compared to sodium fluoride varnish in the treatment of dentine hypersensitivity in periodontal maintenance patients: A randomized controlled clinical study. Photomed Laser Surg 2011;29:721–725.
44. Fernandes-Dias SB, de Marco AC, Santamaria M Jr, Kerbauy WD, Jardini MA, Santamaria MP. Connective tissue graft associated or not with low laser therapy to treat gingival recession: Randomized clinical trial. J Clin Periodontol 2015;42:54–61.
45. Han JS, John V, Blanchard SB, Kowolik MJ, Eckert GJ. Changes in gingival dimensions following connective tissue grafts for root coverage: Comparison of two procedures. J Periodontol 2008;79:1346–1354.
46. Zucchelli G, De Sanctis M. Treatment of multiple recession-type defects in patients with esthetic demands. J Periodontol 2000;71:1506–1514.
47. Mörmann W, Meier C, Firestone A. Gingival blood circulation after experimental wounds in man. J Clin Periodontol 1979;6:417–424.
48. Zucchelli G, Mele M, Mazzotti C, Marzadori M, Montebugnoli L, De Sanctis M. Coronally advanced flap with and without vertical releasing incisions for the treatment of multiple gingival recessions: A comparative controlled randomized clinical trial. J Periodontol 2009;80:1083–1094.
49. Allen EP, Miller PD Jr. Coronal positioning of existing gingiva: Short term results in the treatment of shallow marginal tissue recession. J Periodontol 1989;60:316–319.
50. Grupe H, Warren R. Repair of gingival defects by a sliding flap operation. J Periodontol 1956;27:92–95.
51. Zucchelli G, Cesari C, Amore C, Montebugnoli L, De Sanctis M. Laterally moved, coronally advanced flap: A modified surgical approach for isolated recession-type defects. J Periodontol 2004;75:1734–1741.
52. Zucchelli G, Mounssif I, Stefanini M, Mele M, Montebugnoli L, Sforza NM. Hand and ultrasonic instrumentation in combination with root-coverage surgery: A comparative controlled randomized clinical trial. J Periodontol 2009;80:577–585.
53. Leite FR, Moreira CS, Theodoro LH, Sampaio JE. Blood cell attachment to root surfaces treated with EDTA gel. Braz Oral Res 2005;19:88–92.
54. Bittencourt S, Ribeiro Edel P, Sallum EA, Sallum AW, Nociti FH Jr, Casati MZ. Root surface biomodification with EDTA for the treatment of gingival recession with a semilunar coronally repositioned flap. J Periodontol 2007;78:1695–1701.

Future Perspectives

The incidence and prevalence rates and epidemiologic data of NCCLs and CDH are increasing every year. Most clinicians are not addressing the etiology of CDH but are rather focused on the use of various desensitizing modalities to treat the symptoms. Many of our teenage and younger patients consume an acidic diet, have parafunctional habits, and are under mental stress, all of which contribute to CDH and the formation and progression of NCCLs. These conditions have worsened over the past 10 years and are frequently uncontrolled.

The objective of this book was to present the most recent data about the etiology of CDH and NCCLs and various technologies that can be applied in clinical treatment procedures. Many researchers are working to verify the mechanisms involved in the etiology of both of these pathologies.

In the future, the patient's saliva could be used as a means for the diagnosis and prevention of NCCLs and CDH. More randomized clinical trials need to be carried out to test new treatment agents and restorative materials. Experiments applying new technologies to biomechanical and biochemical studies should also be conducted. And additional tests on the effectiveness of occlusal equilibration in the elimination of CDH should be pursued.

We observe that new technologies in dental materials and bonding interface strategies need to be addressed. Class V restorations present the highest failure levels in adhesive dentistry and need more attention throughout treatment. The opinion leaders and public health organizations throughout the world need to include NCCLs and CDH in their respective public health problems list. For many countries, caries and periodontal disease are still the primary problems in dental health. However, in most of the countries with better economic conditions, NCCLs and CDH affect more people than caries and periodontal diseases. The authors recommend that clinicians maintain their focus on the following risk groups: patients with GERD and gastric diseases, athletes (professional and amateur), patients with an acidic diet, patients who have undergone orthodontics, and mentally stressed patients who brux or clench their teeth.

We encourage our dental industry partners to help us improve the in-office dental agents and effective long-term treatment materials. Patients should be advised that they should not treat themselves, because current desensitizing dentifrices only treat the symptoms. Treatment agents do not remove the causative main factors, namely stress manifested as abfraction and biocorrosion. Students and future professionals must understand that at this time there is no safe, effective, long-term, at-home self-treatment. Recent studies have proven that carefully evaluating the patient's occlusion and then equilibrating eccentric loading points offers the best long-term solution to CDH and NCCLs by eliminating their cause.

Paulo V. Soares
John O. Grippo

Appendix

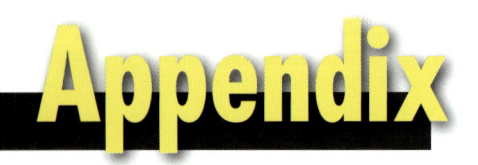

Table 1 Randomized controlled trials evaluating the effectiveness of chemical desensitizers in the management of CDH

Authors (year)	No. of patients	Age (y)	Experimental intervention	Follow-up	Pain stimuli
At-home desensitizing agents					
Miller et al[1] (1969)	23	NA	0.4% stannous fluoride dentifrice, placebo	NA	Thermal, tactile
Minkoff and Axelrod[2] (1987)	61	18–65	10% strontium chloride, placebo	12 weeks	Thermal, tactile
Sharma et al[3] (2012)	30	NA	5% potassium nitrate/sodium fluoride, 3% potassium nitrate/sodium fluoride	4 weeks	Thermal, air
Liu and Hu[4] (2012)	79	20–65	2% strontium chloride/5% potassium nitrate in silica, silica without active ingredient	3 days	Thermal, tactile
Pradeep et al[5] (2012)	149	20–60	5% potassium nitrate, 5% calcium sodium phosphosilicate with silica, 3.85% amine fluoride, placebo	6 weeks	Thermal, air
Uraz et al[6] (2013)	36	27–43	8% arginine/calcium carbonate, 1.23% sodium fluoride gel	4 weeks	Thermal, air, tactile
Elías Boneta et al[7] (2013)	118	18–70	8% arginine in sodium carbonate base + 8% arginine mouthwash, 5% potassium nitrate in silica base + 0.51% potassium chloride mouthwash	8 weeks	Air, tactile
Elías Boneta et al[8] (2013)	75	18–70	8% arginine, 2.4% potassium nitrate, 0.5% sodium fluoride (negative control)	6 weeks	Air, tactile
Hu et al[9] (2013)	90	18–70	8% arginine, placebo	8 weeks	Air, tactile
Neuhaus et al[10] (2013)	151	18–70	15% calcium sodium phosphosilicate, 15% calcium sodium phosphosilicate/2.7% sodium fluoride, placebo	4 weeks	Air, tactile
Sharma et al[11] (2013)	56	NA	1.4% potassium oxalate, control group	5 days	Air, tactile
Kakar and Kakar[12] (2013)	100	NA	5% potassium nitrate/sodium monofluorophosphate, sodium monofluorophosphate (control group)	8 weeks	Air, tactile
Acharya et al[13] (2013)	20	18–65	5% calcium sodium phosphosilicate, 5% potassium nitrate (positive control)	8 weeks	Air
West et al[14] (2013)	80	NA	8% arginine/calcium carbonate, 8% arginine/silica	3 days	Air, tactile
Flecha et al[15] (2013)	62	NA	Cyanoacrylate, low-intensity laser	24 weeks	Thermal, air
Vano et al[16] (2014)	105	20–70	Nanohydroxyapatite 15%, fluoride, placebo	4 weeks	Air, tactile
Samuel et al[17] (2014)	57	20–50	8% arginine paste, 5% glutaraldehyde/HEMA	4 weeks	Thermal, air, tactile
Lee et al[18] (2015)	82	20–65	Nanocarbonate apatite, high-intensity laser	4 weeks	Thermal, air, tactile
In-office desensitizing agents					
Pillon et al[19] (2004)	15	NA	3% potassium oxalate gel, placebo	3 weeks	Home routine
Ritter et al[20] (2006)	19	NA	5% sodium fluoride varnish	24 weeks	Air, thermal
Kobler et al[21] (2008)	142	18–60	Strontium chloride	24 weeks	Air, tactile
Vieira et al[22] (2009)	30	24–68	Potassium oxalate, low-intensity laser, placebo	12 weeks	Air, tactile
Aranha et al[23] (2009)	39	NA	5% glutaraldehyde/HEMA, ditrimethacrylate resin, 3% potassium oxalate, 2.59% sodium fluoride, low-intensity laser	24 weeks	Air
Sethna et al[24] (2011)	250	20–55	5% glutaraldehyde/HEMA, 1% thymol/1% chlorhexidine	12 weeks	Thermal, air, tactile
Craig et al[25] (2012)	19	23–60	38% diamine silver fluoride/potassium iodide, oxalic acid/potassium salt/water	1 week	Thermal, air

Table 1 *(cont)* **Randomized controlled trials evaluating the effectiveness of chemical desensitizers in the management of CDH**

Authors (year)	No. of patients	Age (y)	Experimental intervention	Follow-up	Pain stimuli
Brahmbhatt et al[26] (2012)	25	20–50	2% sodium fluoride, 5% glutaraldehyde/HEMA, iontophoresis with distilled water, 2% sodium fluoride iontophoresis	12 weeks	Thermal, air, tactile
Camilloti et al[27] (2012)	42	18–70	50 mg sodium fluoride, 5% sodium fluoride, 6% sodium fluoride/6% calcium fluoride, 2% sodium fluoride, 3% potassium oxalate, placebo	4 weeks	Thermal, air, tactile
Vora et al[28] (2012)	50	NA	5% glutaraldehyde/HEMA, oxalate, placebo	24 weeks	Air, tactile
Lopes and Aranha[29] (2013)	24	NA	5% glutaraldehyde/HEMA, high-intensity laser, both	24 weeks	Thermal, air, tactile
Raichur et al[30] (2013)	54	25–45	Low-intensity laser, 0.4% stannous fluoride gel, 5% potassium nitrate gel	24 weeks	Air
Neuhaus et al[10] (2013)	151	18–70	15% calcium sodium phosphosilicate/2.7% sodium fluoride, 15% calcium sodium phosphosilicate/fluoride, placebo	4 weeks	Air, tactile
Ding et al[31] (2014)	31	NA	Resin-modified glass ionomer, 5% glutaraldehyde/HEMA	4 weeks	Thermal, air, tactile
Talesara et al[32] (2014)	20	25–55	Potassium binoxalate gel, high-intensity laser	36 weeks	Thermal, air
Purra et al[33] (2014)	NA	20–40	5% potassium nitrate, propolis, water	12 weeks	Thermal
Samuel et al[17] (2014)	57	20–50	8% arginine paste, 5% glutaraldehyde/HEMA	4 weeks	Thermal, air, tactile
Pinna et al[34] (2015)	46	NA	Sodium fluoride varnish, HEMA adhesive system, resin dentin sealant, self-adhering flowable composite	12 weeks	Thermal
Lee et al[18] (2015)	82	20–65	Nanocarbonate apatite, high-intensity laser	4 weeks	Thermal, air, tactile

NA, not available.

References

1. Miller JT, Shannon IL, Kilgore WG, Bookman JE. Use of a water-free stannous fluoride-containing gel in the control of dental hypersensitivity. J Periodontol 1969;40:490–491.
2. Minkoff S, Axelrod S. Efficacy of strontium chloride in dental hypersensitivity. J Periodontol 1987;58:470–474.
3. Sharma S, Shetty NJ, Uppoor A. Evaluation of the clinical efficacy of potassium nitrate desensitizing mouthwash and a toothpaste in the treatment of dentinal hypersensitivity. J Clin Exp Dent 2012;4:e28–e33.
4. Liu H, Hu D. Efficacy of a commercial dentifrice containing 2% strontium chloride and 5% potassium nitrate for dentin hypersensitivity: A 3-day clinical study in adults in China. Clin Ther 2012;34:614–622.
5. Pradeep AR, Agarwal E, Naik SB, Bajaj P, Kalra N. Comparison of efficacy of three commercially available dentifrices on dentinal hypersensitivity: A randomized clinical trial. Aust Dent J 2012;57:429–434 [erratum 2013;58:272].
6. Uraz A, Erol-Şimşek Ö, Pehlivan S, Suludere Z, Bal B. The efficacy of 8% Arginine-CaCO3 applications on dentine hypersensitivity following periodontal therapy: A clinical and scanning electron microscopic study. Med Oral Patol Oral Cir Bucal 2013;18:e298–e305.
7. Elías Boneta AR, Galán Salás RM, Mateo LR, et al. Efficacy of a mouthwash containing 0.8% arginine, PVM/MA copolymer, pyrophosphates, and 0.05% sodium fluoride compared to a commercial mouthwash containing 2.4% potassium nitrate and 0.022% sodium fluoride and a control mouthwash containing 0.05% sodium fluoride on dentine hypersensitivity: A six-week randomized clinical study. J Dent 2013;41(suppl 1):S34–S41.
8. Elías Boneta AR, Ramirez K, Naboa J, et al. Efficacy in reducing dentine hypersensitivity of a regimen using a toothpaste containing 8% arginine and calcium carbonate, a mouthwash containing 0.8% arginine, pyrophosphate and PVM/MA copolymer and a toothbrush compared to potassium and negative control regimens: An eight-week randomized clinical trial. J Dent 2013;41(suppl 1):S42–S49.
9. Hu D, Stewart B, Mello S, et al. Efficacy of a mouthwash containing 0.8% arginine, PVM/MA copolymer, pyrophosphates, and 0.05% sodium fluoride compared to a negative control mouthwash on dentin hypersensitivity reduction. A randomized clinical trial. J Dent 2013;41(suppl 1):S26–S33.
10. Neuhaus KW, Milleman JL, Milleman KR, et al. Effectiveness of a calcium sodium phosphosilicate-containing prophylaxis paste in reducing dentine hypersensitivity immediately and 4 weeks after a single application: A double-blind randomized controlled trial. J Clin Periodontol 2013;40:349–357.

Appendix

11. Sharma D, McGuire JA, Amini P. Randomized trial of the clinical efficacy of a potassium oxalate-containing mouthrinse in rapid relief of dentin sensitivity. J Clin Dent 2013;24:62–67.
12. Kakar A, Kakar K. Measurement of dentin hypersensitivity with the Jay Sensitivity Sensor Probe and the Yeaple probe to compare relief from dentin hypersensitivity by dentifrices. Am J Dent 2013;26(spec no. B):21B–28B.
13. Acharya AB, Surve SM, Thakur SL. A clinical study of the effect of calcium sodium phosphosilicate on dentin hypersensitivity. J Clin Exp Dent 2013;5:e18–e22.
14. West N, Newcombe RG, Hughes N, et al. A 3-day randomised clinical study investigating the efficacy of two toothpastes, designed to occlude dentine tubules, for the treatment of dentine hypersensitivity. J Dent 2013;41:187–194.
15. Flecha OD, Azevedo CG, Matos FR, et al. Cyanoacrylate versus laser in the treatment of dentin hypersensitivity: A controlled, randomized, double-masked and non-inferiority clinical trial. J Periodontol 2013;84:287–294.
16. Vano M, Derchi G, Barone A, Covani U. Effectiveness of nano-hydroxyapatite toothpaste in reducing dentin hypersensitivity: A double-blind randomized controlled trial. Quintessence Int 2014;45:703–711.
17. Samuel SR, Khatri SG, Acharya S. Clinical evaluation of self and professionally applied desensitizing agents in relieving dentin hypersensitivity after a single topical application: A randomized controlled trial. J Clin Exp Dent 2014;6:e339–e343.
18. Lee SY, Jung HI, Jung BY, Cho YS, Kwon HK, Kim BI. Desensitizing efficacy of nano-carbonate apatite dentifrice and Er,Cr:YSGG laser: A randomized clinical trial. Photomed Laser Surg 2015;33:9–14.
19. Pillon FL, Romani IG, Schmidt ER. Effect of a 3% potassium oxalate topical application on dentinal hypersensitivity after subgingival scaling and root planing. J Periodontol 2004;75:1461–1464.
20. Ritter AV, de L Dias W, Miguez P, Caplan DJ, Swift EJ Jr. Treating cervical dentin hypersensitivity with fluoride varnish: A randomized clinical study. J Am Dent Assoc 2006;137:1013–1020.
21. Kobler A, Kub O, Schaller HG, Gernhardt CR. Clinical effectiveness of a strontium chloride-containing desensitizing agent over 6 months: A randomized, double-blind, placebo-controlled study. Quintessence Int 2008;39:321–325.
22. Vieira AH, Passos VF, de Assis JS, Mendonça JS, Santiago SL. Clinical evaluation of a 3% potassium oxalate gel and a GaAlAs laser for the treatment of dentinal hypersensitivity. Photomed Laser Surg 2009;27:807–812.
23. Aranha AC, Pimenta LA, Marchi GM. Clinical evaluation of desensitizing treatments for cervical dentin hypersensitivity. Braz Oral Res 2009;23:333–339.
24. Sethna GD, Prabhuji ML, Karthikeyan BV. Comparison of two different forms of varnishes in the treatment of dentine hypersensitivity: A subject-blind randomised clinical study. Oral Health Prev Dent 2011;9:143–150.
25. Craig GG, Knight GM, McIntyre JM. Clinical evaluation of diamine silver fluoride/potassium iodide as a dentine desensitizing agent. A pilot study. Aust Dent J 2012;57:308–311.
26. Brahmbhatt N, Bhavsar N, Sahayata V, Acharya A, Kshatriya P. A double blind controlled trial comparing three treatment modalities for dentin hypersensitivity. Med Oral Patol Oral Cir Bucal 2012;17:e483–e490.
27. Camilotti V, Zilly J, Busato Pdo M, Nassar CA, Nassar PO. Desensitizing treatments for dentin hypersensitivity: A randomized, split-mouth clinical trial. Braz Oral Res 2012;26:263–268.
28. Vora J, Mehta D, Meena N, Sushma G, Finger WJ, Kanehira M. Effects of two topical desensitizing agents and placebo on dentin hypersensitivity. Am J Dent 2012;25:293–298.
29. Lopes AO, Aranha AC. Comparative evaluation of the effects of Nd:YAG laser and a desensitizer agent on the treatment of dentin hypersensitivity: A clinical study. Photomed Laser Surg 2013;31:132–138.
30. Raichur PS, Setty SB, Thakur SL. Comparative evaluation of diode laser, stannous fluoride gel, and potassium nitrate gel in the treatment of dentinal hypersensitivity. Gen Dent 2013;61:66–71.
31. Ding YJ, Yao H, Wang GH, Song H. A randomized double-blind placebo-controlled study of the efficacy of Clinpro XT varnish and Gluma dentin desensitizer on dentin hypersensitivity. Am J Dent 2014;27:79–83.
32. Talesara K, Kulloli A, Shetty S, Kathariya R. Evaluation of potassium binoxalate gel and Nd:YAG laser in the management of dentinal hypersensitivity: A split-mouth clinical and ESEM study. Lasers Med Sci 2014;29:61–68.
33. Purra AR, Mushtaq M, Acharya SR, Saraswati V. A comparative evaluation of propolis and 5.0% potassium nitrate as a dentine desensitizer: A clinical study. J Indian Soc Periodontol 2014;18:466–471.
34. Pinna R, Bortone A, Sotgiu G, Dore S, Usai P, Milia E. Clinical evaluation of the efficacy of one self-adhesive composite in dental hypersensitivity. Clin Oral Investig 2015;19:1663–1672.

Table 2 Controlled clinical trials evaluating the longevity of composite resin restorations for NCCLs

Authors (year)	Maximum recall	No. of patients	No. of restorations	Adhesive system	Restorative material	Survival rates
Jang et al[1] (2017)	2 years	35	164	Two-step and one-step self-etch	Microhybrid composite resin	Just three restorations were dislodged over 24 months, all from the two-step self-etch group
Lopes et al[2] (2016)	6 months	31	124	Universal adhesive with etch-and-rinse and self-adhesive methods	Nanohybrid composite resin	Retention rates were between 90.3% and 96.8% for etch-and-rinse and 80.7% for self-etch
Loguercio et al[3] (2015)	18 months	30	60	One-step self-etch	Nanohybrid composite resin	Restoration retention rate of 73%
Araújo et al[4] (2015)	2 years	22	126 NCCLs	Two types of self-etch adhesive system (with or without chlorhexidine gluconate)	Microhybrid composite resin	Restoration retention rates were 82% (with chlorhexidine) and 97% (without chlorhexidine)
Dall'Orologio and Lorenzi[5] (2014)	8 years	50	150 NCCLs	Two-step etch-and-rinse	Nanofilled ormocer (organic-inorganic hybrid polymers) or microhybrid composite resin	Cumulative loss rate of 7% for both restorative materials; annual failure lower than 1%
Torres et al[6] (2014)	5 years	30	136 NCCLs	Two-step etch-and-rinse with or without deproteinization (10% NaOCl gel)	Microfilled composite resin	Restoration retention rates were 77% (conventional) and 68% (with deproteinization)
Oginni and Adeleke[7] (2014)	2 years	89	287 NCCLs	Two-step etch-and-rinse	Microhybrid resin composite	Retention rates in NCCLs with and without occlusal wear facets were 63.9% and 74.4%, respectively
Moretto et al[8] (2013)	3 years	30	175 NCCLs	HEMA-rich one-step self-etch or HEMA-free one-step self-etch	Composite resin	Retention rate of 93.8% for HEMA-rich and 98.8% for HEMA-free
Tuncer et al[9] (2013)	2 years	24	123 NCCLs	Two-step etch-and-rinse or all-in-one self-etching	Nanohybrid resin composite	Restoration retention rates of 69% for two-step etch-and-rinse and 49% for all-in-one self-etching system
Qin et al[10] (2013)	2 years	46	116 NCCLs	Two types of two-step self-etch adhesive system	Nanohybrid and nanoparticulated composite resin	Retention rates of 100% for nanohybrid and 91.38% for nanoparticulated composite resin
Stojanac et al[11] (2013)	2 years	30	90 NCCLs	Two-step etch-and-rinse (1), two-step self-etch (2), or one-step self-etch (3)	Microfilled composite resin (1), nanohybrid composite (2), or compomer Dyract (3)	Retention rates were 80% (microfilled), 83.7% (nanohybrid), and 83.7% (compomer)
Van Dijken et al[12] (2012)	7 years	60	139 NCCLs	One-step self-etch	Hybrid composite resin or polyacid-modified composite resin	Cumulative loss rate for 7 years was 23%, independent of curing technique or restorative material
Karaman et al[13] (2012)	2 years	21	134 NCCLs	One-step self-etch	Nanohybrid composite resin or flowable composite resin	Restoration retention rates of 60% (nanohybrid) and 54% (flowable)
Burrow[14] (2011)	3 years	13	41 NCCLs	HEMA-free all-in-one adhesive	Hybrid resin composite	Cumulative retention rate of 85%
Van Landuyt et al[15] (2011)	3 years	52	276 NCCLs	HEMA-free one-step or three-step etch-and-rinse	Microhybrid composite	Retention rates of 94.74% (one-step self-etch) and 94.03% (three-step etch-and-rinse)
Peumans et al[16] (2010)	8 years	29	100 NCCLs	Two-step self-etch with or without selective acid etching of enamel cavity margins with 40% phosphoric acid	Composite resin	Retention rate of 97% in both groups
Kubo et al[17] (2010)	3 years	22	98 NCCLs	All-in-one self-etch	Hybrid composite resin or flowable composite resin	Retention rates of 100% (hybrid) and 94% (flowable)

Appendix

Table 2 *(cont)* Controlled clinical trials evaluating the longevity of composite resin restorations for NCCLs

Authors (year)	Maximum recall	No. of patients	No. of restorations	Adhesive system	Restorative material	Survival rates
Brackett et al[18] (2010)	2 years	14	80 NCCLs	Two-step self-etch or all-in-one self-etch	Hybrid composite resin	Retention rate of 81%–84% for both groups
Santiago et al[19] (2010)	2 years	30	70 NCCLs	Two-step etch-and-rinse	Composite resin or resin-modified glass-ionomer cement	Restoration retention rates of 78.8% (composite resin) and 100% (glass ionomer)
Van Dijken et al[20] (2007)	13 years	119	337 NCCLs	Three-step etch-and-rinse, two-step etch-and-rinse, or two-step self-etch	Composite resin	Cumulative loss rates of 60.3% with significantly different failure rates for the different systems (26.3%–94.7%)
Peumans et al[21] (2007)	7 years	71	142 NCCLs	Two types of three-step etch-and-rinse adhesive	Two types of microhybrid composite resin	Retention rates were between 87% and 92%
Çelik et al[22] (2007)	2 years	37	252 NCCLs	Two-step etch-and-rinse	Three different flowable composite resins and one hybrid composite resin	The survival rate for all materials was 92%
Onal and Pamir[23] (2005)	2 years	30	130 NCCLs	Resin-modified glass-ionomer primer (1), polyacid-modified resin-based composite primer and adhesive (2), three-step etch-and-rinse adhesive (3)	Resin-modified glass ionomer (1), two types of polyacid-modified resin-based composite (2), resin-based composite (3)	Retention rates were 100% (resin-modified glass ionomer), 67% and 68% (polyacid-modified resin-based composite), and 70% (resin-based composite)
Van Meerbeek et al[24] (1993)	2 years	NA	306 NCCLs	Clearfil New Bond adhesive (two-step etch-and-rinse) or Scotchbond 2 (two-step etch-and-rinse)	Clearfil Ray composite resin or Silux Plus composite resin	Restoration retention rates were between 21% and 99% for Clearfil New Bond and between 13% and 100% for Scotchbond 2; the lower rates were for NCCLs without an enamel bevel or acid etching and with a butt-joint cavity

NA, not available.

References

1. Jang JH, Kim HY, Shin SM, et al. Clinical effectiveness of different polishing systems and self-etch adhesives in Class V composite resin restorations: Two-year randomized controlled clinical trial. Oper Dent 2017;42:19–29.
2. Lopes LS, Calazans FS, Hidalgo R, et al. Six-month follow-up of cervical composite restorations placed with a new universal adhesive system: A randomized clinical trial. Oper Dent 2016;41:465–480.
3. Loguercio AD, Luque-Martinez I, Lisboa AH, et al. Influence of isolation method of the operative field on gingival damage, patients' preference, and restoration retention in noncarious cervical lesions. Oper Dent 2015;40:581–593.
4. Araújo MS, Souza LC, Apolonio FM, et al. Two-year clinical evaluation of chlorhexidine incorporation in two-step self-etch adhesive. J Dent 2015;43:140–148.
5. Dall'Orologio GD, Lorenzi R. Restorations in abrasion/erosion cervical lesions: 8-year results of a triple blind randomized controlled trial. Am J Dent 2014;27:245–250.
6. Torres CRG, Barcellos DC, Batista GR, et al. Five-year clinical performance of the dentine deproteinization technique in non-carious cervical lesions. J Dent 2014;42:816–823.
7. Oginni AO, Adeleke AA. Comparison of pattern of failure of resin composite restorations in non-carious cervical lesions with and without occlusal wear facets. J Dent 2014;42:824–830.
8. Moretto SG, Russo EM, Carvalho RC, et al. 3-year clinical effectiveness of one-step adhesives in non-carious cervical lesions. J Dent 2013;41:675–682.
9. Tuncer D, Yazici AR, Özgünaltay G, Dayangac B. Clinical evaluation of different adhesives used in the restoration of non-carious cervical lesions: 24-month results. Aust Dent J 2013;58:94–100.
10. Qin W, Song Z, Ye YY, Lin ZM. Two-year clinical evaluation of composite resins in non-carious cervical lesions. Clin Oral Investig 2013;17:799–804.
11. Stojanac IL, Premovic MT, Ramic BD, Drobac MR, Stojsin IM, Petrovic LM. Noncarious cervical lesions restored with three different tooth-colored materials: Two-year results. Oper Dent 2013;38:12–20.
12. van Dijken JW, Pallesen U. A 7-year randomized prospective study of a one-step self-etching adhesive in non-carious cervical lesions. The effect of curing modes and restorative material. J Dent 2012;40:1060–1067.
13. Karaman E, Yazici AR, Ozgunaltay G, Dayangac B. Clinical evaluation of a nanohybrid and a flowable resin composite in non-carious cervical lesions: 24-month results. J Adhes Dent 2012;14:485–492.
14. Burrow MF. Clinical evaluation of non-carious cervical lesion restorations using a HEMA-free adhesive: Three-year results. Aust Dent J 2011;56:401–405.

15. Van Landuyt KL, Peumans M, De Munck J, Cardoso MV, Ermis B, Van Meerbeek B. Three-year clinical performance of a HEMA-free one-step self-etch adhesive in non-carious cervical lesions. Eur J Oral Sci 2011;119:511–516.
16. Peumans M, De Munck J, Van Landuyt KL, Poitevin A, Lambrechts P, Van Meerbeek B. Eight-year clinical evaluation of a 2-step self-etch adhesive with and without selective enamel etching. Dent Mater 2010;26:1176–1184.
17. Kubo S, Yokota H, Yokota H, Hayashi Y. Three-year clinical evaluation of a flowable and a hybrid resin composite in non-carious cervical lesions. J Dent 2010;38:191–200.
18. Brackett MG, Dib A, Franco G, Estrada BE, Brackett WW. Two-year clinical performance of Clearfil SE and Clearfil S3 in restoration of unabraded non-carious class V lesions. Oper Dent 2010;35:273–278.
19. Santiago SL, Passos VF, Vieira AH, Navarro MF, Lauris JR, Franco EB. Two-year clinical evaluation of resinous restorative systems in non-carious cervical lesions. Braz Dent J 2010;21:229–234.
20. Van Dijken JW, Sunnegårdh-Grönberg K, Lindberg A. Clinical long-term retention of etch-and-rinse and self-etch adhesive systems in non-carious cervical lesions. A 13 years evaluation. Dent Mater 2007;23:1101–1117.
21. Peumans M, De Munck J, Van Landuyt KL, et al. Restoring cervical lesions with flexible composites. Dent Mater 2007;23:749–754.
22. Çelik C, Ozgünaltay G, Attar N. Clinical evaluation of flowable resins in non-carious cervical lesions: Two-year results. Oper Dent 2007;32:313–321.
23. Onal B, Pamir T. The two-year clinical performance of esthetic restorative materials in noncarious cervical lesions. J Am Dent Assoc 2005;136:1547–1555.
24. Van Meerbeek B, Braem M, Lambrechts P, Vanherle G. Evaluation of two dentin adhesives in cervical lesions. J Prosthet Dent 1993;70:308–314.

Index

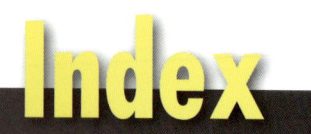

Page numbers followed by "f" indicate figures; those followed by "t" indicate tables; those followed by "b" indicate boxes

A

Abfractions
- biocorrosive, 36f–37f, 40f, 77, 87f
- definition of, 6, 34
- description of, 61
- illustration of, 11f
- occlusal loading as cause of, 96f

Abfractive lesions
- biomechanical behavior of, 38
- description of, 34
- illustration of, 87f
- stress concentration and, 80

Ablations, 6

Abrasion
- biocorrosion effects on, 47, 61
- from dentifrices, 44f, 44–45, 48
- description of, 43
- from toothbrushing. See Toothbrushing.

Abrasivity
- of dentifrices, 45, 45t
- of whitening toothpastes, 46, 47t

Acellular dermal matrix, 168
Acetylsalicylic acid, 58
Acid(s)
- citric, 55
- dentin affected by, 52
- enamel affected by, 52, 52f
- endogenous. See Endogenous acids.
- exogenous. See Exogenous acids.
- historical writings about, 5
- salivary flow affected by, 53
- smear layer removal caused by, 52

Acid dissociation constant value, 51–52
Acidulated sodium fluoride, 107
Acquired pellicle, 53–54
Additive occlusal therapy, 99
Adhesive/adhesive systems
- air drying of, 128
- antimicrobial monomers added to, 126
- application of, 128
- cavity preparation contraindications for, 127
- etch-and-rinse, 126–128, 127f
- evidence-based bonding protocols for, 126–129
- field isolation for, 126
- fillers added to, 126
- history of, 125
- hydrophobic resin coating used with, 128
- initiators, 126
- layers created using, 127f
- light curing of, 129
- monomers, 125–126
- rubber dam uses in, 126
- self-etch, 126–128, 127f, 137f
- solvents, 126
- types of, 127, 127f
- universal, 127–128

Afibrillar cementum, 25
Air drying, of adhesives, 128
Air indexing, 88, 88f
Alcohol, 56
Aluminum oxide, 149
Alveolar bone, 24
Anterior guidance, 99
Antimicrobial monomers, 126
Arginine, 109, 109f
Articulating foils, 98
Articulating paper, 97, 97f, 100f
Articulator
- centric relation recording on, 100
- occlusal mapping on, 101, 101f
- occlusal therapy uses of, 98, 98f–99f

Ascorbic acid, 58
Athletes, 58–59
Attached gingiva, 25
Attrition
- description of, 43, 62
- in gastroesophageal reflux disease and bruxism, 63f

B

Bacteria, dentinal surface colonization by, 6, 6f–7f
Biocorrosion
- abfractive lesions caused by, 36f–37f, 40f, 77, 87f
- abrasion affected by, 47, 61
- in athletes, 58–59
- in bulimia nervosa patients, 62, 64
- chemical degradation in. See Chemical degradation.
- "cupping" associated with, 60, 61f, 87f
- of dentin, 53, 53f
- dentinal wear caused by, 24
- drug use and, 58
- of enamel, 52–53
- erosion versus, 6
- exercise and, 57
- exogenous acid as cause of. See Exogenous acids.
- experimental studies of, 7f
- in gastroesophageal reflux disease patients, 62, 63f
- in hyperthyroidism, 64
- illicit drug use and, 58
- in lactovegetarians, 55
- lesion location and, 88
- lifestyle factors, 57–58
- management of, 66
- mechanism of action, 51
- medications as cause of, 58
- mouthrinses as cause of, 58
- nutritional habits as cause of, 56–57, 57b
- in posterior teeth, 60, 61f
- in pregnancy, 64
- prevention of, 66
- radiotherapy as risk factor for, 59, 59f
- in rumination syndrome, 64
- saliva's protective effects against, 53–54, 54b, 54f
- sodium fluoride effects on, 65
- stages of, 52–53
- stress-biocorrosion, 37, 37f, 61
- in swimmers, 59
- toothbrushing considerations in, 48

Bioglass, 108–109, 109f
Bis-GMA, 129

Index

Bleaching, tooth
  agents for, 46-47
  tooth sensitivity caused by, 119
Bone deflection, 39
Breakage strain, 33
Bromelain, 46
Brushing. *See* Toothbrushing.
Bruxism, 34-35, 62, 63f, 86
Buffering capacity, 60
Bulimia nervosa, 62, 64
Bulk-fill composite resins, 131

C

CAF. *See* Coronally advanced flap.
Calcium carbonate, 44f, 45, 46f
Calcium oxalates, 105-106
Calcium sodium phosphosilicate, 108
Camphorquinone, 126, 130
Canine guidance, 99, 102, 103f
Carbonic acid, 55
Caries
  chemoparasitic theory of, 4
  erosion and, 3
  in interproximal contact areas, 6
Casein phosphopeptide-amorphous calcium phosphate, 108
Cavity preparation
  for adhesive systems, 127
  for composite resins, 147-148, 148
CDH. *See* Cervical dentin hypersensitivity.
CEJ. *See* Cementoenamel junction.
Cementoenamel junction, 21f, 25f, 25-26, 80, 80f, 87
Cementum, 24-25, 25f
Centric occlusion
  description of, 87
  occlusal adjustment in, 100f-103f, 100-102
Centric prematurities, 100
Centric relation
  articulator recording of, 100
  description of, 87
  maximal intercuspal position and, 100, 100f
Ceramic fragments, 134, 134f
Ceramic restorations, indirect technique for, 156-157, 157f-158f, 159t
Ceramics, 132, 132f. *See also* Glass-ceramics.
Cervical dentin hypersensitivity
  age of onset, 10
  air indexing for, 88, 88f
  case report of, 110f-111f
  characteristics of, 88
  definition of, 9
  dental whitening and, 47
  dentifrices and, 12
  detection methods, 10
  diagnosis of, 88-89. *See also* Diagnosis.
  in drug addicts, 58
  etiology of
    biocorrosion. *See* Biocorrosion.
    friction. *See* Friction.
    historical descriptions of, 9-10
    pathologies associated with, 86
    stress. *See* Stress.
  frictional dental hypersensitivity as cause of, 10, 10t
  historical descriptions of, 3-4
  hydrodynamic theory of, 9, 9f, 24, 115
  nomenclature of, 9-10
  noncarious cervical lesions and, 10-11
  pain associated with, 9, 9f, 85, 88
  in postorthodontic patients, 39f
  prevalence of, 10, 10t
  root coverage for, 177-178, 179f-181f
  toothbrushing and, 12
  treatment of
    chemical therapy. *See* Chemical therapy.
    laser therapy. *See* Laser therapy.
    occlusal therapy. *See* Occlusal therapy.
  T-Scan occlusal analysis for, 89, 89f
Cervical erosions, 6
Cervical gingival notch, 6
Cervical region
  dentin in, 33
  enamel in, 33
  stress concentration in, 33, 35, 38
Cervical root caries, 12
C-factor, 135, 135f
Chemical degradation. *See also* Biocorrosion.
  acids as cause of. *See* Acid(s).
  acquired pellicle's effect on, 53
  in athletes, 58-59
  of dentin, 53, 53f
  of enamel, 52f, 52-53
  in factory workers manufacturing acidic products, 59
  mechanisms of, 51-53
  medications as cause of, 58
  mouthrinses as cause of, 58
  nutritional habits as cause of, 56-57, 57b
  occupational, 58-59
  saliva's protective effect against, 53-54, 54b, 54f
  in swimmers, 59
  in winemakers/wine tasters, 59
Chemical desensitizers, 112t, 184t-185t. *See also* Chemical therapy.
Chemical therapy
  arginine, 109, 109f
  bioglass, 108-109, 109f
  case report of, 110f-111f
  casein phosphopeptide-amorphous calcium phosphate, 108
  fluorides, 107-108
  glutaraldehyde, 106f, 106-107
  laser therapy and, combined protocol using, 118b, 118-119
  microapplicators used in, 111f
  neural agents, 104-105, 105b, 105f, 112t
  oxalates, 105-106
  potassium, 104-105, 105b, 105f
  potassium oxalate, 106, 109, 109f
  protocol for, 110, 111f
  recommendations for, 112t
  strontium, 106
  tubule-occluding agents, 105-109, 105f-109f, 112t
  varnishes, 107
Chemico-abrasion, 5
Chief complaint, 85-86
Chlorhexidine, 107
Citric acid, 55
Class V composite inlays, 144
Class V restorations
  cementation of, 152-153, 153f-154f
  description of, 135, 135f
  direct, 135, 135f-143f, 144t
  direct-indirect, 144t, 144-156, 146f-155f
  finishing of, 154f, 154-155
  polishing of, 154-155, 155f
  precementation surface treatment of, 150-151, 151f
Clenching, 34-35, 91
Clinical examination, 86-87
CO_2 laser, 117
Composite resins
  application of, 148-149, 149f
  bulk-fill, 131
  cavity preparation for, 147-148, 148
  classification of, 130
  description of, 125
  direct technique with, 135, 135f-143f
  direct-indirect technique

Index

description of, 143-144
    steps involved in, 146-155, 147f-155f
extraoral finishing and polishing of, 149-150, 150f
fillers in, 129-130
flowable, 131
gingiva-colored, 147, 147f
hybrid, 130, 142f
initiators of, 130
light activation of, 149, 149f-150f
monomers in, 129
nanofilled, 130, 137f-139f
optical properties of, 146-147
packable, 131
shade of, 146
silane, 130
tooth-colored, 147, 148f
Compressive stress, 31, 32f
Concave noncarious cervical lesions, 76, 77f, 82f
Connective tissue graft
    harvesting of, 168
    subepithelial
        description of, 168
        illustration of, 176f
        modified envelope with, 168-169, 169t
Coronal wall, 75, 76f
Coronally advanced flap, 168, 170-174, 171f-173f
Crown, 35
"Cupping," 60, 61f, 87f

D

Degree of saturation, 60
Dental compression syndrome, 6
Dental materials, 159t
Dentin
    acids' effect on, 52
    bacterial colonization of surface of, 6, 6f-7f
    in cervical region, 33
    chemical degradation of, 53, 53f
    demineralization of, 53
    endogenous acids' effect on, 65-66
    fracture strength of, 24
    gastric enzymes' effect on, 65-66
    hardness of, 24
    high-power laser effects on, 117-118
    hypersensitive, 24
    mineral composition of, 48
    Nd:YAG laser effects on, 116, 117f
    reactionary, 23, 23f, 36, 114
    sclerotic, 80-81, 127
    structural composition of, 22, 23f
    ultimate compressive strength of, 34, 34f
    ultimate tensile strength of, 34, 34t
    viscoelasticity of, 23-24
    wear of, 24
Dentin hypersensitivity, 9
"Dentin island," 87, 87f
Dentin sclerosis, 23
Dentinal tubules
    acidic beverages' effect on, 116
    adhesive sealing of, 119, 119f
    description of, 33
    high-power laser obliteration of, 115, 116f
    occlusion of
        occluding agents for, 105f-109f, 105-109, 112t
        protein coagulation for, 115
Dentinoenamel junction, 18, 18f, 20, 20f
Dentin-pulp complex
    biomechanical behavior of, 23-24
    structural composition of, 22-23, 23f

Dentifrices
    abrasive agents in, 44f, 44-45
    abrasivity of, 45, 45t, 48
    cervical dentin hypersensitivity and, 12
    cleaning efficacy of, 45, 46f
    composition of, 44
    detergents in, 48
    pH, 45
    whitening, 46-47, 47t
Diagnosis
    case report of, 89-91, 90f-91f
    chief complaint in, 85-86
    clinical examination in, 86-87
    extraoral examination in, 86
    full-mouth radiographic analysis in, 86
    intraoral examination in, 86-87
    lesion analysis in, 87-88
    location in, 88
    morphology in, 87-88
    occlusal examination in, 87
    patient history in, 85-86, 86b
    periodontal examination in, 87
    supplementary examinations in, 87
Diet, acids from, 37, 54-57, 55f-56f, 56t, 57b
Direct-indirect Class V restoration, 144t, 144-156, 146f-155f

E

Ecstasy, 58
EDTA. See Ethylenediaminetetraacetic acid.
Elastic deformation of teeth, 5, 5f
Elastic modulus, 19f, 19-20
Elastic strain, 31, 32f
Elasticity of enamel, 19, 19f
EMD. See Enamel matrix derivative.
Enamel
    acids' effect on, 52, 52f
    biomechanical behavior of, 19f-21f, 19-21
    in cervical region, 33
    chemical degradation of, 52f, 52-53
    composition of, 17, 18f
    cracks in, 20-21, 21f, 31f, 80, 91f, 119f
    demineralization-remineralization process of, 22
    dentinoenamel junction, 18, 18f, 20, 20f
    dissolution of, 7
    elasticity of, 19f, 19-20
    fracture resistance by, 21
    fracture toughness of, 20
    hardness of, 19-20
    microcracks in, 80
    permeability of, 17
    physical characteristics of, 17-18, 18f
    radial cracks in, 20, 21f
    stress concentration effects on, 80
    structural composition of, 17, 18f
    surface roughness of, 87
    thickness of, 18
    ultimate compressive strength of, 34, 34f
    ultimate tensile strength of, 34, 34t
    wear of, 24
Enamel fracture
    illustration of, 19f
    resistance to, 21
    types of, 20, 21f
Enamel matrix derivative, 168, 172f–176f
Enamel prisms, 33, 33f
Enamel rods, 17, 20
Endogenous acids
    bulimia nervosa as source of, 62, 64
    demineralization caused by, 65, 65f
    exposed dentin affected by, 65-66
    gastroesophageal reflux disease as source of, 62, 63f

hyperthyroidism as source of, 64
rumination syndrome as source of, 64
stomach as source of, 62
Energy drinks, 55, 56t
Envelope flaps with paramarginal incisions, 174–176, 175f–176f
Er,Cr:YSGG laser, 117, 118f
Erosion
    biocorrosion versus, 6
    caries and, 3
    historical writings about, 3–5
Er:YAG laser, 117, 118f
Etch-and-rinse adhesive systems, 126–128, 127f
Ethylenediaminetetraacetic acid, 127
Exercise, 57
Exogenous acids
    alcohol, 56
    buffering capacity of, 60
    chemical parameters of, 59–60
    degree of saturation of, 60
    dentinal tubules affected by, 116
    dietary sources of, 37, 54–56, 55f–56f, 56t, 57b
    energy drinks, 55, 56t
    fruits and fruit juices, 55
    hydrogen potential of, 59–60
    mechanism of action, 51–52, 52f
    noncarious cervical lesions caused by, 60, 61f
    soft drinks, 55, 56t
    sources of, 37, 54–57, 55f–56f, 56t
    strength of, 51–52
    titratable acidity of, 60
Extraoral examination, 86

F
Feldspar, 132
Feldspathic ceramics, 132
Feldspathic porcelain, 132, 133f
Fillers
    in adhesive systems, 126
    in composite resins, 129–130
Flowable composite resins, 131
Fluoridated hydroxyapatite, 107
Fluoride, 107–108, 110
Fluorosilicates, 108
Fracture toughness, 20
Frankfort plane, 98, 98f
Friction
    classification of, 43
    definition of, 11–12
    lesion location and, 88
    noncarious cervical lesions caused by, 43–48
    toothbrushing as cause of, 48
Frictional dental hypersensitivity, 10
Fruit juices, 55
Fruits, 55
Fulcrum point, 39, 40f
Full-mouth radiographic analysis, 86

G
Gastric enzymes, 65–66
Gastroesophageal reflux disease, 4, 22, 62, 63f
GERD. See Gastroesophageal reflux disease.
Gingiva, 25f, 25–26
Gingiva recession
    defects caused by
        coronally advanced flap for, 168, 170–174, 171f–173f
        envelope flaps with paramarginal incisions for, 174–176, 175f–176f
        laterally positioned flap for, 173–174
        Miller classification of, 167–168
        modified envelope with subepithelial connective tissue graft for, 168–169, 169f, 169t
    description of, 25f, 25–26, 40f, 87

Gingiva-colored composite resins, 147, 147f
Gingival crevicular fluid, 5
Gingival margin finishing, 145
Gingival wall, 75, 76f
Glass-ceramics
    classification of, 132
    leucite-reinforced, 132, 134f
    lithium disilicate-reinforced, 133, 156, 158f
Glass-ionomer cements, 131
Glutaraldehyde, 106f, 106–107
Glycerolphosphate dimethacrylate, 129
Grinding, of premature occlusal contacts, 101f, 102

H
Hard-bristle toothbrushes, 44
Hardness
    dentin, 24
    enamel, 19–20
Heartburn, 62
Helium-neon laser, 114
HEMA. See Hydroxyethyl methacrylate.
High-power lasers, 114t, 115–118, 116f
History-taking, 85–86, 86b
Hybrid composite resins, 130, 142f
Hybrid layer, 126
Hydrochloric acid, 69
Hydrodynamic theory, 9, 9f, 24, 115
Hydrogen potential, 59–60
Hydroxyapatite
    chemical degradation of, 51, 59
    description of, 17, 18f
    fluoridated, 107
    Nd:YAG laser effects on, 116
Hydroxyethyl methacrylate, 106, 126
Hypersensitive dentin, 24
Hyperthyroidism, 64
Hypochlorous acid, 69
Hyposalivation, 62

I
Illicit drugs, 58
Indirect technique for ceramic restorations, 156–157, 157f–158f, 159t
Initiators
    of adhesive systems, 126
    of composite resins, 130
Interdental septum, 24
International Organization for Standardization, 45
Interproximal contact areas, 6
Intertubular dentin, 23, 23f
Intraoral examination, 86–87
Intratubular dentin, 81
Irregular noncarious cervical lesions, 76–77, 77f

K
Ka. See Acid dissociation constant value.

L
Lactic acid, 86
Lactovegetarians, 55, 58
Laminate veneers, 156
Laser therapy
    chemical therapy and, combined protocol using, 118b, 118–119
    CO_2 laser, 117
    desensitizing effects of, 113
    Er,Cr:YSGG laser, 117, 118f
    Er:YAG laser, 117, 118f
    high-power lasers used in, 114t, 115–118, 116f
    literature review regarding, 113–114
    low-power lasers used in, 114t, 114–115, 115f

Index

Nd:YAG laser, 116, 117f
  occlusal therapy versus, 113
Lateral excursion prematurities, occlusal adjustment for, 102–104, 103f
Laterally positioned flap, 173–174
Leucite-reinforced glass-ceramics, 132, 134f
Levers, 36
Light curing, 129
Light-curing units, 134–135
Light-emitting diode curing lights, 129
Lithium disilicate-reinforced glass-ceramics, 133, 156, 158f
Loading
  historical writings about, 5
  horizontal, 5
  nonaxial loads, 34
  occlusal. *See* Occlusal loading.
Low-power lasers, 114t, 114–115, 115f
L-shaped coronally advanced flap, 170–172, 172f

M

Macrofilled composites, 130
Macromorphology. *See also* Morphology.
  depth, 78f, 78–79
  form/geometry, 75–77, 76f–78f, 82t
  location, 80, 80f, 88
Matrix metalloproteinases, 64, 65t
Maximal intercuspal position, 100, 100f
MDP. *See* 10-Methacryloyloxydecyl dihydrogenphosphate.
Mechanoreceptors, 9
Medications, chemical degradation caused by, 58
Methacrylate methacryloyloxydecylpyridinium bromide, 126
Methacrylate monomers, 125
10-Methacryloyloxydecyl dihydrogenphosphate, 126
Microapplicators, 111f
Microfilled composites, 130
Micromorphology, 80–81, 81f
Miller classification, of gingival recession defects, 167–168
MIP. *See* Maximal intercuspal position.
Modified envelope with subepithelial connective tissue graft, 168–169, 169t
Modified Stillman technique, 43
Modulus of elasticity, 130
Monomers
  in adhesive systems, 125–126
  in composite resins, 129
Morphology, of noncarious cervical lesions
  classifications for, 76, 76f–77f, 79f
  composition, 80–81, 81f
  concave, 76, 77f, 82f
  depth, 78f, 78–79
  description of, 36–37, 36f–37f, 60
  etiologic factors and, relationship between, 82
  form/geometry, 75–77, 76f–78f, 82t
  location, 80, 80f, 88
  macromorphology, 75–80, 76f–78f, 80f
  micromorphology, 80–81, 81f
  textures, 81, 81f
  wedge-shaped, 35–36, 36f, 76–77, 76f–77f, 88, 90f
Mouthrinses, 58, 109
Mouthwash
  fluoride in, 108
  potassium nitrate in, 105
Mucogingival junction, 167

N

Nanofilled composites, 130, 137f–139f
NCCLs. *See* Noncarious cervical lesions.
Nd:YAG laser, 116, 117f
Neural activity, 104–105, 105f
Neural agents, 104–105, 105b, 105f, 112t
Nonaxial loads, 34

Noncarious cervical lesions
  aggressive, 63f
  on buccal surfaces, 37
  case report of, 89–91, 90f–91f
  in cattle, 82, 83f
  cavitation of, 147f
  cervical dentin hypersensitivity and, 10–11
  cervical root caries versus, 12
  classification of, 6, 75f–79f, 76, 82b
  common sites of, 7
  concave, 76, 77f, 82f
  depth of, 78f, 78–79
  diagnosis of. *See* Diagnosis.
  in drug addicts, 58
  early-stage, 60, 61f
  enzymatic action in progression of, 64–66, 65t
  etiology/etiologic factors of
    biocorrosion. *See* Biocorrosion.
    friction. *See* Friction.
    historical studies of, 3–7
    interaction among, 47–48
    morphology and, relationship between, 82
    multifactorial, 10–12, 11b, 47, 87
    pathologies associated with, 86
    premature occlusal contacts, 21, 21f, 34
    stress. *See* Stress.
  exogenous biocorrosion as cause of, 60, 61f
  form of, 76–77, 76f–77f
  historical descriptions of, 3–7, 4t
  intermediate-stage, 60, 61f
  irregular, 76–77, 77f
  location of, 80, 80f, 88
  morphology of. *See* Morphology, of noncarious cervical lesions.
  nonaxial loads associated with, 34
  occlusal factors, 34–35
  in posterior teeth, 88
  in postorthodontic patients, 38–39, 39f
  precementation surface treatment of, 151–152, 152f–153f
  prevalence of, 7–9, 8t, 31
  progression of, 64–66, 65t
  rounded, 76, 76f
  scanning electron microscopic studies of, 6
  severe, 60
  shape of, 76, 76f
  subgingival, 80, 80f
  supragingival, 80, 80f
  surface roughness of, 81, 81f
  texture of, 81, 81f
  treatment of
    chemical therapy. *See* Chemical therapy.
    laser therapy. *See* Laser therapy.
    occlusal therapy. *See* Occlusal therapy.
    restorations. *See* Restorations.
  wedge-shaped, 35–36, 36f, 76–77, 76f–77f, 88, 90f
Nutritional habits, 56–57, 57b

O

Occlusal adjustment, selective
  in centric occlusion, 100f–103f, 100–102
  definition of, 99
  indications for, 100
  for lateral excursion prematurities, 102–104, 103f
  in protrusion, 104, 104f
Occlusal examination, 87
Occlusal imbalance, 96
Occlusal loading
  abfractive process caused by, 96f
  muscular adaptation to, 96
  periodontal supporting structures affected by, 39
  stress concentration affected by, 35–37, 35f–37f

Occlusal therapy
    additive, 99
    choices for, 99
    description of, 95–96
    indications for, 96
    laser therapy versus, 113
    recording media for
        articulating foils, 98
        articulating paper, 97, 97f, 100f
        articulators, 98, 98f–99f
        occlusal wax indicators, 97f, 97–98
        overview of, 96–97
    selective occlusal adjustment. See Occlusal adjustment, selective.
    subtractive, 99
    T-scan digital analysis applications, 98–99
Occlusal wax indicators, 97f, 97–98
Occlusion
    in canine guidance, 102, 103f
    centric
        description of, 87
        occlusal adjustment in, 100f–103f, 100–102
Occupational chemical degradation, 58–59
Odontoblast processes, 18f
Orthodontic treatment, 38–39
Oxalates, 105–106, 109

P
Packable composite resins, 131
Pain, cervical dentin hypersensitivity-related
    description of, 9, 9f, 85, 88
    laser therapy for, 114
Parafunctional habits
    history-taking about, 86b
    stress concentration caused by, 37, 37f
    wear facets associated with, 87
Patient history, 85–86, 86b
Pellicle
    acquired, 53–54
    description of, 12
Pepsin, 65–66
Periodontal examination, 87
Periodontal ligament, 25, 39
Periodontium
    alveolar bone, 24
    cementum, 24–25, 25f
    gingiva, 25, 25f
    periodontal ligament, 25
Peritubular dentin, 23
pH, dentifrice, 45
Plastic strain, 31, 32f
Polyacrylic acid, 126
Polyalkenoic acid, 131
Polychromatic method, 147
Polymerization shrinkage, 145
Porcine resorbable collagen matrix, 168
Posterior teeth
    biocorrosion in, 60, 61f
    noncarious cervical lesions in, 88
Potassium, 104–105, 105b, 105f
Potassium nitrate, 105, 110
Potassium oxalate, 106, 109, 109f
Pregnancy, 64
Premature occlusal contacts
    noncarious cervical lesions caused by, 21, 34
    selective grinding of, 102
Protein coagulation, 115
Proteoglycans, 24
Protrusion, occlusal adjustment in, 104, 104f
Pulp, 23, 23f
Pulp wall, 75, 76f

Q
Quartz tungsten halogen light-curing units, 134

R
Radioactive dentin abrasion, 45, 45t, 47t, 48
Radiotherapy, 59, 59f
RDA. See Radioactive dentin abrasion.
Reactionary dentin, 23, 23f, 36, 114
Recording media, for occlusal therapy
    articulating foils, 98
    articulating paper, 97, 97f, 100f
    articulators, 98, 98f–99f
    occlusal wax indicators, 97f, 97–98
    overview of, 96–97
Reparative tertiary dentin, 23
Resin composites. See Composite resins.
Resin-modified glass ionomers, 131
Restorations
    adhesive systems. See Adhesive/adhesive systems.
    ceramic, indirect technique for, 156–157, 157f–158f, 159t
    ceramics, 132, 132f
    composite resins, 125, 129–131
    connective tissue graft with coronally advanced flap for root coverage after, in noncarious cervical lesions, 177, 178f
    dental materials recommended for, 159t
    glass-ionomer cements, 131
    indications for, 38, 38f
    precementation surface treatment of, 150–151, 151f
Retraction cords, 148, 149f, 151
Root caries, 12
Root coverage
    case reports of, 177–180, 178f–181f
    in cervical dentin hypersensitivity, 177–178, 179f–181f
    connective tissue graft for, 168
    coronally advanced flap for, 168, 170–174, 171f–173f
    envelope flaps with paramarginal incisions for, 174–176, 175f–176f
    modified envelope with subepithelial connective tissue graft for, 168–169, 169f, 169t
    in restored noncarious cervical lesions, 177–180, 178f–181f
    root decontamination with, 177
Root decontamination, 177
Rubber dam, 126
Rumination syndrome, 64

S
Saliva, 53–54, 54b, 54f, 57
Sclerotic dentin, 80–81, 127
SCTG. See Subepithelial connective tissue graft.
Selective occlusal adjustment. See Occlusal adjustment, selective.
Self-etch adhesive systems, 126–128, 127f, 137f
Shear stress, 31, 32f
Silanation, 150
Silane, 130
Smear layer, 12, 48, 52
Smith and Knight tooth wear index, 79, 79t
Sodium bicarbonate, 46
Sodium fluoride, 65, 110. See also Fluoride.
Soft drinks, 55, 56t
Soft-bristle toothbrushes, 44
Solvents, 126
Stannous fluoride, 65, 107
Strain
    breakage, 33
    definition of, 31
    types of, 31, 32f
Stress
    attrition and, 62
    in cervical region, 12, 33–35
    classification of, 31, 32f
    definition of, 31

description of, 6, 7f
dissipation of, 32f
on periodontal ligament, 39
stress-strain, 31-33, 32f-33f
Stress concentration
  abfractive lesions and, 80
  biocorrosive abfractions resulting from, 40f
  in cervical region, 33, 35, 38
  eccentric loading effects on, 36
  enamel cracks caused by, 80
  fulcrum point changes in, 36
  in noncarious cervical lesions, 77, 78f
  occlusal load direction effects, 35-37, 35f-37f
  orthodontic movement effects on, 38, 38f
  parafunctional habit as cause of, 37, 37f
  tongue-thrusting forces as cause of, 37, 37f
Stress-biocorrosion, 37, 37f, 61-62
Strontium, 106
Subepithelial connective tissue graft
  description of, 168
  illustration of, 176f
  modified envelope with, 168-169, 169t
Subgingival noncarious cervical lesions, 80, 80f
Subtractive occlusal therapy, 99
Supragingival noncarious cervical lesions, 80, 80f
Swimmers, 59

T
Teeth
  elastic deformation of, 5, 5f
  wasting of, 4-5
Temporomandibular disorders, 86b
Tensile stress, 6, 31, 32f-33f
Titanium tetrafluoride, 65
Titratable acidity, 60
Tongue-thrusting forces, 37, 37f
Tooth enamel. *See* Enamel.
Tooth erosion. *See* Erosion.
Tooth wear index, 79, 79t
Tooth whitening
  tooth sensitivity caused by, 119
  toothpastes for, 46-47, 47f
Toothbrushes, 44
Toothbrushing
  benefits of, 43
  of biocorroded tooth, 48
  cervical dentin hypersensitivity and, 12
  dentifrices used in, 44f, 44-45, 45t
  enamel scratches caused by, 81
  friction during, 48
  historical writings about, 4-5
  incorrect technique of, 43, 44f
  modified Stillman technique, 43
  technique of, 43-44, 44f
Toothpastes
  abrasivity of, 45, 45t
  arginine in, 109, 109f
  bioglass in, 108-109
  calcium sodium phosphosilicate in, 109
  cleaning efficacy of, 45, 46f
  fluoride in, 108
  potassium nitrate in, 105
  strontium in, 106
  whitening, 46-47, 47f
Trypsin, 66
T-Scan occlusal analysis
  articulating papers and, 97
  description of, 89, 89f, 98-99

U
UDMA, 129
Ultimate compressive strength, 34, 34f
Ultimate tensile strength, 34, 34t

V
Varnishes, 107
VAS. *See* Visual analog scale.
Visual analog scale, 88

W
Wasting of teeth, 4-5
Wear
  dentin, 24
  enamel, 24
  in gastroesophageal reflux disease and bruxism, 62
  occlusal, 235
  tooth wear index, 79, 79t
Wear facets, 87, 87f, 91f
Wedge-shaped noncarious cervical lesions, 35-36, 36f, 76-77, 76f-77f, 88, 90f
Whitening toothpastes, 46-47, 47f
Winemakers/wine tasters, 59